the SMARTPOINTS® *cookbook*

FEEL GREAT, LOSE WEIGHT, AND EAT WELL WITH 150 SCRUMPTIOUS RECIPES

WEIGHT WATCHERS PUBLISHING GROUP

VP Content/Editor in Chief **Theresa DiMasi**

Creative Director **Ed Melnitsky**

Associate Managing Editor **Katerina Gkionis**

Food Editor **Eileen Runyan**

Project Editor **Alice K. Thompson**

Contributing Editors **Lisa Chernick, Leslie Fink, MS, RD**

Photo Director **Marybeth Dulany**

Nutrition Consultant **Ariella Sieger**

Production Manager **Alan Biederman**

Art/Design Director **Daniela A. Hritcu**

Art/Production Assistant **Rebecca Kollmer**

Photographer **John Kernick**

Food Stylist **Simon Andrews**

Prop Stylist **Alistair Turnbull**

SKU #12030

Printed in the USA

Front cover:
Philly Chicken Cheese Steaks, page 51

Back cover:
Shakshouka (Tomato-and-Egg Stew), page 8; Turkey BLTs on Ciabatta, page 77;
Grilled Flank Steak with Marjoram Salsa Verde, page 90

ABOUT WEIGHT WATCHERS INTERNATIONAL, INC.

Weight Watchers International, Inc. is the world's leading commercial provider of weight-management services, operating globally through a network of company-owned and franchise operations. Weight Watchers holds more than 36,000 meetings each week, at which members receive group support and learn about healthy eating patterns, behavior modification, and physical activity. Weight Watchers provides innovative digital weight-management products through its websites, mobile sites, and apps. Weight Watchers is the leading provider of online subscription weight-management products in the world. In addition, Weight Watchers offers a wide range of products, publications, and programs for those interested in weight loss and weight control.

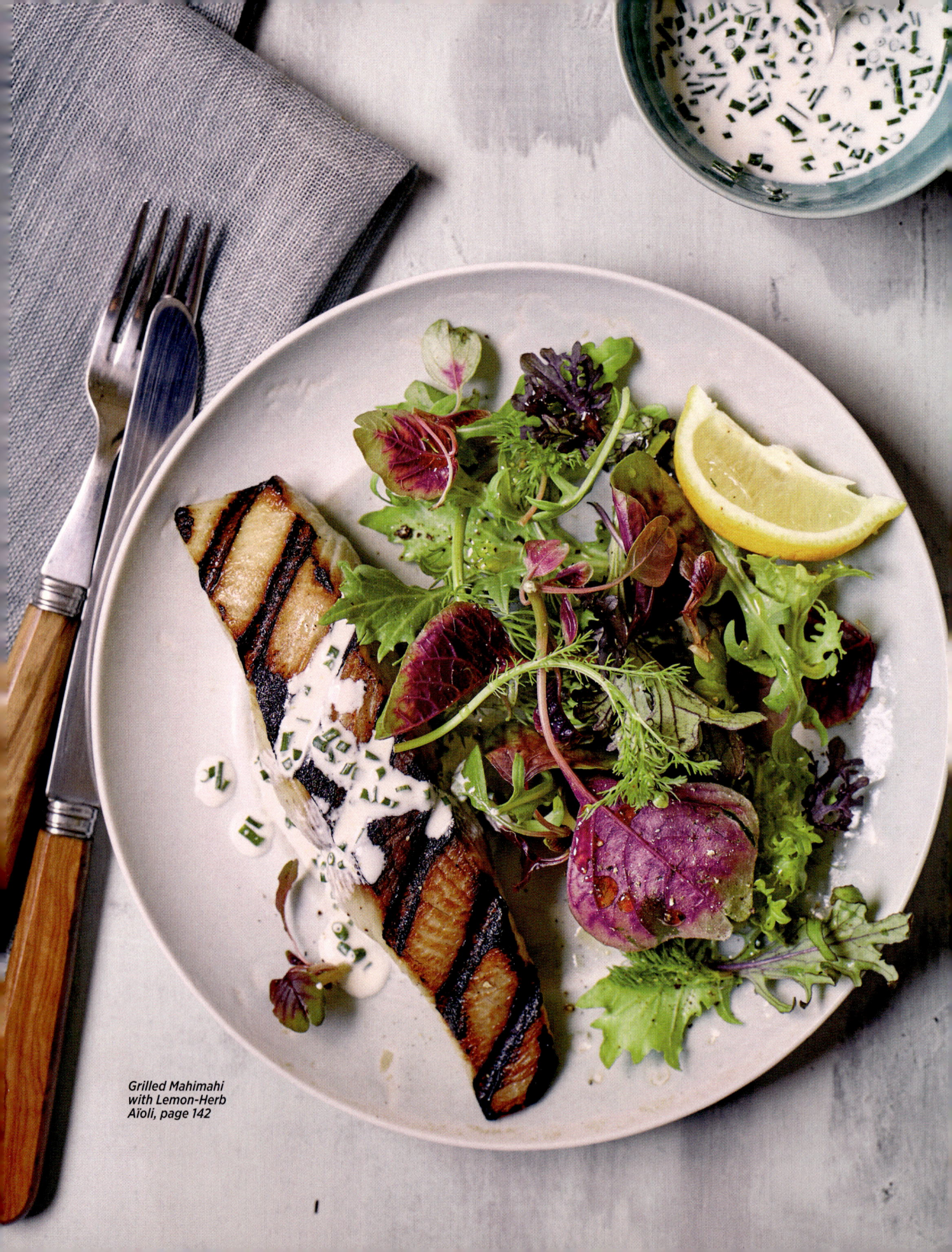

*Grilled Mahimahi
with Lemon-Herb
Aïoli, page 142*

CONTENTS

ABOUT OUR RECIPES

While losing weight isn't only about what you eat, Weight Watchers realizes the critical role it plays in your success and overall good health. That's why our philosophy is to offer great-tasting, easy recipes that are nutritious as well as delicious. We create most of our recipes with the healthy and filling foods we love: lots of fresh fruits and vegetables, most of which have 0 SmartPoints® value, and satisfying lean proteins, which are low in SmartPoints. We also try to ensure that our recipes fall within the recommendations of the U.S. Dietary Guidelines for Americans so they support a diet that promotes health and reduces the risk for disease. If you have special dietary needs, consult with your health-care professional for advice on a diet that is best for you, then adapt these recipes to meet your specific nutritional needs.

GET STARTED, KEEP GOING, AND ENJOY GOOD NUTRITION

At Weight Watchers, we believe that eating well makes life better, no matter where you are in your weight-loss journey. These delicious recipes are ideal, whether you're just getting started or have already reached your goals on the SmartPoints plan. Unlike other weight-loss programs, which focus solely on calories, the SmartPoints plan guides you toward healthier foods that are lower in sugar and saturated fat and higher in protein. But this isn't a diet—all food is "in." Eating well should be fun, energizing, and delicious so that healthy food choices become second nature. To get maximum satisfaction, we suggest you keep the following information in mind while preparing our recipes:

● SmartPoints values are given for each recipe. The SmartPoints assigned for each ingredient is based on the number of calories and the amount of saturated fat, sugar, and protein per the ingredient quantity. The SmartPoints for each ingredient are then added together and divided by the number of servings, and the result is rounded.

● Recipes include approximate nutritional information: They are analyzed for Calories (Cal), Total Fat, Saturated Fat (Sat Fat), Sodium (Sod), Total Carbohydrates (Total Carb), Sugar, Dietary Fiber (Fib), and Protein (Prot). The nutritional values are obtained from the Weight Watchers database, which is maintained by registered dietitians.

● To boost flavor, we often include fresh herbs or a squeeze of citrus instead of increasing the salt. If you don't need to restrict your sodium intake, feel free to add a touch more salt as desired.

● Recipes in this book that are designated gluten free do not contain any wheat (in all forms, including kamut, semolina, spelt, and triticale), barley, or rye, or any products that are made from these ingredients, such as breads, couscous, pastas, seitan, soy sauce, beer, malt vinegar, and malt beverages. Other foods such as salad dressings, Asian-style sauces, salsa and tomato sauce, shredded cheese, yogurt, and sour cream may be sources of gluten. Check ingredient labels carefully on packaged foods that recipes call for, as different brands of the same premade food product may or may not contain gluten. If you are following a gluten-free diet because you have celiac disease, please consult your health-care professional.

● *Cook's Tip* and *Up the Protein* suggestions have a SmartPoints value of 0 unless otherwise stated.

● For information about the science behind lasting weight loss and more, please visit WeightWatchers.com/science.

CALCULATIONS NOT WHAT YOU EXPECTED?

SmartPoints for the recipes in this book are calculated without counting any fruits and most vegetables, but the nutrition information does include the nutrient content from fruits and vegetables. This means you may get a different SmartPoints value if you calculate the SmartPoints based on the nutrition. To allow for your "free" fruits and veggies, use the SmartPoints assigned to the recipes. Also, please note, when fruits and veggies are liquefied or pureed (as in a smoothie), their nutrient content is incorporated into the recipe calculations. These nutrients can increase the SmartPoints.

Alcohol is included in our SmartPoints calculations. Because alcohol information is generally not included on nutrition labels, it's not an option you can include when using the handheld or online calculator or the Weight Watchers Mobile app. But since we include the alcohol information that we get from our database in our recipes, you might notice discrepancies between the SmartPoints you see here in our recipes and the values you get using the calculator. The SmartPoints listed for our recipes are the most accurate values.

SIMPLY FILLING (THE NO-COUNT OPTION)

If counting SmartPoints isn't your thing, try Simply Filling, a no-count technique. To follow it, eat just until satisfied, primarily from the list of Simply Filling foods found in your *Pocket Guide*. For more information see your member guidebook. A list of recipes in this book that work with the Simply Filling technique is included on page 249.

CHOOSING INGREDIENTS

As you learn to eat healthier and add more wholesome foods to your meals, consider the following to help you choose foods wisely:

LEAN MEATS AND POULTRY

Purchase lean meats and poultry, and trim them of all visible fat before cooking. When poultry is cooked with the skin on, we recommend removing the skin before eating. Nutritional information for recipes that include meat, poultry, and fish is based on cooked, skinless boneless portions (unless otherwise stated) with the fat trimmed.

SEAFOOD

Whenever possible, our recipes call for seafood that is sustainable and deemed the most healthful for human consumption so that your choice of seafood is not only good for the oceans but also good for you. For more information about the best seafood choices and to download a pocket guide, go to the Environmental Defense Fund at seafood.edf.org or seafoodwatch.org.

PRODUCE

For best flavor, maximum nutrient content, and the lowest prices, buy fresh local produce such as vegetables, leafy greens, and fruits in season. Rinse them thoroughly before using, and keep a supply of cut-up vegetables and fruits in your refrigerator for convenient healthy snacks.

WHOLE GRAINS

Explore your market for whole-grain products such as whole wheat and whole-grain breads and pastas, brown rice, bulgur, barley, cornmeal, whole wheat couscous, oats, and quinoa to enjoy with your meals.

READ THE RECIPE

Take a couple of minutes to read through the ingredients and directions before you start to prepare a recipe. This will prevent you from discovering midway through that you don't have an important ingredient or that a recipe requires several hours of marinating. It's also a good idea to assemble all ingredients and utensils within easy reach before you begin cooking.

WEIGHING AND MEASURING

The success of any recipe depends on accurate weighing and measuring. The effectiveness of the Weight Watchers Program and the accuracy of the nutritional analysis depend on correct measuring as well. Use the following techniques:

● Weigh foods such as meat, poultry, and fish on a food scale.

● To measure liquids, use a standard glass or plastic measuring cup placed on a level surface. For amounts less than ¼ cup, use standard measuring spoons.

● To measure dry ingredients, use metal or plastic measuring cups that come in ¼-, ⅓-, ½-, and 1-cup sizes. Fill the appropriate cup and level it with the flat edge of a knife or spatula. For amounts less than ¼ cup, use standard measuring spoons.

WHY CHOOSE PROTEIN?
BECAUSE IT WORKS!

Protein is powerful. It's vital to building, maintaining, and repairing every major system in our bodies. It helps fuel our activity and gives us energy—not instantly, the way the caffeine in a cup of coffee or the sugar in a glass of juice might, but over the long run, for the sustained strength and vitality we need to work, play, and enjoy everyday life. It even helps our brains function efficiently, and some studies suggest it enhances our mood.

But there's more: Protein is particularly important during weight loss. Eating enough protein contributes to maintaining muscle (which burns calories) while helping us to lose fat. It also aids us in feeling full and satisfied, a boon to those looking to make wise food choices.

These reasons and more are why protein is a key element in the SmartPoints formula. Higher amounts of protein can help lower the amount of SmartPoints a food or recipe serving clocks in at. And, as we'll show you throughout this book, that can lead to some very delicious math!

There are other components of SmartPoints, and we've paid close attention to those as well. Lowering the amount of added sugar and saturated fat will also reduce the SmartPoints value of a dish, so we've designed our recipes with that in mind. And not all protein sources are created equal: We focus on lean, trimmed animal proteins and high-quality plant-based proteins so that you'll get the most from your daily SmartPoints target.

How much protein do you need? The amount varies from individual to individual depending on factors such as age, physical activity, and health goals. Current recommended daily allowances from the Health and Medicine Division is 46 grams a day for women and 56 grams a day for men; you can get a more customized calculation by multiplying your weight in pounds by .36. Recent studies suggest that consuming 20 grams or more at each meal may be beneficial. But we don't want you to have to focus too heavily on these numbers. That's one reason we've given you *Up the Protein* tips throughout our recipes. Take a look at these simple suggestions anytime you feel that your meals might not be giving you as much protein as you'd benefit from.

Here at Weight Watchers, good food and the joy of sharing it is something we're passionate about. We're thrilled that *The SmartPoints Cookbook* brings together the latest weight-loss science with the foods and recipes our members adore.

ENJOY!

PROTEIN STANDBYS

How much protein do some of our favorite, most convenient foods pack? Take a look! Refer to this list anytime you think your meal or snack could use a little boost.

FOOD	PROTEIN	SMARTPOINTS
EGGS AND DAIRY		
1 large hard-cooked egg	6 grams	2 SmartPoints
1 large egg white	4 grams	0 SmartPoints
1 cup fat-free milk	8 grams	3 SmartPoints
½ cup fat-free cottage cheese	8 grams	2 SmartPoints
½ cup fat-free Greek yogurt	11 grams	1 SmartPoints
1 ounce reduced-fat Cheddar cheese	7 grams	3 SmartPoints
1 scoop (2 tablespoons) whey protein powder	17 grams	2 SmartPoints
MEAT AND SEAFOOD		
3 ounces cooked skinless boneless chicken breast	26 grams	2 SmartPoints
½ cup (2 ounces) cooked diced skinless turkey breast	17 grams	1 SmartPoints
3 ounces trimmed lean cooked flank steak	18 grams	3 SmartPoints
1 (1-ounce) slice roast beef	7 grams	1 SmartPoints
½ cup (2 ounces) diced extra lean low-sodium ham	10 grams	2 SmartPoints
2 ounces smoked salmon	10 grams	1 SmartPoints
3 ounces peeled, cooked shrimp	27 grams	1 SmartPoints
½ can (2.75 ounces) tuna in water	18 grams	1 SmartPoints
BEANS AND SOY		
½ cup cooked black beans	7 grams	3 SmartPoints
½ cup cooked chickpeas	9 grams	3 SmartPoints
½ cup cooked green peas	4 grams	2 SmartPoints
½ cup cooked lentils	9 grams	3 SmartPoints
½ cup cooked, shelled edamame	9 grams	3 SmartPoints
1 cup plain unsweetened soy milk	7 grams	2 SmartPoints
½ cup drained firm tofu	10 grams	2 SmartPoints
NUTS AND SEEDS		
2 tablespoons whole almonds	4 grams	2 SmartPoints
2 tablespoons unsweetened almond butter	7 grams	6 SmartPoints
1 cup plain unsweetened almond milk	2 grams	1 SmartPoints
2 tablespoons peanut butter	7 grams	6 SmartPoints
1 tablespoon dry-roasted peanuts	2 grams	2 SmartPoints
12 pistachios	2 grams	1 SmartPoints
2 tablespoons chopped walnuts	2 grams	3 SmartPoints
1 tablespoon green pumpkin seeds	2 grams	1 SmartPoints
1 tablespoon chia seeds	2 grams	2 SmartPoints
VEGGIES AND GRAINS		
8 spears asparagus	3 grams	0 SmartPoints
1 cup cooked broccoli florets	4 grams	0 SmartPoints
1 cup cooked green beans	2 grams	0 SmartPoints
1 cup sliced raw mushrooms	2 grams	0 SmartPoints
½ cup cooked brown rice	2 grams	4 SmartPoints
½ cup cooked quinoa	4 grams	3 SmartPoints
½ cup cooked rolled oats	3 grams	2 SmartPoints

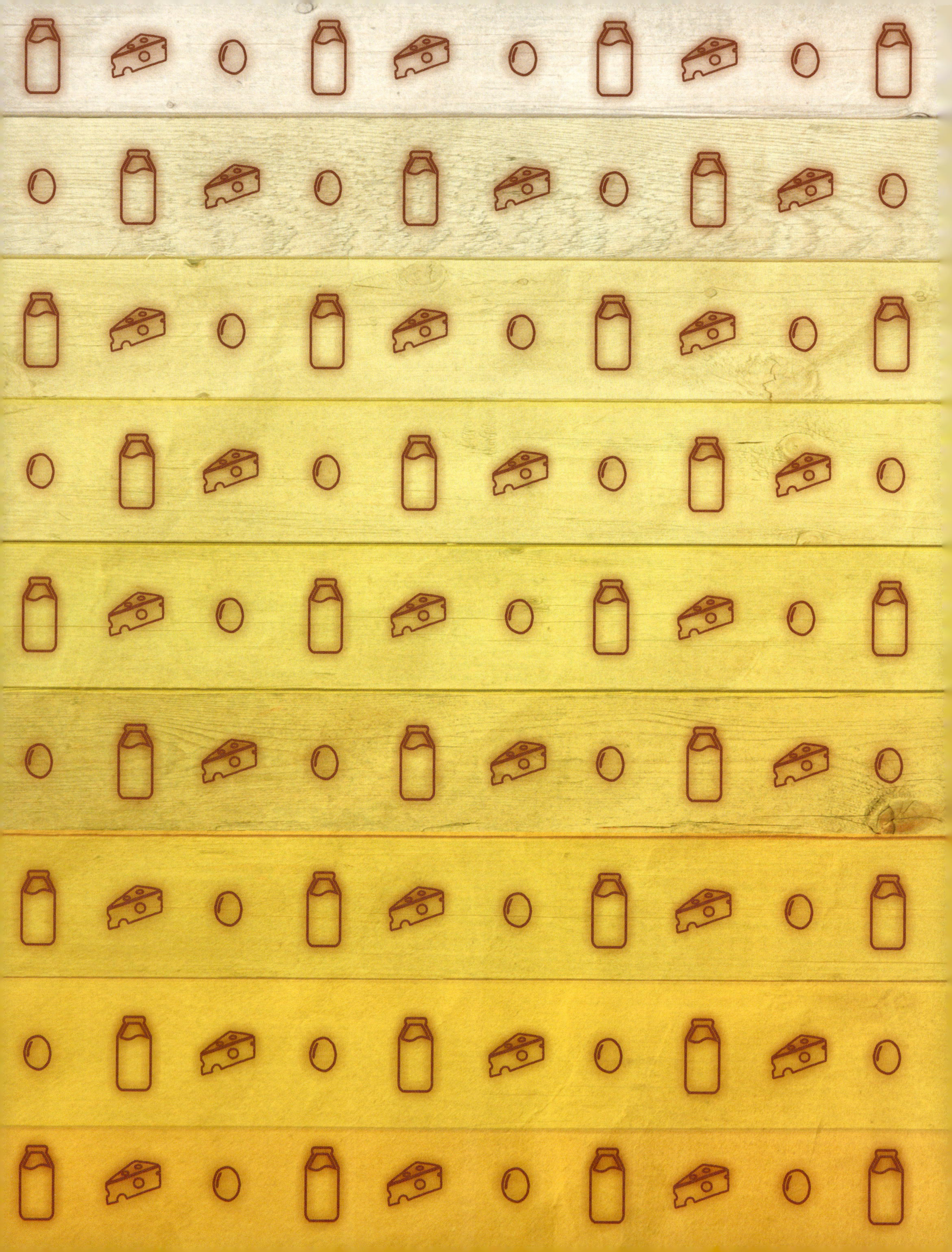

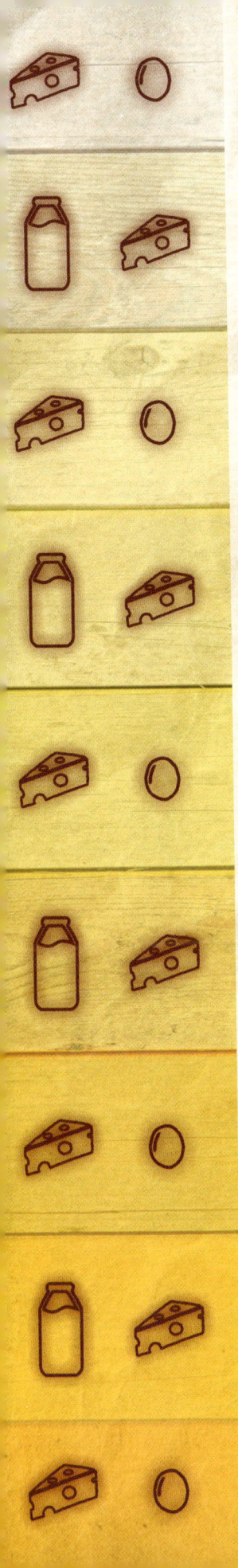

EGGS MILK YOGURT & CHEESE

HEALTHIER EGGS BENEDICT WITH CANADIAN BACON

SERVES 4

1 tablespoon white-wine vinegar

4 large eggs, at room temperature

4 slices Canadian bacon

¼ cup reduced-calorie mayonnaise

¼ cup plain fat-free Greek yogurt

1 teaspoon Dijon mustard

½ teaspoon finely grated lemon zest

1 teaspoon lemon juice

2 teaspoons unsalted butter, softened

2 light whole-grain English muffins, split and toasted

4 thick slices tomato

2 tablespoons chopped fresh chives

1 Fill large skillet halfway with water and bring to boil. Add vinegar; reduce heat so water barely simmers.

2 One at a time, break eggs into small cup, then slide into water. Cook eggs until whites set, about 4 minutes; with slotted spoon, transfer eggs to paper towels to drain.

3 Pour out water and wipe skillet dry; add bacon and cook over medium-high heat, turning once, until bacon is heated through, about 1 minute per side.

4 To make sauce, whisk mayonnaise, yogurt, mustard, lemon zest, and lemon juice together in small microwavable bowl; microwave on High until hot, about 30 seconds, then stir in butter until melted.

5 Top each toasted muffin half with 1 slice tomato, 1 slice bacon, 1 egg, and about 2 tablespoons sauce; sprinkle with chives.

7 SmartPoints value

Per serving (1 open-face sandwich): 228 Cal, 13 g Total Fat, 4 g Sat Fat, 534 mg Sod, 14 g Total Carb, 2 g Sugar, 3 g Fib, 16 g Prot.

COOK'S TIP

If you want to poach the eggs ahead, take them out of the poaching water about 1 minute earlier and slip them into a bowl of ice water. Refrigerate them in the water up to 1 day; reheat them gently in simmering water.

HOMEMADE TURKEY SAUSAGE WITH SCRAMBLED EGG WHITES

SERVES 4 • GLUTEN FREE

3 teaspoons olive oil

2 red or yellow bell peppers, thinly sliced

¾ teaspoon salt

¾ pound ground skinless turkey breast

¼ cup finely chopped onion

4 tablespoons chopped fresh parsley

½ teaspoon fennel seeds

½ teaspoon dried sage

¼ teaspoon black pepper

⅛ teaspoon red pepper flakes

8 large egg whites

1 tablespoon fat-free milk

1 Heat 1 teaspoon oil in large nonstick skillet over medium heat. Add bell peppers and ¼ teaspoon salt and cook, stirring frequently, until peppers soften, about 8 minutes. Transfer to platter and keep warm.

2 Meanwhile, combine turkey, onion, 2 tablespoons parsley, fennel seeds, sage, ¼ teaspoon salt, ⅛ teaspoon black pepper, and red pepper flakes in medium bowl. With damp hands, shape mixture into 8 (½-inch-thick) patties.

3 Wipe out skillet peppers cooked in. Place skillet over medium heat and add 1 teaspoon oil. Place patties in skillet and cook, turning once, until cooked through and browned, 4–5 minutes per side. Place on platter with peppers.

4 Whisk egg whites, remaining 2 tablespoons parsley, milk, remaining ¼ teaspoon salt, and remaining ⅛ teaspoon black pepper together in large bowl. Wipe out skillet patties cooked in; add remaining 1 teaspoon oil and place over medium heat. Add egg white mixture and cook, stirring frequently, just until set, 2–3 minutes. Serve eggs with patties and bell peppers.

3 SmartPoints value

Per serving (2 sausage patties, ⅓ cup eggs, and about ½ cup bell pepper): 191 Cal, 7 g Total Fat, 1 g Sat Fat, 599 mg Sod, 5 g Total Carb, 3 g Sugar, 2 g Fib, 27 g Prot.

UP THE PROTEIN

Craving cheese? If you like, mix ¾ cup shredded low-fat Cheddar into the egg whites in the last minute of cooking and increase the per-serving SmartPoints value by 1.

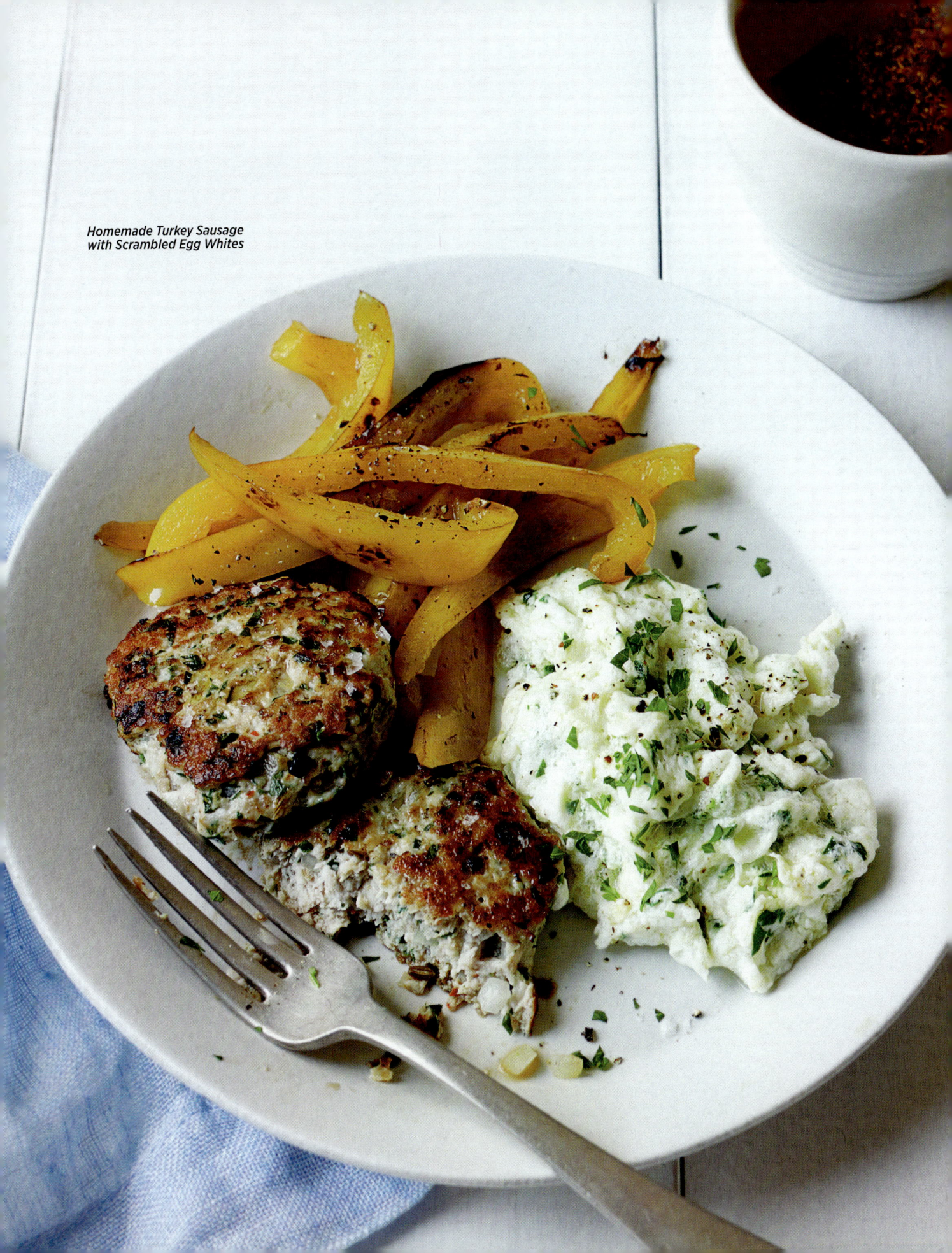

*Homemade Turkey Sausage
with Scrambled Egg Whites*

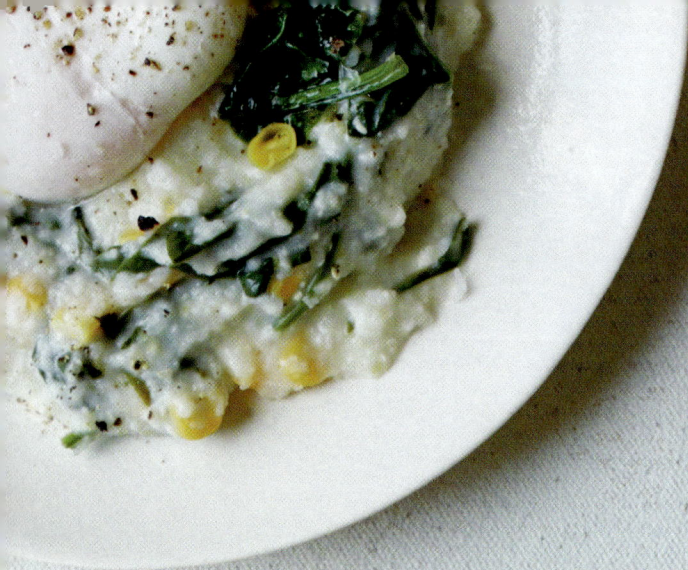

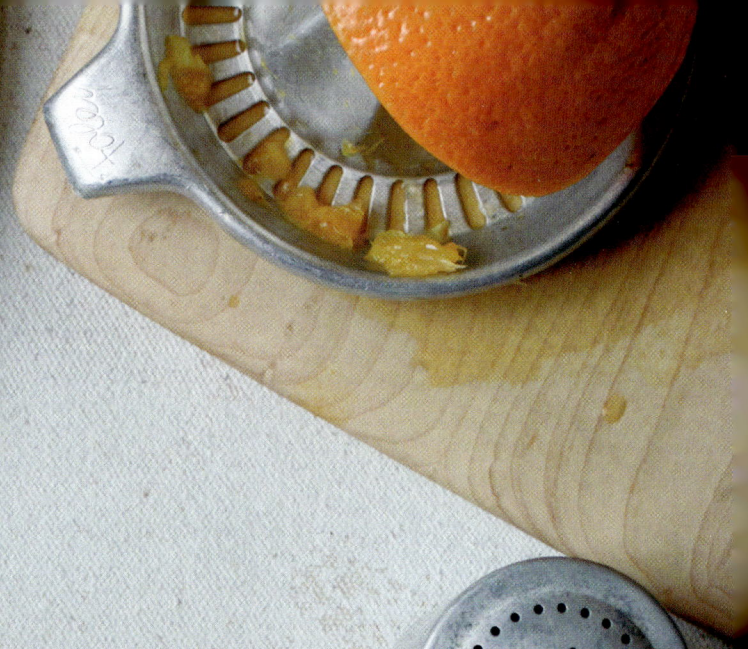

Spinach-Garlic Grits with Poached Eggs

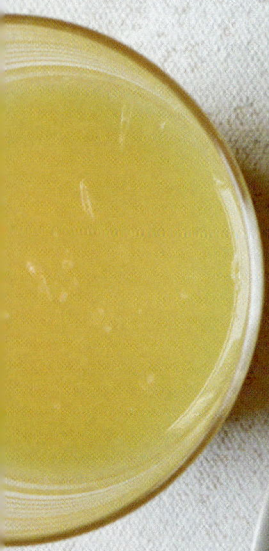

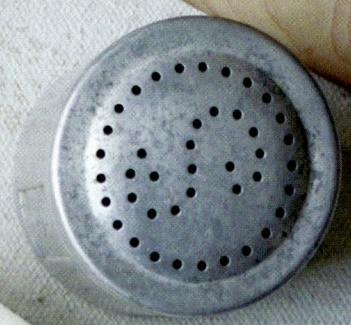

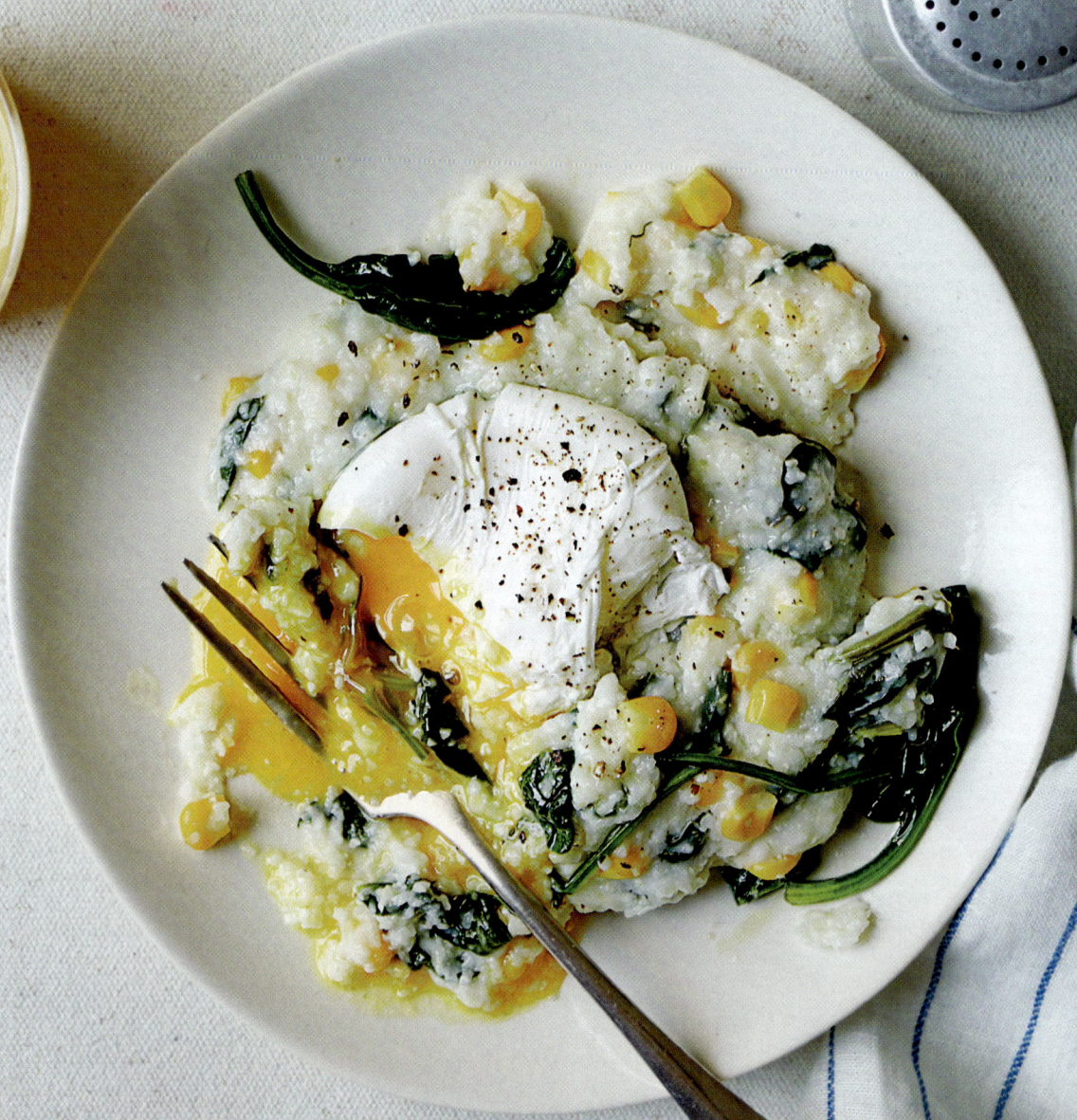

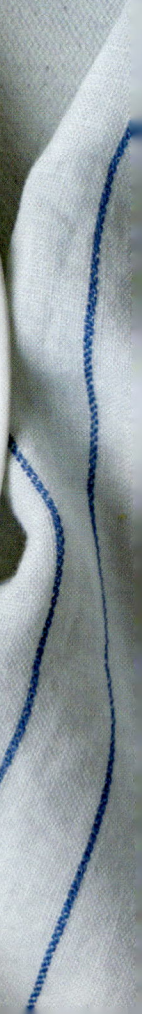

SPINACH-GARLIC GRITS WITH POACHED EGGS

SERVES 4 • GLUTEN FREE • VEGETARIAN

2½ cups water

¼ teaspoon salt

½ cup quick-cooking grits

2 teaspoons olive oil

2 garlic cloves, minced

3 cups coarsely chopped fresh spinach

¾ cup fresh or frozen corn kernels, thawed

2 tablespoons fat-free cream cheese

⅛ teaspoon black pepper

2 teaspoons apple cider vinegar

4 large eggs

1 Combine water and salt in large saucepan; bring to boil over medium-high heat. Slowly pour in grits in thin, steady stream, stirring constantly. Reduce heat and cook, covered, stirring often, until grits are softened and creamy, about 15 minutes.

2 Meanwhile, heat oil in large nonstick skillet over medium heat. Add garlic and cook, stirring constantly, until fragrant, about 30 seconds. Add spinach and corn and cook, stirring frequently, until spinach wilts, 1–2 minutes.

3 Add spinach mixture, cream cheese, and pepper to grits; stir until well blended. Cover and keep warm.

4 Fill another large skillet halfway with water and bring to boil over high heat. Add vinegar and reduce heat until water is simmering. Carefully break eggs into water. Simmer until whites are opaque and yolks are set, 3–4 minutes.

5 Divide grits mixture evenly among 4 shallow bowls. Using slotted spoon, top each serving of grits with an egg. Sprinkle with more salt and pepper if desired and serve at once.

6 SmartPoints value

Per serving (¾ cup grits and 1 egg): 208 Cal, 8 g Total Fat, 2 g Sat Fat, 285 mg Sod, 25 g Total Carb, 2 g Sugar, 2 g Fib, 11 g Prot.

COOK'S TIP

Get a jump start on this recipe by making the grits ahead: Prepare as directed through Step 3 and transfer the grits to a microwavable container; cool and refrigerate overnight or up to 2 days. Reheat in the microwave on High until hot, 1 to 2 minutes.

SHAKSHOUKA (TOMATO-AND-EGG STEW)

SERVES 6 • GLUTEN FREE • VEGETARIAN

1 tablespoon olive oil

3 garlic cloves, chopped

½ onion, diced

1 cup sliced mushrooms

3 cups lightly packed baby spinach

1½ teaspoons ground cumin

1 (28-ounce) can diced tomatoes

2 tablespoons tomato paste

1 teaspoon hot pepper sauce

½ teaspoon salt

6 large eggs

1 tablespoon chopped fresh parsley

1 Heat oil in large skillet over medium heat. Add garlic and onion and cook, stirring, until soft, about 3 minutes. Add mushrooms and cook, stirring often, until mushrooms brown, 3–5 minutes. Add spinach and cumin and cook just until spinach wilts.

2 Stir in tomatoes, tomato paste, hot pepper sauce, and salt; bring to simmer. One at a time, break eggs into small cup and gently slide into skillet. Leave space between eggs so they remain separate.

3 Cover skillet and reduce heat to low; simmer until eggs are just set, 12–15 minutes. Remove from heat; garnish with parsley.

3 SmartPoints value

Per serving (1 egg and ⅔ cup sauce): 133 Cal, 7 g Total Fat, 2 g Sat Fat, 530 mg Sod, 9 g Total Carb, 5 g Sugar, 2 g Fib, 9 g Prot.

UP THE PROTEIN

This flavorful Middle Eastern dish is often served for breakfast, but it makes a speedy and satisfying lunch or dinner as well. Serve it with protein- and fiber-rich quinoa to make it a full meal; ½ cup cooked quinoa per serving will increase the SmartPoints value by 3.

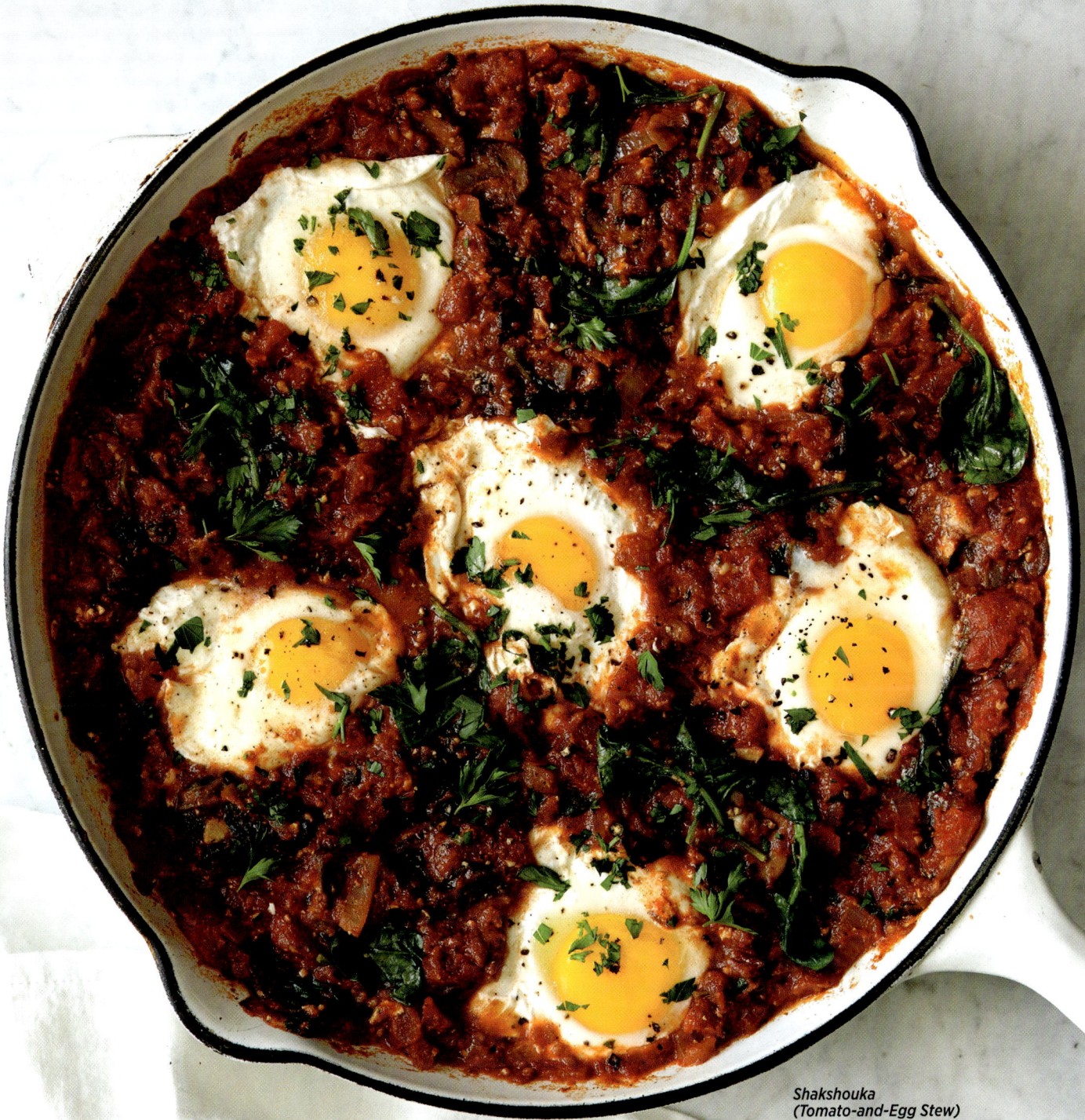

Shakshouka
(Tomato-and-Egg Stew)

BROCCOLINI AND GOAT CHEESE FRITTATA

SERVES 4 • GLUTEN FREE • VEGETARIAN

½ bunch Broccolini (Asparation), thick stems trimmed, stalks cut into 1-inch pieces

1½ cups fat-free egg substitute

1 tablespoon chopped fresh marjoram or parsley

½ teaspoon salt

¼ teaspoon black pepper

1 tablespoon olive oil

4 scallions, thinly sliced

2 small plum tomatoes, thinly sliced

½ cup crumbled low-fat goat cheese

1 Put Broccolini in steamer basket and set in saucepan over 1 inch boiling water. Cover tightly and steam until crisp-tender, 4–5 minutes.

2 Meanwhile, preheat broiler. Whisk egg substitute, marjoram, salt, and pepper together in medium bowl. Set aside.

3 Heat oil in large ovenproof skillet over medium heat. Add scallions and cook, stirring frequently, until softened, about 2 minutes. Stir in Broccolini. Pour egg mixture over vegetable mixture. Cook until eggs are almost set, 3–4 minutes.

4 Arrange tomato slices in single layer on top of frittata and sprinkle with goat cheese. Place frittata under broiler and broil 5 inches from heat until center is set and cheese is gooey, about 3 minutes. Let stand 2 minutes before serving. Cut into 4 wedges.

3 SmartPoints value

Per serving (1 wedge): 166 Cal, 8 g Total Fat, 3 g Sat Fat, 500 mg Sod, 11 g Total Carb, 4 g Sugar, 3 g Fib, 15 g Prot.

COOK'S TIP

When preparing Broccolini, be sure to trim off and discard the thick woody lower part of the stem, similar to the way you would trim asparagus stalks. You can usually snap the tough stem off with your fingers just below where the first leaves start.

GREEK FRITTATA WITH FETA AND DILL

SERVES 4 • GLUTEN FREE • VEGETARIAN

2 cups fat-free egg substitute

⅔ cup crumbled feta

2 tablespoons finely chopped fresh dill

½ teaspoon kosher salt

⅛ teaspoon black pepper

1 medium onion, diced

5 ounces baby spinach

½ cup diced drained water-packed roasted red bell pepper

2 plum tomatoes, seeded and diced

1 Preheat oven to 350°F. Whisk egg substitute, feta, dill, salt, and black pepper together in medium bowl; set aside.

2 Spray 10-inch ovenproof skillet with nonstick spray and set over medium-high heat. When hot, add onion and cook, stirring frequently, until softened, 5–7 minutes.

3 Add spinach, in batches, stirring and tossing until wilted. Add roasted pepper and tomatoes and cook, stirring, 1 minute.

4 Pour egg mixture into skillet and cook until underside begins to set, about 5 minutes. Transfer skillet to oven and bake until center is set, 15–20 minutes. Remove from oven, cut into 4 wedges, and serve warm.

4 SmartPoints value

Per serving (1 wedge): 171 Cal, 6 g Total Fat, 4 g Sat Fat, 877 mg Sod, 14 g Total Carb, 6 g Sugar, 2 g Fib, 18 g Prot.

COOK'S TIP

Dill and feta are a classic combo, but you can opt for basil, parsley, or oregano instead of dill.

Mozzarella, Basil, and
Roasted Pepper Omelette

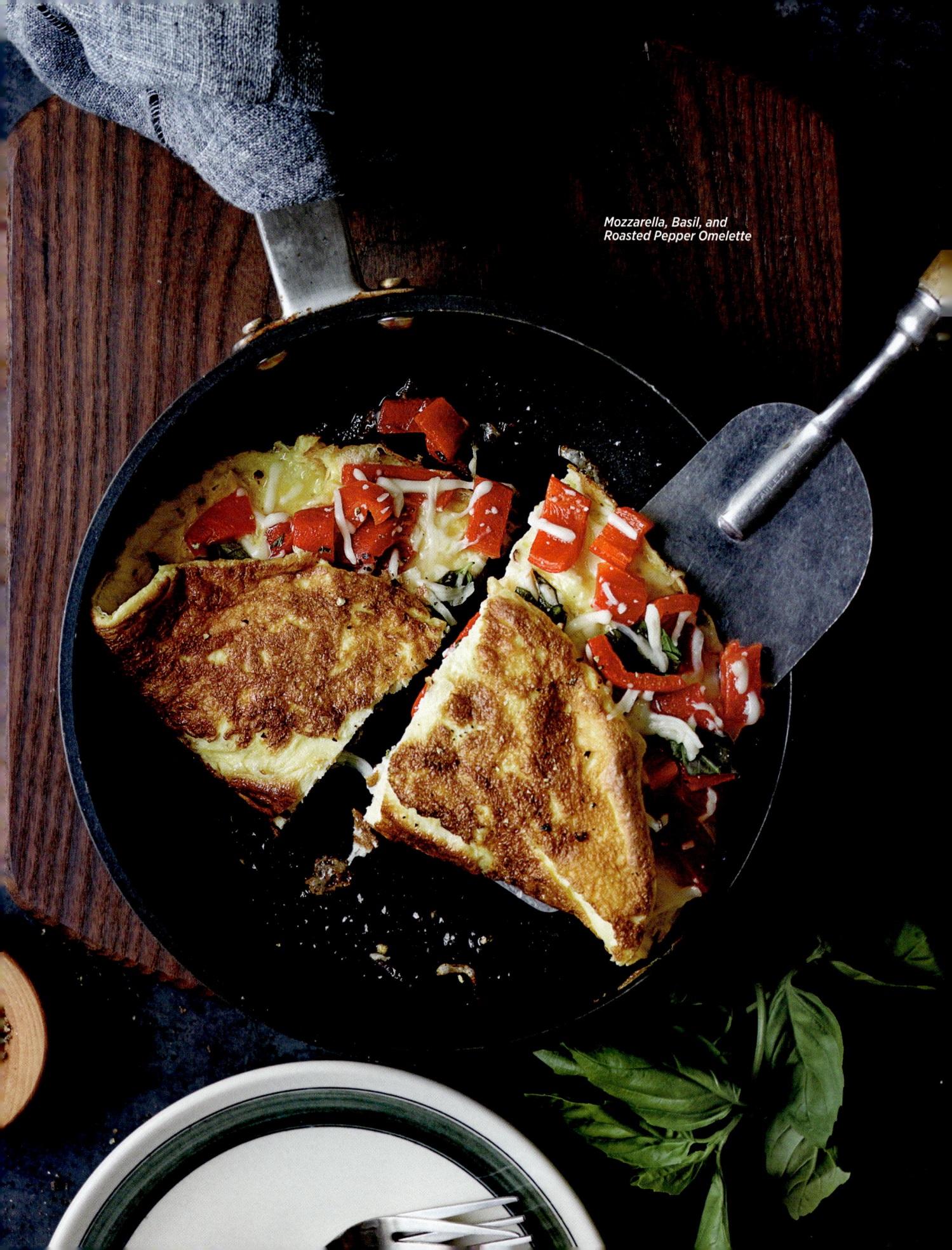

MOZZARELLA, BASIL, AND ROASTED PEPPER OMELETTE

SERVES 2 • GLUTEN FREE • VEGETARIAN • UNDER 20 MINUTES

¼ cup chopped drained water-packed roasted red bell pepper

2 large eggs

2 large egg whites

1 tablespoon fat-free milk

¼ teaspoon salt, or to taste

¼ teaspoon black pepper

1 teaspoon olive oil

⅓ cup shredded fat-free mozzarella

1 tablespoon chopped fresh basil

1 Pat roasted pepper dry with paper towels. Beat eggs, egg whites, milk, salt, and black pepper in medium bowl until frothy.

2 Heat oil in medium nonstick skillet over medium heat. Pour in egg mixture. Cover and cook until almost set, about 2 minutes.

3 Sprinkle mozzarella, roasted pepper, and basil evenly over half of omelette. With heatproof rubber spatula, fold other half of omelette over filling and continue to cook until filling is heated through and eggs are set, about 1 minute longer.

4 Cut omelette in half and slide each half onto plate.

3 SmartPoints value

Per serving (½ omelette): 154 Cal, 7 g Total Fat, 2 g Sat Fat, 648 mg Sod, 7 g Total Carb, 2 g Sugar, 0 g Fib, 16 g Prot.

UP THE PROTEIN

Ham lovers can add ½ cup (2 ounces) diced, lean, low-sodium ham along with the cheese in Step 3 for an additional 2 SmartPoints per serving.

BREAKFAST VEGGIE CASSEROLES

SERVES 4 ● VEGETARIAN

---

4 slices whole wheat bread
½ teaspoon canola oil
½ cup diced red onion
½ cup diced red bell pepper
½ cup diced zucchini
½ teaspoon salt
4 large eggs
4 large egg whites
¼ teaspoon black pepper
½ cup reduced-fat Mexican cheese blend

1 Preheat oven to 400°F. Lightly spray 4 (8-ounce) ramekins or ovenproof bakers with nonstick spray. Cut 4-inch circle from each slice bread and firmly press 1 into bottom of each ramekin; set aside. Discard scraps or save for another use.

2 Heat oil in medium skillet over medium-high heat. Add onion, bell pepper, zucchini, and ¼ teaspoon salt; cook, stirring occasionally, until vegetables soften and onion is translucent, 3–5 minutes. Remove from heat and set aside.

3 Whisk eggs, egg whites, remaining ¼ teaspoon salt, and black pepper together in medium bowl until frothy; stir in cooked vegetables and ¼ cup cheese blend. Divide mixture evenly among ramekins. Sprinkle each with 1 tablespoon remaining cheese.

4 Place ramekins on small baking sheet and bake until knife inserted into center of each casserole comes out clean, about 20 minutes. Remove from oven and cool 5–10 minutes before serving.

5 SmartPoints value

Per serving (1 casserole): 191 Cal, 8 g Total Fat, 3 g Sat Fat, 436 mg Sod, 13 g Total Carb, 3 g Sugar, 2 g Fib, 16 g Prot.

COOK'S TIP

You can make the casseroles ahead, cool them completely, cover each with plastic wrap, and refrigerate up to 3 days. Reheat in the microwave on High until hot, 1 to 1½ minutes.

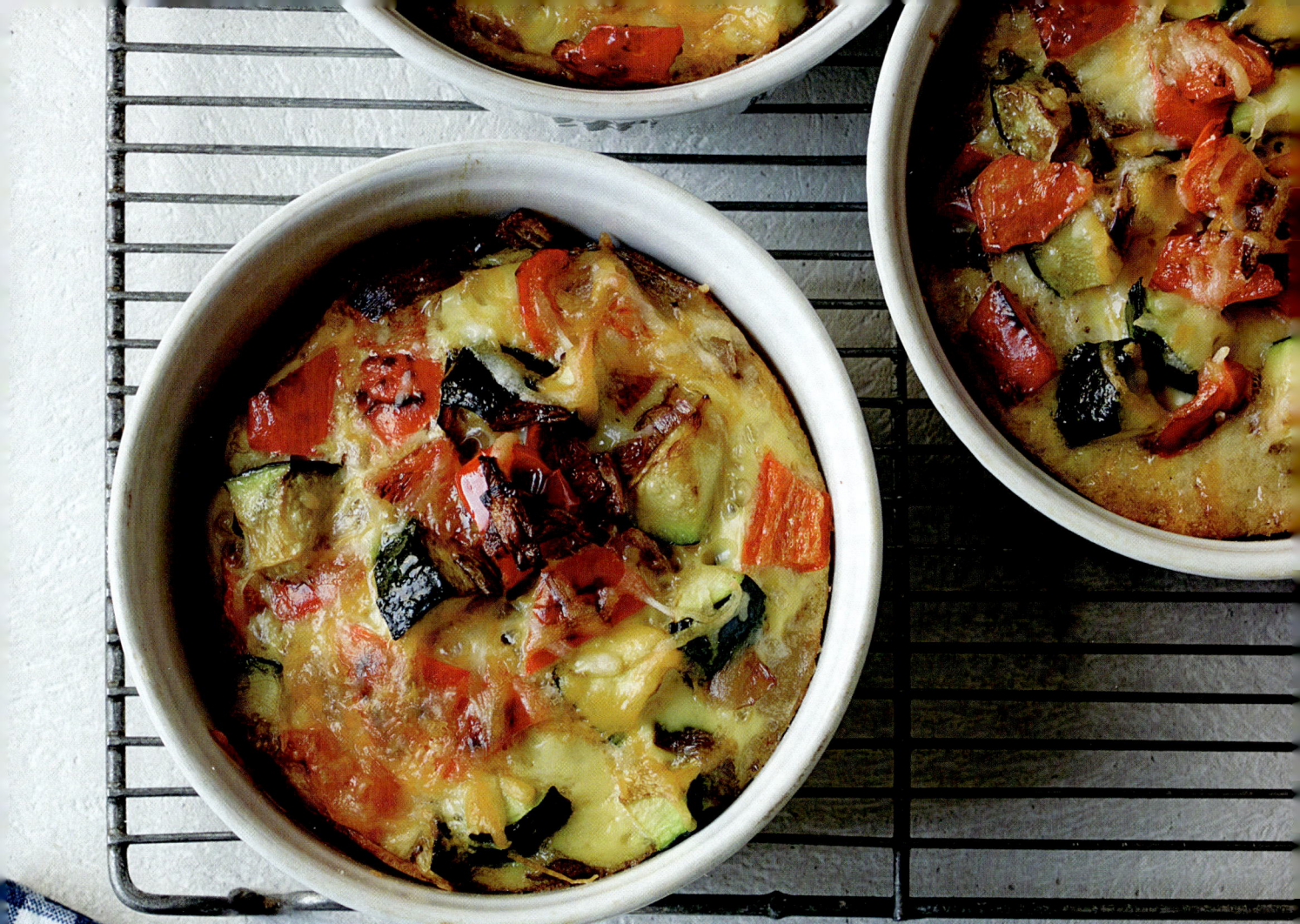

*Breakfast Veggie
Casseroles*

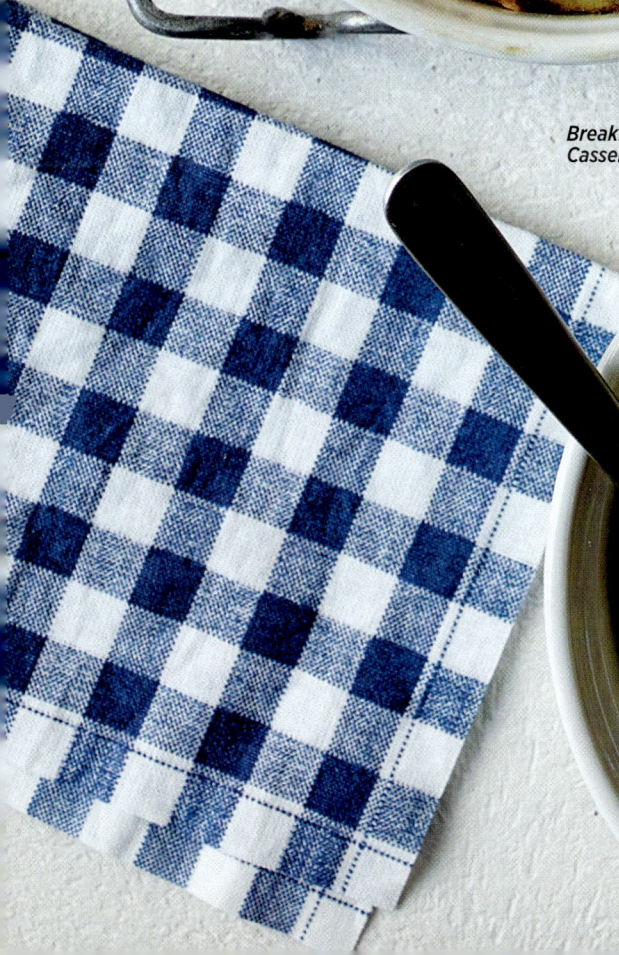

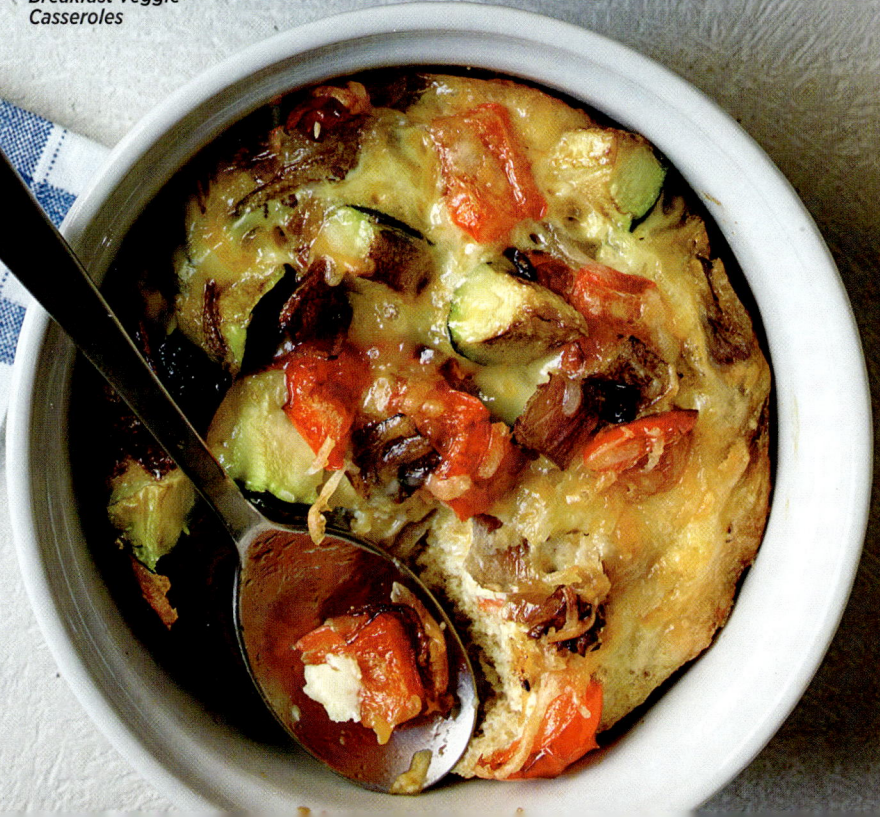

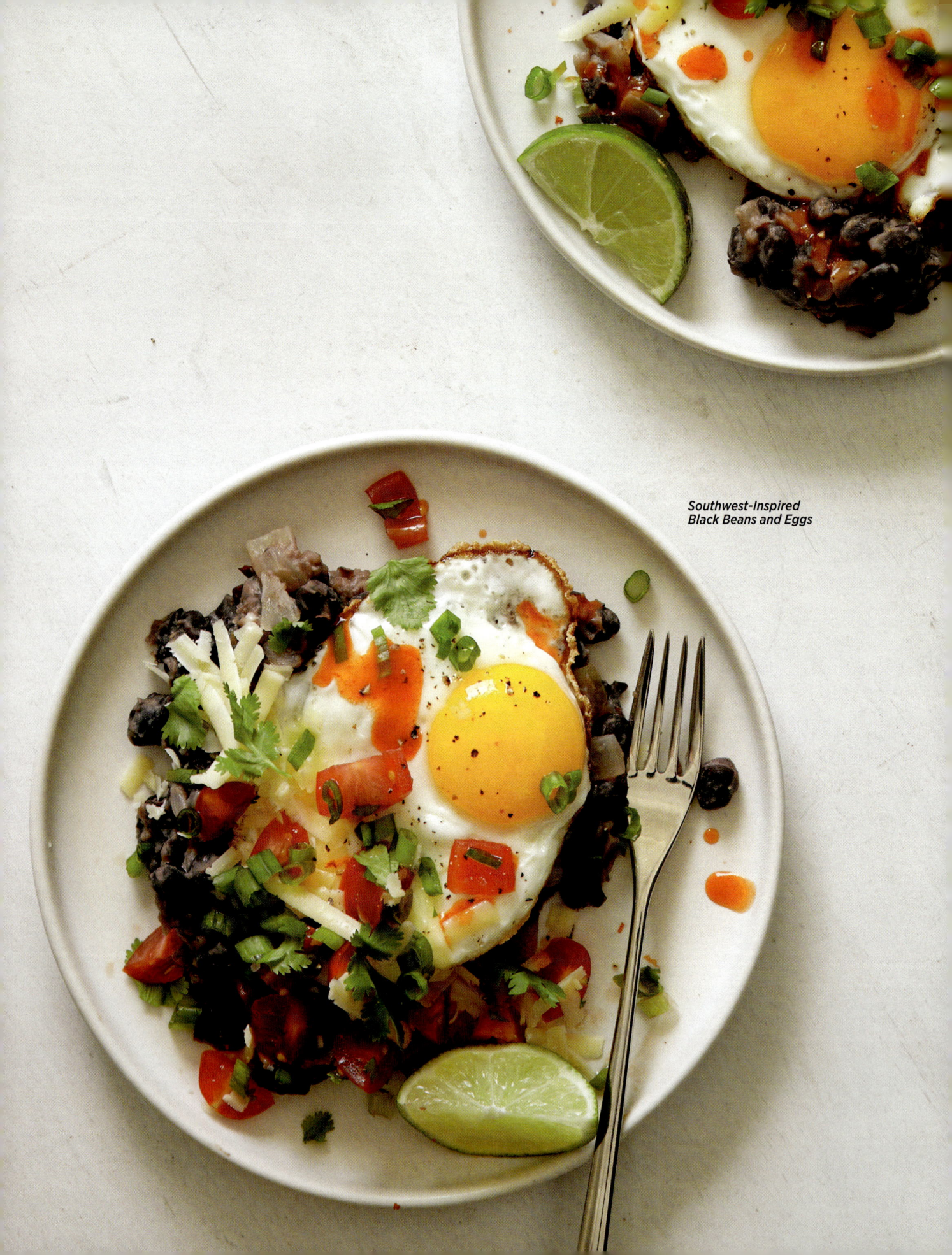

*Southwest-Inspired
Black Beans and Eggs*

SOUTHWEST-INSPIRED BLACK BEANS AND EGGS

SERVES 6 • GLUTEN FREE • VEGETARIAN

2 teaspoons olive oil

1 large onion, diced

1 small jalapeño pepper, seeded and diced

2 (15-ounce) cans black beans, rinsed and drained

¼ cup water

4 teaspoons lime juice

1 garlic clove, finely chopped

½ teaspoon salt

½ teaspoon ground cumin

6 large eggs

2 cups grape tomatoes, chopped

3 scallions, sliced

¼ cup shredded sharp Cheddar

¼ cup chopped fresh cilantro

1 lime, cut into 6 wedges

1 Heat 1½ teaspoons oil in large skillet over medium-high heat. Add onion and jalapeño and cook, stirring often, until softened, 7–10 minutes. Add beans, water, lime juice, garlic, salt, and cumin; stir and heat through. Remove skillet from heat; lightly mash beans and cover to keep warm.

2 Brush large nonstick skillet with remaining ½ teaspoon oil and place over medium heat. When hot, break eggs into skillet and cook until set, flipping eggs if desired.

3 Divide bean mixture among 6 plates and top each with an egg. Sprinkle with tomatoes, scallions, Cheddar, and cilantro; serve with lime wedges.

6 SmartPoints value

Per serving (1 egg, ½ cup bean mixture, 2 teaspoons Cheddar, and ⅓ cup vegetables): 260 Cal, 9 g Total Fat, 3 g Sat Fat, 838 mg Sod, 30 g Total Carb, 3 g Sugar, 11 g Fib, 17 g Prot.

COOK'S TIP

Serve these eggs with a refreshing side of sliced mango or papaya sprinkled with lime juice and sliced mint leaves.

AMAZING COCONUT PANCAKES

SERVES 6 • GLUTEN FREE • VEGETARIAN • UNDER 20 MINUTES

⅔ cup coconut flour

1¼ teaspoons baking powder

¼ teaspoon salt

4 large eggs

1 cup fat-free milk

¼ cup packed light brown sugar

¼ teaspoon vanilla extract

1½ tablespoons melted coconut oil

1 Whisk coconut flour, baking powder, and salt together in small bowl. Whisk eggs, milk, brown sugar, vanilla, and 1 tablespoon coconut oil together in medium bowl. Whisk flour mixture into egg mixture. Let batter sit 5 minutes to thicken.

2 Heat heavy skillet or griddle over medium heat. Brush with some of remaining coconut oil. Working in batches, pour pancake batter by scant ¼ cupfuls onto pan. Cook until pancakes are very brown on undersides and tops begin to set, about 4 minutes. Flip pancakes and cook until other side is browned, 2–3 minutes more; pancakes will be difficult to flip if tops aren't firm, so don't rush. Lower heat if pancakes brown too quickly, and brush pan with more oil between batches as needed.

8 SmartPoints value

Per serving (2 pancakes): 174 Cal, 8 g Total Fat, 5 g Sat Fat, 285 mg Sod, 19 g Total Carb, 14 g Sugar, 4 g Fib, 7 g Prot.

COOK'S TIP

Top these superb gluten-free pancakes with your favorite fresh fruit for natural sweetness.

*Amazing Coconut
Pancakes*

SPELT BLINTZES WITH RICOTTA AND BERRIES

SERVES 4 • VEGETARIAN

1 cup plus 2 tablespoons
low-fat (1%) milk

1 large egg

2 teaspoons unsalted
butter, melted

¼ teaspoon salt

½ cup spelt flour

½ cup all-purpose flour

1 teaspoon canola oil

1 cup fat-free ricotta

2 teaspoons honey

1 teaspoon finely grated
orange zest

4 cups mixed berries

1 Whisk milk, egg, butter, and salt together in large bowl. Add spelt flour and all-purpose flour and whisk until smooth.

2 Brush medium nonstick skillet with some of the oil and set over medium heat. When hot, pour scant ¼ cup batter onto skillet and swirl to make thin, circular layer of batter. Cook until underside is set, 1–2 minutes. Flip and cook through, about 30 seconds longer. Transfer to plate. Brush skillet again with oil. Repeat with remaining batter, stacking crêpes between layers of wax paper and making total of 8.

3 Stir ricotta, honey, and zest together in small bowl. For each blintz, spread 2 tablespoons ricotta mixture on a crêpe; sprinkle with ⅓ cup berries and roll up. Repeat to make total of 8 blintzes. Serve with remaining 1⅓ cups berries.

8 SmartPoints value

Per serving (2 filled blintzes and about ⅓ cup berries): 327 Cal, 7 g Total Fat, 2 g Sat Fat, 323 mg Sod, 52 g Total Carb, 18 g Sugar, 7 g Fib, 17 g Prot.

COOK'S TIP

Spelt is an ancient grain that contains a higher amount of protein than wheat and has a light, nutty, slightly sweet flavor. It's in the same family as wheat, so it's a good replacement for whole wheat flour in recipes.

CREAMY FRUIT-TOPPED WAFFLES

SERVES 4 • VEGETARIAN • UNDER 20 MINUTES

1 cup low-fat (1%)
cottage cheese

1 peach, chopped, or
1 cup chopped frozen
unsweetened peaches

¾ cup chopped fresh pineapple
or drained canned
pineapple in juice

4 low-fat waffles

4 teaspoons honey

¼ teaspoon cinnamon

1 Place cottage cheese in small food processor or blender; pulse until almost smooth. Transfer to small bowl and stir in peach and pineapple.

2 Prepare waffles according to package directions. Spoon about ½ cup fruit mixture over each waffle, drizzle with honey, and sprinkle with cinnamon.

5 SmartPoints value

Per serving (1 topped waffle and 1 teaspoon honey): 182 Cal, 2 g Total Fat, 1 g Sat Fat, 425 mg Sod, 32 g Total Carb, 15 g Sugar, 3 g Fib, 10 g Prot.

UP THE PROTEIN

Customize these waffles with a healthy, crunchy garnish of your choice: 1 tablespoon chopped walnuts or chia seeds per serving will add 2 SmartPoints, while 1 tablespoon of either ground flaxseed or sliced almonds per serving will add 1 SmartPoints.

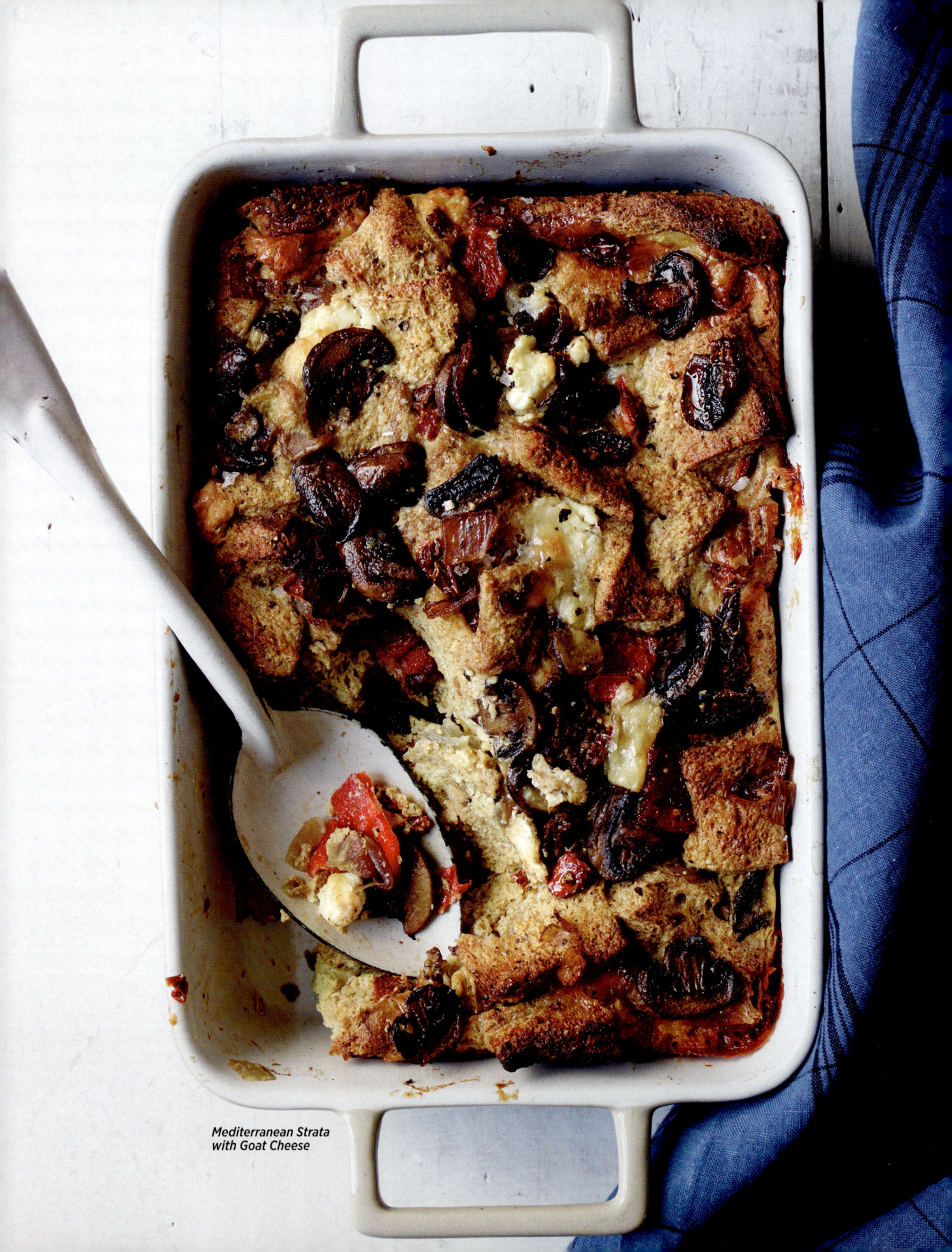

*Mediterranean Strata
with Goat Cheese*

MEDITERRANEAN STRATA WITH GOAT CHEESE

SERVES 6 • VEGETARIAN

1 tablespoon unsalted butter

1 large red onion, chopped

8 ounces cremini mushrooms, thinly sliced

1 teaspoon kosher salt

⅛ teaspoon black pepper

1 teaspoon salt-free Italian seasoning

½ cup water-packed roasted red peppers, rinsed, drained, and coarsely chopped

½ cup sun-dried tomatoes in oil, drained and coarsely chopped

10 slices reduced-calorie wheat bread, crusts removed, bread cubed

2 ounces goat cheese, crumbled

3 cups egg substitute

1 Preheat oven to 350°F.

2 Melt butter in large nonstick skillet over medium heat. Add onion, mushrooms, salt, and black pepper; cook, stirring frequently, until water from mushrooms is released and evaporates and mushrooms begin to brown, 15–20 minutes. Remove skillet from heat; stir in Italian seasoning, roasted peppers, and tomatoes. Add bread cubes and toss gently to combine.

3 Spray 1½-quart casserole dish with nonstick spray. Spoon in bread mixture and sprinkle with goat cheese. Pour egg substitute over top.

4 Bake, uncovered, until center is set, about 1 hour. Let stand 10 minutes; cut into 6 pieces and serve.

6 SmartPoints value

Per serving (⅙ of strata): 244 Cal, 7 g Total Fat, 4 g Sat Fat, 805 mg Sod, 25 g Total Carb, 5 g Sugar, 5 g Fib, 22 g Prot.

COOK'S TIP

If you like, you can prepare the strata through Step 3 the night before, cover, and refrigerate. Uncover, bring to room temperature, and bake as directed above.

QUINOA AND APPLE BREAKFAST CEREAL

SERVES 6 • GLUTEN FREE • VEGETARIAN

1 cup quinoa

1 tablespoon salted butter

2 apples, cored and chopped

2 cups water

½ teaspoon cinnamon

3 tablespoons packed brown sugar

½ cup fat-free milk

1 Rinse quinoa well under cold running water. Set aside.

2 Spray large skillet with nonstick spray; set over medium heat. When skillet is hot, add ½ tablespoon butter and cook until melted and beginning to sizzle. Add apples and cook, turning occasionally, until apples are soft and begin to caramelize, 5–10 minutes depending on variety; set aside.

3 Add quinoa and water to medium saucepan and bring to boil over medium-high heat; boil 1 minute. Reduce heat to low, cover tightly, and simmer for 10 minutes. When quinoa is cooked (a white spiral will appear on each grain), remove from heat and fluff with fork. Add remaining ½ tablespoon butter, cinnamon, brown sugar, and milk; stir to combine and fold in apples. Divide among 6 bowls.

6 SmartPoints value®

Per serving (about ⅔ cup): 187 Cal, 4 g Total Fat, 1 g Sat Fat, 32 mg Sod, 35 g Total Carb, 14 g Sugar, 4 g Fib, 5 g Prot.

UP THE PROTEIN

Topping each serving with ½ cup plain fat-free Greek yogurt will increase the SmartPoints value by 1.

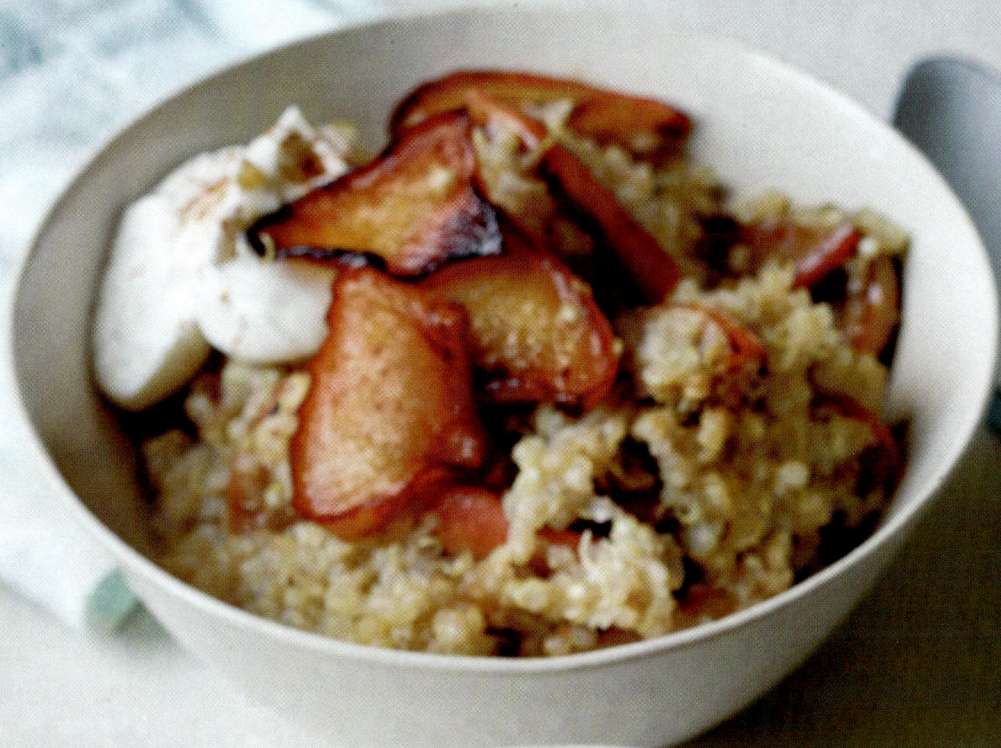

*Quinoa and Apple
Breakfast Cereal*

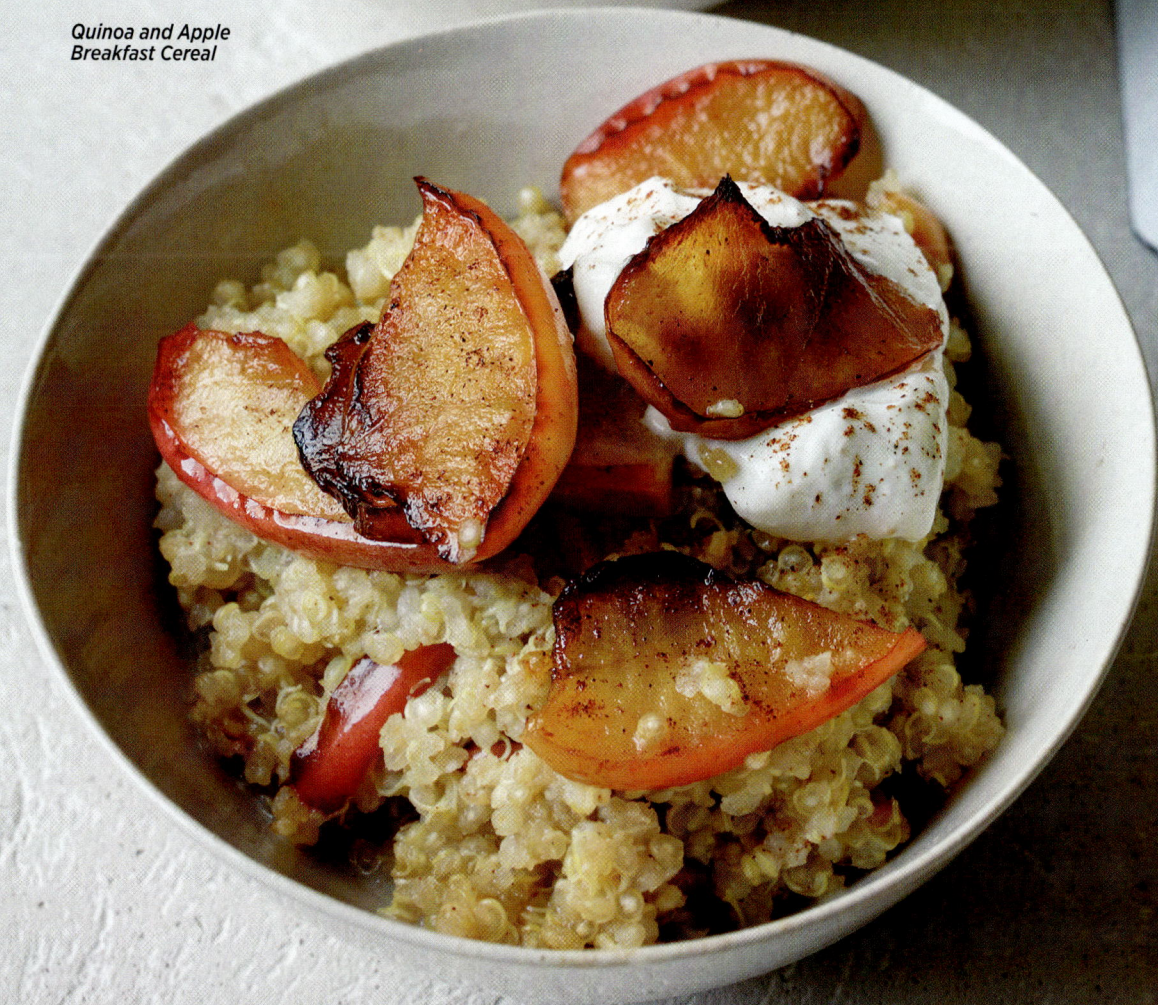

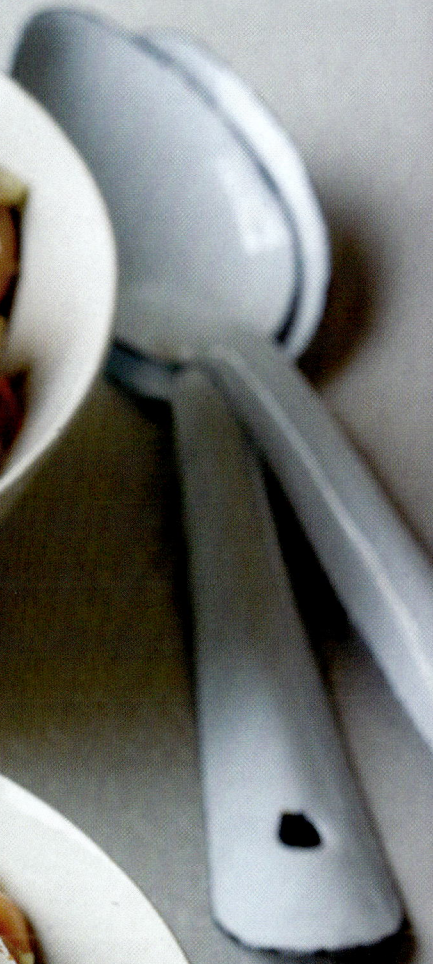

ORANGE-PECAN COUSCOUS BREAKFAST PUDDING

SERVES 6 • VEGETARIAN

1½ cups water
1 cup whole wheat couscous
Pinch salt
3 cups low-fat (1%) milk
1½ tablespoons honey
½ teaspoon grated orange zest
1 large egg white
¼ cup toasted wheat germ
¾ teaspoon vanilla extract
3 tablespoons chopped pecans, toasted

1 Bring water to boil in large saucepan over high heat. Stir in couscous and salt. Reduce heat and simmer until water is absorbed, about 2 minutes. Remove from heat and fluff couscous with fork. Cover and let stand 5 minutes.

2 Whisk milk, honey, and orange zest into couscous. Bring to boil over medium-high heat, whisking frequently to break up any lumps. Reduce heat to medium-low and cook, stirring frequently, until mixture is slightly thickened, about 5 minutes. Remove from heat.

3 Whisk ½ cup couscous mixture and egg white together in small bowl. Add egg mixture to saucepan and cook over low heat, stirring, until pudding is thick and creamy, about 5 minutes.

4 Stir in wheat germ and vanilla. Spoon pudding evenly into 6 bowls and sprinkle evenly with pecans.

8 SmartPoints value

Per serving (generous ¾ cup pudding and ½ tablespoon pecans): 218 Cal, 5 g Total Fat, 1 g Sat Fat, 116 mg Sod, 35 g Total Carb, 13 g Sugar, 4 g Fib, 10 g Prot.

COOK'S TIP

Top each serving of the pudding with a handful of fresh blueberries, raspberries, or strawberries for more natural sweetness without additional SmartPoints.

BACON-AND-SWISS QUICHE

SERVES 8

2 sheets phyllo, each cut into 3 strips

3 large eggs

¼ cup fat-free egg substitute

1 cup evaporated fat-free milk

½ teaspoon salt

¼ teaspoon black pepper

¼ teaspoon ground nutmeg

Pinch cayenne

½ cup shredded low-fat Swiss cheese

4 ounces turkey bacon, cooked until crisp, and crumbled

1 Preheat oven to 350°F. Spray 9-inch pie plate with nonstick spray.

2 Lay phyllo in pie plate, one piece at a time, spraying each layer with nonstick spray; dough should cover bottom and sides of plate in overlapping layers. Fold in any overhanging corners.

3 Whisk eggs, egg substitute, milk, salt, black pepper, nutmeg, and cayenne together in small bowl.

4 Sprinkle Swiss cheese and bacon over phyllo. Pour in egg mixture and place plate on baking sheet. Bake until firm, 30–35 minutes. Cool at least 5 minutes before cutting into 8 wedges.

4 SmartPoints value

Per serving (1 wedge): 142 Cal, 7 g Total Fat, 2 g Sat Fat, 565 mg Sod, 7 g Total Carb, 4 g Sugar, 0 g Fib, 12 g Prot.

COOK'S TIP

If you want more veggies in your quiche, add 1 cup chopped steamed broccoli florets to the pie plate along with the cheese and bacon in Step 4.

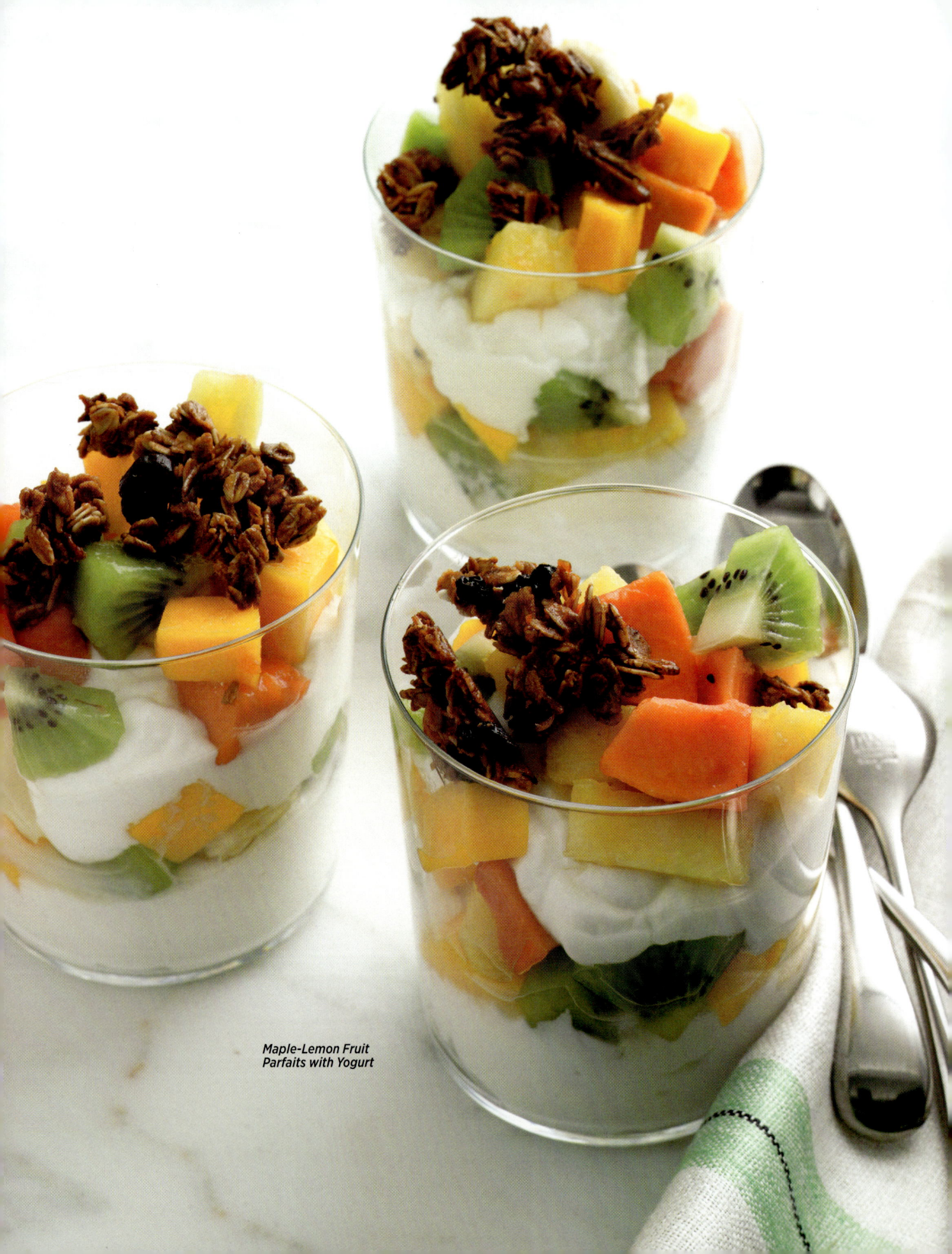

*Maple-Lemon Fruit
Parfaits with Yogurt*

MAPLE-LEMON FRUIT
PARFAITS WITH YOGURT

SERVES 4 • VEGETARIAN • UNDER 20 MINUTES • NO COOK

2 cups diced pineapple

1 large mango, peeled, pitted, and cubed

1 small banana, cubed

1 teaspoon grated lemon zest

1 tablespoon lemon juice

2 cups plain low-fat Greek yogurt

2 teaspoons maple syrup

4 tablespoons low-fat granola

1 Stir pineapple, mango, banana, lemon zest, and lemon juice together in medium bowl. Combine yogurt and maple syrup in another medium bowl.

2 Spoon ¼ cup yogurt into each of 4 parfait glasses or 4 small lidded jars (such as mason jars). Top each with ½ cup fruit mixture. Repeat layering once. Serve at once, or refrigerate overnight or up to 12 hours. Sprinkle parfaits evenly with granola before serving.

3 SmartPoints value

Per serving (1 parfait): 241 Cal, 2 g Total Fat, 2 g Sat Fat, 60 mg Sod, 45 g Total Carb, 33 g Sugar, 4 g Fib, 14 g Prot.

COOK'S TIP

Maple and lemon accentuate the flavor of most fruit, so you can use whatever is in season to make these parfaits. Use berries for color and flavor, kiwifruit for a tropical touch, or cherries for summery deliciousness.

TOMATOES STUFFED WITH TABBOULEH EGG SALAD

SERVES 4 • VEGETARIAN

1 cup water

¾ teaspoon salt

⅓ cup bulgur

4 large hard-cooked eggs, peeled and chopped

½ cup chopped fresh parsley

½ red bell pepper, chopped

2 tablespoons chopped red onion

1 tablespoon lemon juice

1½ teaspoons red-wine vinegar

1 tablespoon olive oil

⅛ teaspoon black pepper

4 large tomatoes

1 Bring water and ¼ teaspoon salt to boil in medium saucepan. Stir in bulgur and remove from heat. Cover and let stand 25 minutes. Drain bulgur in colander, pressing out excess liquid with back of spoon.

2 Transfer bulgur to large bowl. Stir in eggs, parsley, bell pepper, onion, lemon juice, vinegar, oil, remaining ½ teaspoon salt, and black pepper; set aside.

3 Cut each tomato crosswise about one-third from the top; reserve top as a "cap." Remove and discard seeds from tomato bottoms. With grapefruit spoon or small knife, scoop pulp from each tomato, leaving a ¼-inch-thick shell. Chop pulp and stir into bulgur mixture. Spoon mixture evenly into tomato shells and top with caps.

4 SmartPoints value

Per serving (1 stuffed tomato): 183 Cal, 9 g Total Fat, 2 g Sat Fat, 525 mg Sod, 18 g Total Carb, 6 g Sugar, 5 g Fib, 10 g Prot.

UP THE PROTEIN

Stir 2 extra hard-cooked chopped egg whites (but no extra yolks) into the filling mixture for no additional SmartPoints.

INDIVIDUAL BAKED ZITIS

SERVES 12 • VEGETARIAN

1 pound whole wheat ziti

¼ cup grated Parmesan

1½ cups shredded part-skim mozzarella

½ cup part-skim ricotta

2½ cups canned crushed tomatoes

1 tablespoon tomato paste

1 tablespoon chopped fresh basil, plus extra for garnish

1 small garlic clove, minced

½ teaspoon Italian seasoning

½ teaspoon red pepper flakes, or to taste

½ teaspoon kosher salt

¼ teaspoon black pepper

1 large egg white

1 tablespoon water

1 Preheat oven to 375°F.

2 Cook pasta according to package directions until barely tender; drain and pat dry.

3 Meanwhile, generously spray 12 extra-large (6-ounce) muffin cups or 6-ounce ramekins with nonstick spray. Sprinkle ½ teaspoon Parmesan in bottom of each and tilt ramekins or muffin pan to cover bottoms evenly.

4 Transfer warm pasta to large bowl; immediately stir in ¾ cup mozzarella and the ricotta. Add tomatoes, tomato paste, basil, garlic, Italian seasoning, red pepper flakes, salt, and black pepper.

5 Combine egg white and water in small bowl; whisk until smooth. Add egg mixture to pasta; stir to combine.

6 Divide pasta mixture evenly among prepared muffin cups and press down lightly with spoon to pack; sprinkle each cup with 1 tablespoon remaining mozzarella. Bake, uncovered, until mozzarella is melted and noodles begin to brown at edges, 12–15 minutes. Remove from oven and let cool for a few minutes; sprinkle remaining 2 tablespoons Parmesan over tops. Remove zitis from muffin pan; garnish with basil.

6 SmartPoints value

Per serving (1 baked ziti): 203 Cal, 5 g Total Fat, 2 g Sat Fat, 305 mg Sod, 31 g Total Carb, 2 g Sugar, 3 g Fib, 11 g Prot.

COOK'S TIP

To freeze extra zitis, cool them, wrap them first in freezer wrap and then foil. They'll keep up to 3 months and can be reheated in the microwave.

CRUNCHY-TOP MAC-AND-CHEESE

SERVES 4 • VEGETARIAN

1 teaspoon olive oil

⅓ cup panko (Japanese bread crumbs)

1 (20-ounce) package peeled and cut-up butternut squash

¾ cup vegetable broth

1 cup shredded reduced-fat sharp Cheddar

2 tablespoons grated pecorino

2 tablespoons light cream cheese (Neufchâtel)

1 teaspoon Dijon mustard

¾ teaspoon salt

⅛ teaspoon cayenne

1¼ cups (4 ounces) mini pasta shells

2 cups small cauliflower florets

1 Preheat oven to 400°F. Spray 8-inch square baking dish with nonstick spray. Bring large saucepan of salted water to boil.

2 Meanwhile, heat oil in medium skillet over medium heat. Add panko and cook, stirring occasionally, until toasted, about 4 minutes; set aside.

3 Add squash to boiling water; cover and return to boil. Cook, uncovered, until squash is very tender, about 10 minutes.

4 Meanwhile, combine broth, Cheddar, pecorino, cream cheese, mustard, salt, and cayenne in blender. With slotted spoon, transfer cooked squash to blender and puree. (Leave water in pan.)

5 Bring water back to boil. Cook pasta half the time directed on package; add cauliflower during last minute of cooking time. Drain; return to pot. Stir in puree and toss to coat. Spread pasta mixture in prepared baking dish; top with crumb mixture and spray with nonstick spray. Bake until top is golden and casserole is bubbling, about 25 minutes.

7 SmartPoints value

Per serving (about 1¼ cups): 303 Cal, 7 g Total Fat, 3 g Sat Fat, 833 mg Sod, 48 g Total Carb, 5 g Sugar, 10 g Fib, 15 g Prot.

COOK'S TIP

If you like, dress up the crumb topping by tossing the toasted panko with 1 teaspoon chopped fresh thyme in Step 2.

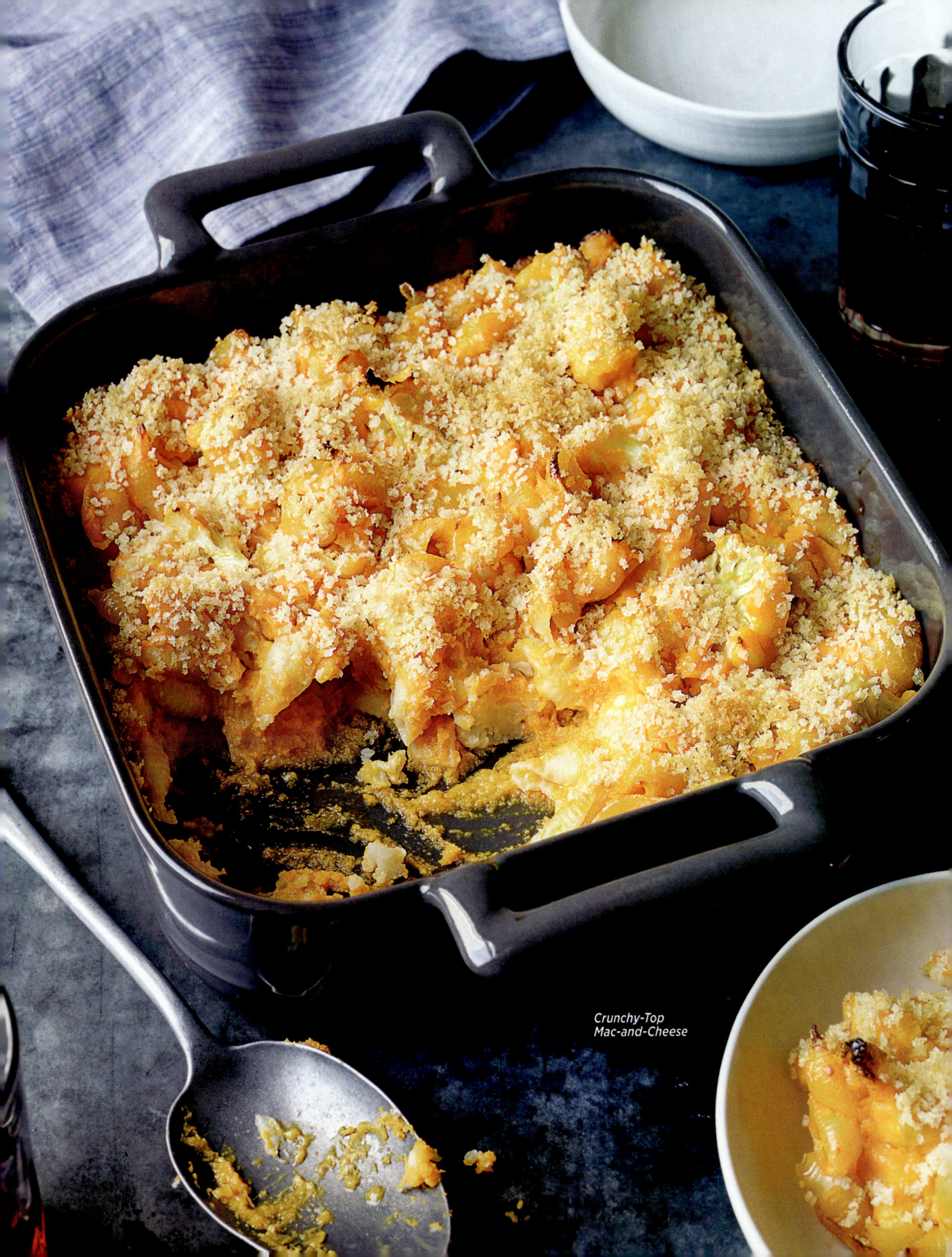

Crunchy-Top
Mac-and-Cheese

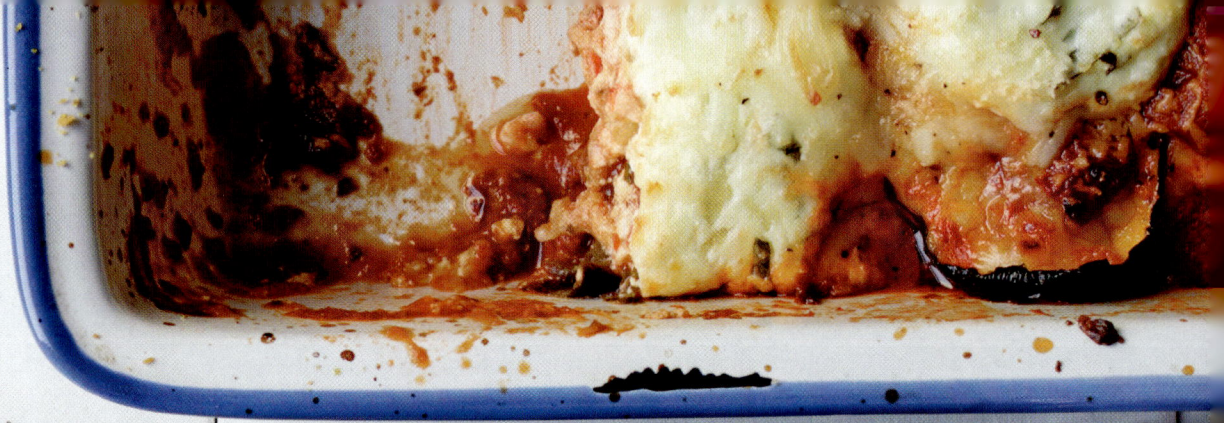

*No-Noodle
Vegetable
Lasagna*

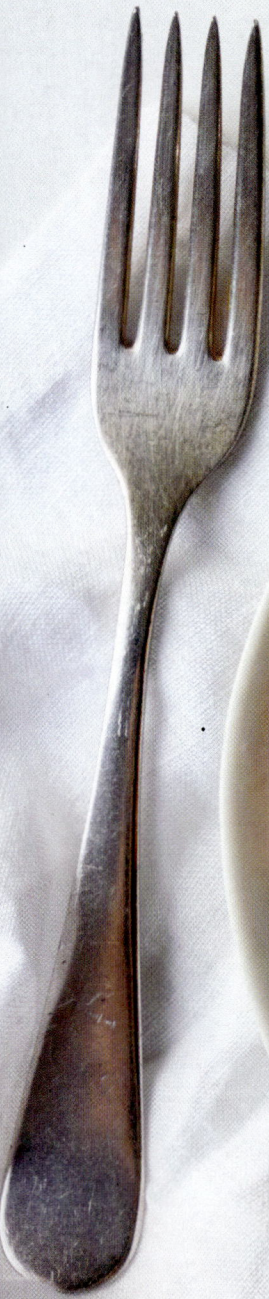

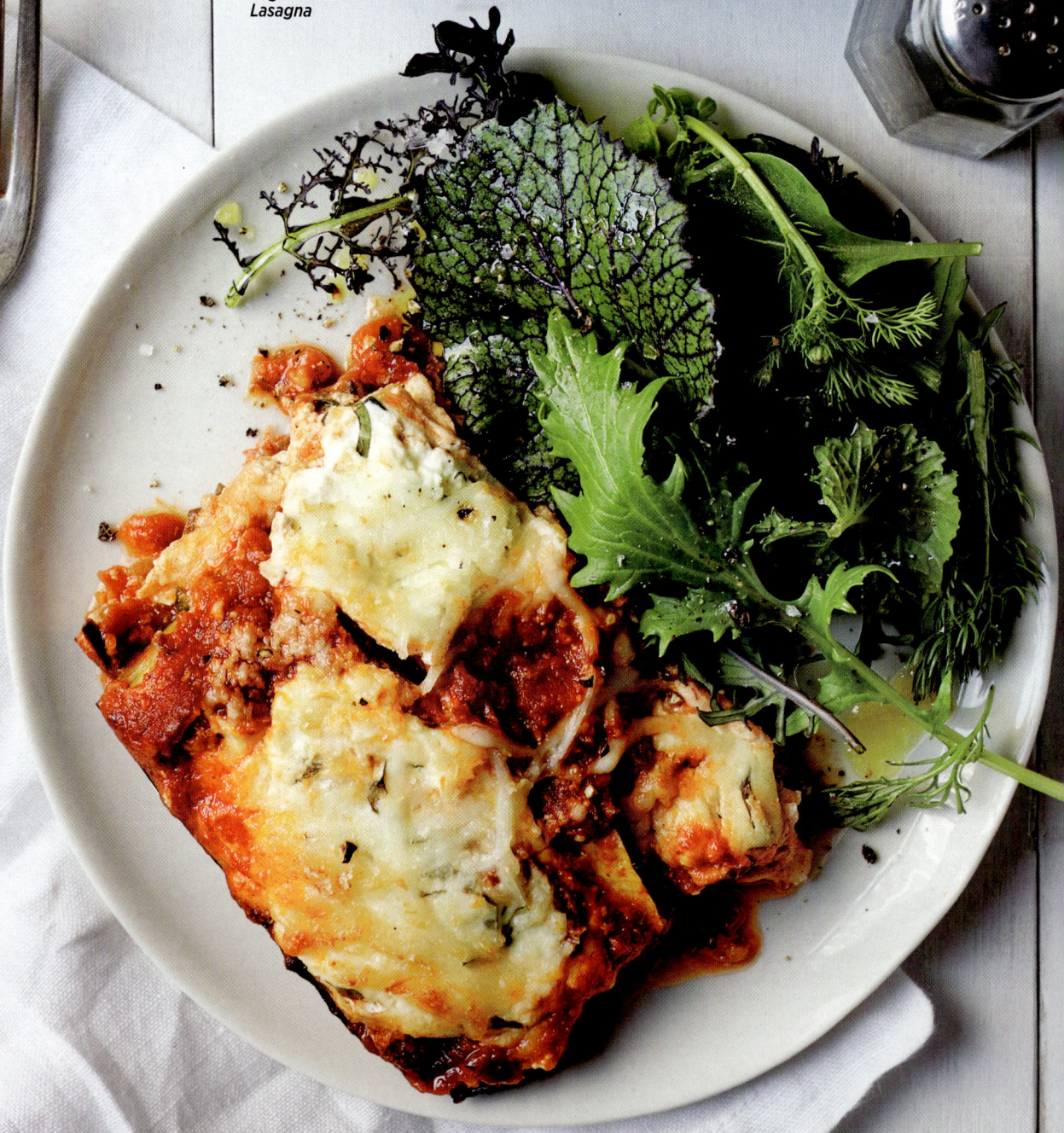

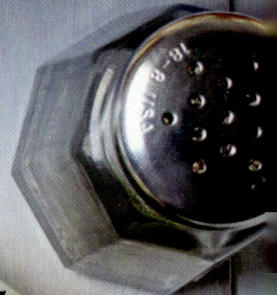

NO-NOODLE VEGETABLE LASAGNA

SERVES 12 • GLUTEN FREE • VEGETARIAN

1 medium eggplant, trimmed, sliced lengthwise into ¼-inch-thick slices

2 large zucchini, trimmed, sliced lengthwise into ¼-inch-thick slices

¾ pound part-skim ricotta

1 large egg, beaten

¼ cup fresh basil leaves, cut into thin strips

½ cup grated Parmesan

4 cups prepared marinara sauce

8 ounces shredded part-skim mozzarella

1 Preheat oven to 400°F. Spray 2 baking sheets with nonstick spray. Place eggplant on one baking sheet and zucchini on other baking sheet; spray vegetables with nonstick spray. Roast 8 minutes; turn vegetables and roast 7–10 minutes more, until vegetables are tender but not mushy. Remove vegetables from oven; reduce temperature to 350°F.

2 While vegetables roast, combine ricotta, egg, basil, and ¼ cup Parmesan in medium bowl; set aside.

3 To assemble lasagna, spray bottom and sides of 14 x 8-inch or 9 x 13-inch baking dish with nonstick spray. Spread thin layer of marinara sauce (¼–⅓ cup) on bottom of dish. Layer eggplant over sauce (use all slices, overlapping if necessary). Cover eggplant with half of remaining sauce and spread half of ricotta mixture on top; sprinkle with half of mozzarella. Top with zucchini and cover zucchini with remaining sauce; spread with remaining ricotta mixture and then sprinkle with remaining mozzarella and remaining Parmesan.

4 Bake until lasagna begins to bubble, 35–40 minutes. Remove from oven and let rest at least 15 minutes before cutting into 12 equal pieces.

5 SmartPoints value

Per serving (1 piece): 178 Cal, 9 g Total Fat, 4 g Sat Fat, 569 mg Sod, 13 g Total Carb, 6 g Sugar, 3 g Fib, 12 g Prot.

COOK'S TIP

Serve the lasagna with a simple salad of mixed baby greens tossed with white-wine vinegar and salt and pepper to taste.

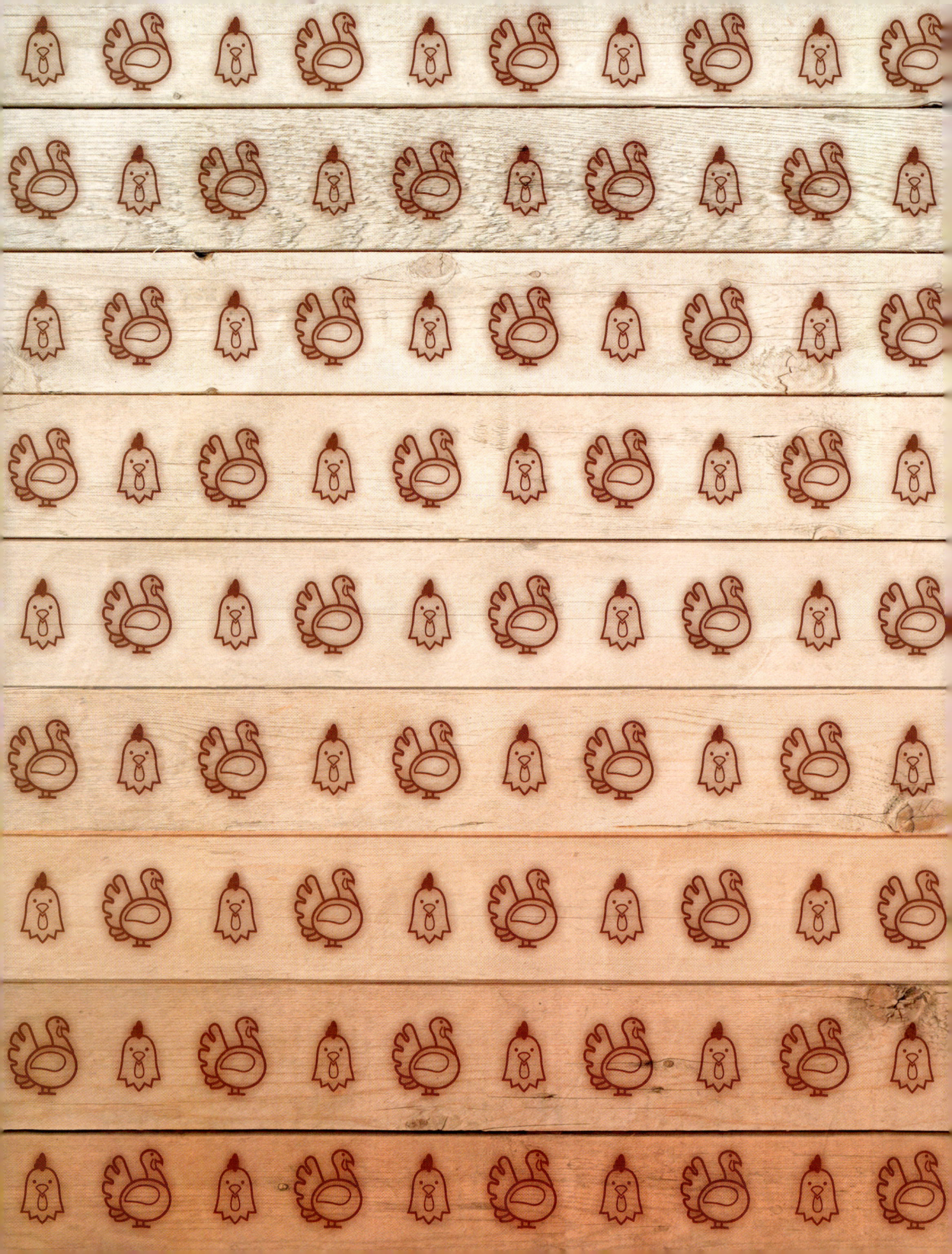

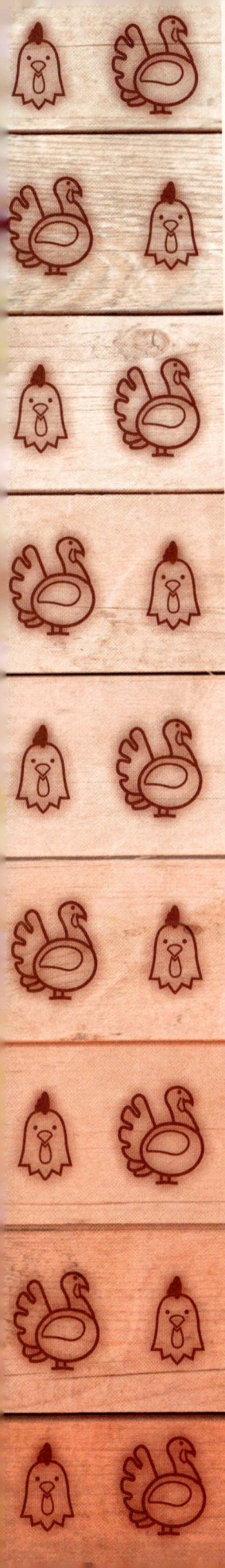

CHICKEN TURKEY & DUCK

CHICKEN BREAST SAUTÉ
PUTTANESCA STYLE

SERVES 4 • GLUTEN FREE

1 teaspoon olive oil

4 (5-ounce) skinless boneless chicken breasts

½ teaspoon salt

½ teaspoon black pepper

2 teaspoons unsalted butter

3 garlic cloves, finely chopped

½ teaspoon red pepper flakes, or to taste

10 black olives, sliced

1 tablespoon capers, drained and chopped

1 (14½-ounce) can diced tomatoes

1 Heat oil in large nonstick skillet over medium heat. Sprinkle chicken with salt and black pepper and add to skillet. Cook until golden brown and cooked through, about 5 minutes per side. Transfer chicken to plate and set aside.

2 Melt butter in same skillet over medium heat. Add garlic and red pepper flakes and cook, stirring, 30 seconds. Stir in olives and capers; pour in tomatoes. Bring to simmer, scraping up any browned bits on bottom of skillet. Reduce heat to low and simmer gently, just until slightly reduced, about 3 minutes.

3 Return chicken and any accumulated juices to skillet; cook just until warmed through, about 2 minutes.

4 SmartPoints value

Per serving (1 chicken breast and about ⅓ cup sauce): 219 Cal, 8 g Total Fat, 2 g Sat Fat, 724 mg Sod, 6 g Total Carb, 3 g Sugar, 2 g Fib, 31 g Prot.

COOK'S TIP

Browning the chicken well before making the sauce is key to this dish's delectably deep flavor, so don't rush the chicken out of the skillet.

PERUVIAN CHICKEN WITH AVOCADO AND RED ONION SALAD

SERVES 6 • GLUTEN FREE

2 tablespoons white-wine vinegar

1 tablespoon paprika

1 tablespoon ground cumin

5 garlic cloves, minced

1 teaspoon canola oil

⅛ teaspoon cayenne

1¾ teaspoons salt

1 (3½-pound) whole chicken, skin and wings removed and discarded

1 heart romaine lettuce, thinly sliced (about 6 cups)

½ small red onion, thinly sliced

½ small avocado, pitted, peeled, and thinly sliced

Juice of ½ lime

Lime wedges for serving

1 Preheat oven to 400°F. Spray roasting rack with nonstick spray and place in roasting pan.

2 Stir vinegar, paprika, cumin, garlic, oil, cayenne, and 1½ teaspoons salt together in small bowl. Rub spice mixture all over meat and inside cavity of chicken. Tie legs together with kitchen string. Place chicken, breast side up, on prepared rack in pan. Roast until instant-read thermometer inserted into thickest part of thigh (not touching bone) registers 165°F, about 1 hour. Transfer chicken to cutting board and let stand 10 minutes.

3 Combine romaine and onion on serving platter. Top with avocado; sprinkle with lime juice and remaining ¼ teaspoon salt.

4 Carve chicken into 6 pieces and serve with salad and lime wedges on the side.

4 SmartPoints value

Per serving (1 piece chicken and 1 cup salad): 211 Cal, 8 g Total Fat, 2 g Sat Fat, 826 mg Sod, 6 g Carb, 1 g Sugar, 3 g Fib, 28 g Prot.

COOK'S TIP

If you think a chicken roasted without the skin will be dry or flavorless, think again. This recipe's combination of bright spices and a touch of canola oil results in a delicious roast bird. Just make sure you don't overcook it.

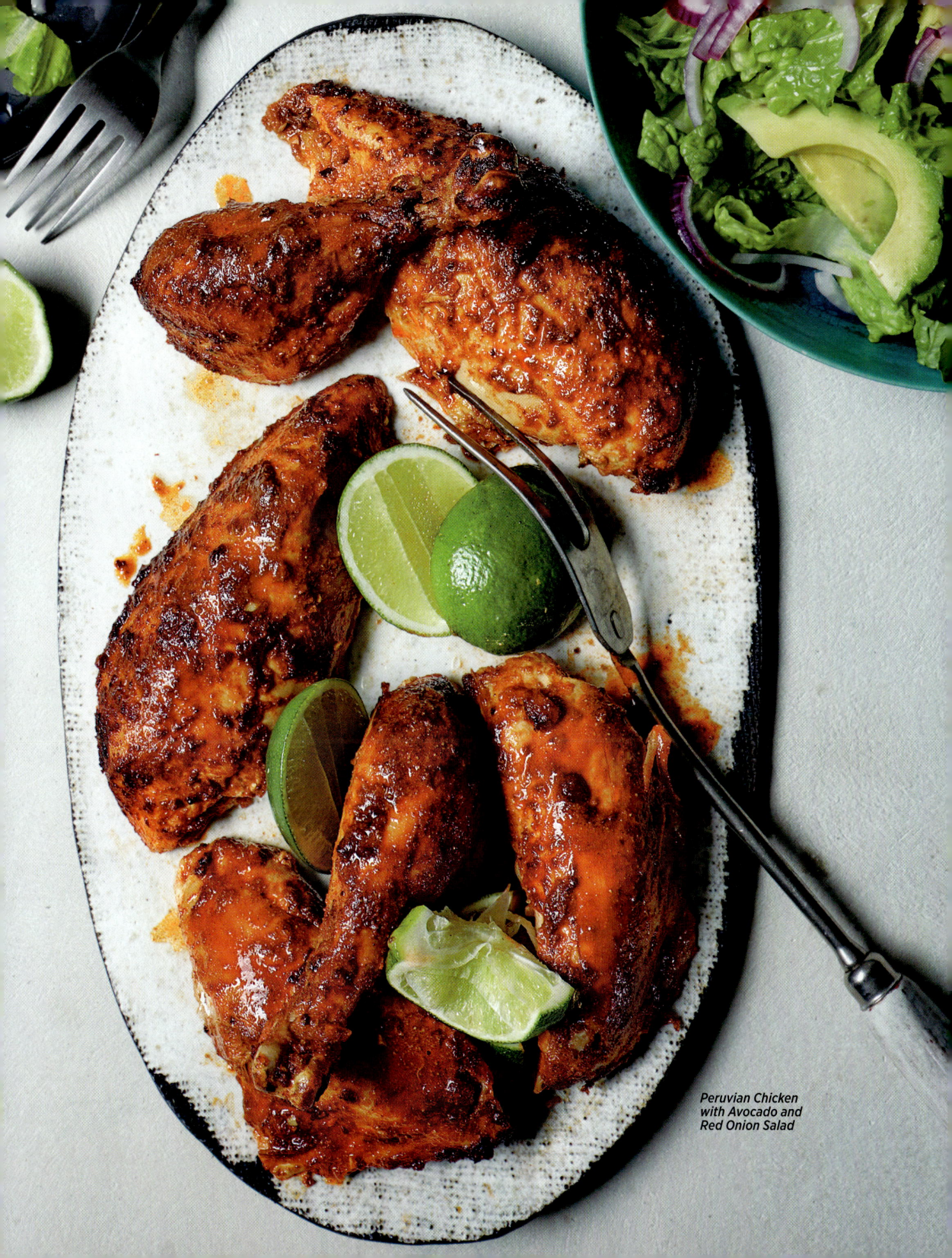

Peruvian Chicken with Avocado and Red Onion Salad

Grilled Chicken with Minty Melon-Feta Salad

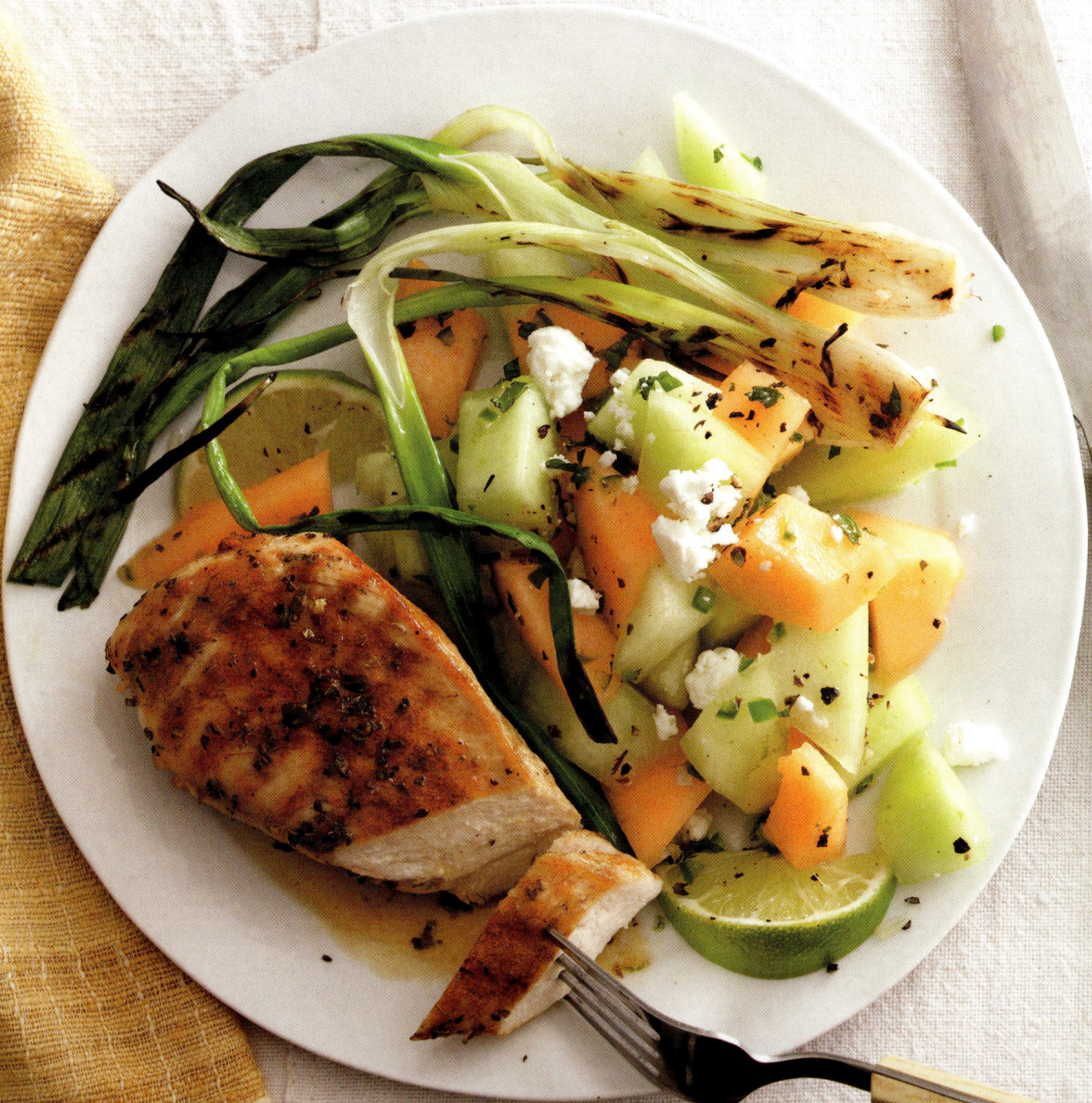

GRILLED CHICKEN WITH MINTY MELON-FETA SALAD

SERVES 4 ● GLUTEN FREE

1 tablespoon olive oil

1 tablespoon minced fresh oregano, or 1 teaspoon dried

1¼ teaspoons grated lime zest

1 garlic clove, minced

½ teaspoon salt

¼ teaspoon black pepper

4 (7-ounce) skinless bone-in chicken breasts

2½ cups diced cantaloupe

2½ cups diced honeydew

2 tablespoons chopped fresh mint

1½ tablespoons lime juice

1 jalapeño pepper, seeded and minced

½ cup crumbled reduced-fat feta

Lime wedges

1 Spray grill rack or nonstick grill pan with nonstick spray. Preheat grill to medium or prepare medium fire, or place grill pan over medium heat.

2 Combine oil, oregano, 1 teaspoon lime zest, garlic, ¼ teaspoon salt, and pepper in large bowl; add chicken and turn to coat. Place chicken on grill rack or in pan; grill, turning occasionally, until chicken is cooked through, about 25 minutes.

3 Meanwhile, to make salad, stir cantaloupe, honeydew, mint, lime juice, jalapeño, remaining ¼ teaspoon salt, and remaining ¼ teaspoon lime zest together in large bowl. Add feta and toss to combine. Serve chicken with salad and lime wedges.

4 SmartPoints value

Per serving (1 chicken breast and 1 cup salad): 301 Cal, 10 g Total Fat, 3 g Sat Fat, 521 mg Sod, 20 g Total Carb, 15 g Sugar, 2 g Fib, 34 g Prot.

COOK'S TIP

Bone-in skinless breasts are a great cut for grilling since the rib bones insulate the meat on one side, helping it stay moist. But if you like you can use 5-ounce skinless boneless breasts. Just decrease the cooking time by about half.

SESAME CHICKEN AND BROCCOLI STIR-FRY

SERVES 4

½ cup chicken broth

3 tablespoons soy sauce

2 tablespoons ketchup

1 tablespoon dark brown sugar

2 teaspoons sambal oelek
or Asian chili sauce

2 teaspoons cornstarch

2 teaspoons sesame oil

1 pound skinless boneless
chicken breast, cut
into cubes

1 tablespoon minced
peeled fresh ginger

2 garlic cloves, minced

4 cups small broccoli florets

1 bunch scallions, white and
light green parts, sliced

2 teaspoons toasted
sesame seeds

1 Whisk broth, soy sauce, ketchup, brown sugar, sambal oelek, and cornstarch together in small bowl; set aside.

2 Heat oil in large skillet or wok over medium-high heat. Add chicken and cook, stirring, just until cooked through, 3–4 minutes. Remove with slotted spoon and set aside.

3 Add ginger and garlic to skillet and cook, stirring, 1 minute. Add broccoli and toss to coat.

4 Add chicken broth mixture to skillet, raise heat to high, cover, and cook until broccoli is crisp-tender, about 5 minutes. Stir in chicken, scallions, and sesame seeds and cook, uncovered, until sauce is thick, about 3 minutes.

4 SmartPoints value

Per serving (1 cup): 238 Cal, 6 g Total Fat, 1 g Sat Fat, 994 mg Sod, 17 g Total Carb, 7 g Sugar, 3 g Fib, 29 g Prot.

UP THE PROTEIN

Love cashews? Chop ¼ cup toasted cashews and add them to the stir-fry with the sesame and increase the SmartPoints value per serving by 2.

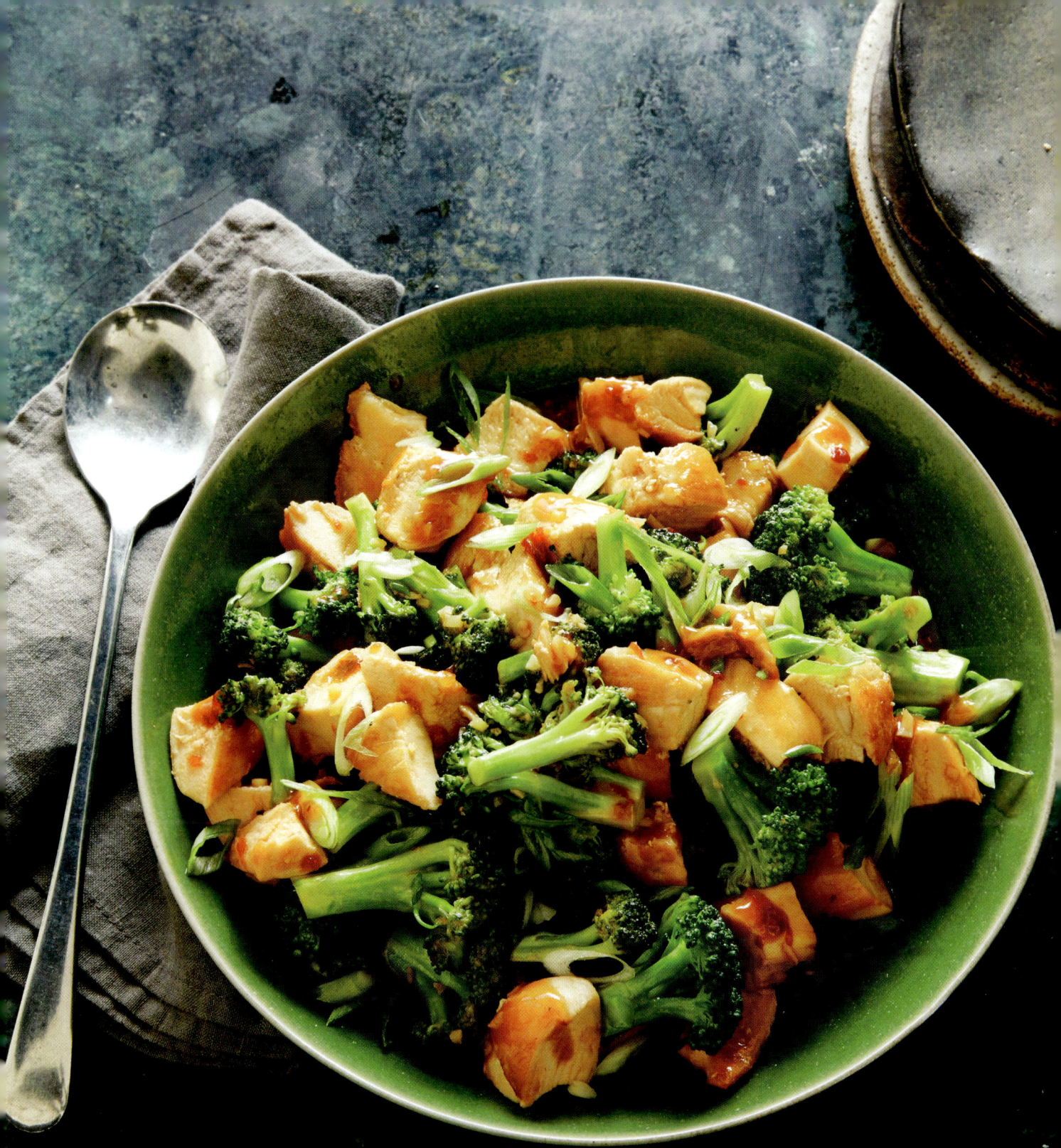

*Sesame Chicken and
Broccoli Stir-Fry*

*Spicy Chicken
Soft Tacos with
Goat Cheese*

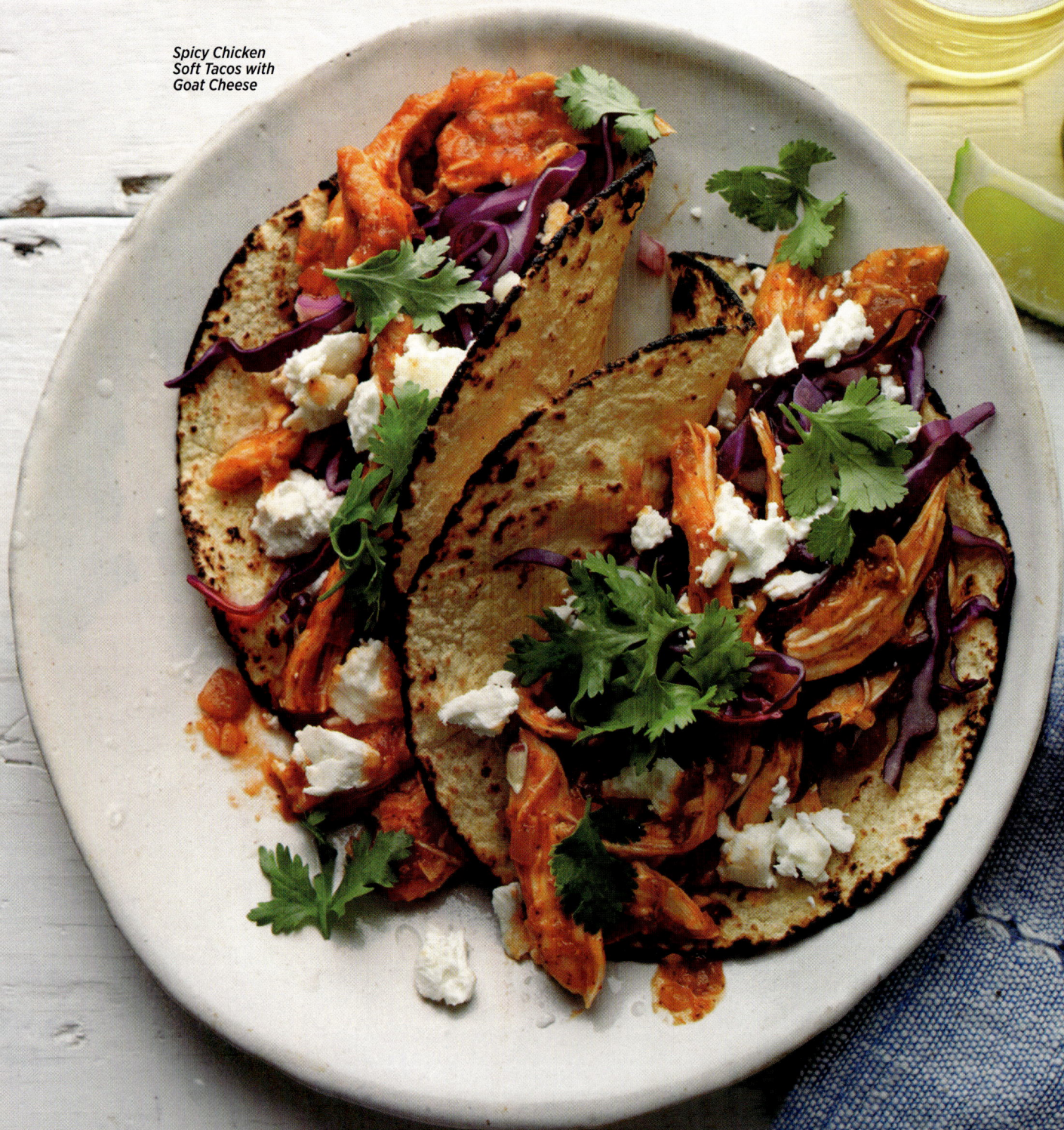

SPICY CHICKEN SOFT TACOS WITH GOAT CHEESE

SERVES 4 • GLUTEN FREE

1 cup canned tomato sauce

1 cup diced onion

1 jalapeño pepper, seeded and minced

1 garlic clove, finely chopped

1 teaspoon chili powder

½ teaspoon ground cumin

1 teaspoon kosher salt

1 pound skinless boneless chicken breast

8 small corn tortillas, warmed

1 cup shredded cabbage

¼ cup crumbled goat cheese

½ cup chopped fresh cilantro leaves

4 lime wedges

1 Combine tomato sauce, onion, jalapeño, garlic, chili powder, cumin, and salt in medium bowl; set aside.

2 Spray medium saucepan with nonstick spray and place over medium-high heat. Add chicken and cook, flipping once, until browned, about 2 minutes per side.

3 Add tomato mixture to pan and pour in as much water as needed to just cover chicken, about ¼ cup. Reduce heat to low and bring to simmer; cook, covered, until chicken is cooked through, about 30 minutes. Transfer chicken to plate.

4 Increase heat to high and cook sauce, stirring a few times, until sauce reduces and thickens, about 5 minutes.

5 Meanwhile, finely shred chicken using 2 forks; add chicken to reduced sauce and heat through. To serve, top each tortilla with about ½ cup chicken, 2 tablespoons cabbage, ½ tablespoon goat cheese, and 1 tablespoon cilantro. Place 2 tacos on each plate and serve with lime wedges.

7 SmartPoints value

Per serving (2 tacos): 334 Cal, 9 g Total Fat, 4 g Sat Fat, 1,012 mg Sod, 32 g Total Carb, 6 g Sugar, 6 g Fib, 32 g Prot.

COOK'S TIP

To up the heat in this dish, stir some canned chipotles en adobo, chopped serrano peppers, or cayenne into the tomato sauce while it reduces. And for crispier tortillas, use tongs to hold each tortilla over the flame or burner of your stove until browned.

CHICKEN TIKKA MASALA

SERVES 4 ● GLUTEN FREE

1¼ pounds skinless boneless chicken breast, cut into ¾-inch cubes

¾ teaspoon salt

2 teaspoons canola oil

1 small onion, chopped

½–1 serrano pepper, stemmed and seeded

3 garlic cloves, finely chopped

1 teaspoon minced peeled fresh ginger

½ cup water

½ cup tomato puree

½ teaspoon garam masala

¼ teaspoon ground turmeric

½ teaspoon sugar

⅓ cup half-and-half

Fresh cilantro for garnish

1 Sprinkle chicken with ¼ teaspoon salt. Heat oil in large nonstick skillet over medium-high heat. Add half of chicken and cook, stirring frequently, until lightly browned, about 5 minutes. Transfer to plate. Repeat with remaining chicken.

2 Meanwhile, combine onion, serrano, garlic, ginger, and water in blender and puree. Return chicken to skillet. Pour onion mixture over chicken and bring to boil. Stir in tomato puree, garam masala, turmeric, sugar, and remaining ½ teaspoon salt. Reduce heat and simmer, partially covered, until flavors blend, 6–8 minutes. Stir in half-and-half; remove from heat and sprinkle with cilantro.

4 SmartPoints value

Per serving (¾ cup): 223 Cal, 7 g Total Fat, 2 g Sat Fat, 739 mg Sod, 7 g Total Carb, 4 g Sugar, 1 g Fib, 32 g Prot.

COOK'S TIP

Cooking rice to serve with this dish? Consider cooking up a large batch so that subsequent meals come together more quickly. Refrigerate cooked rice up to 4 days. A ½-cup portion of cooked brown rice has a SmartPoints value of 4.

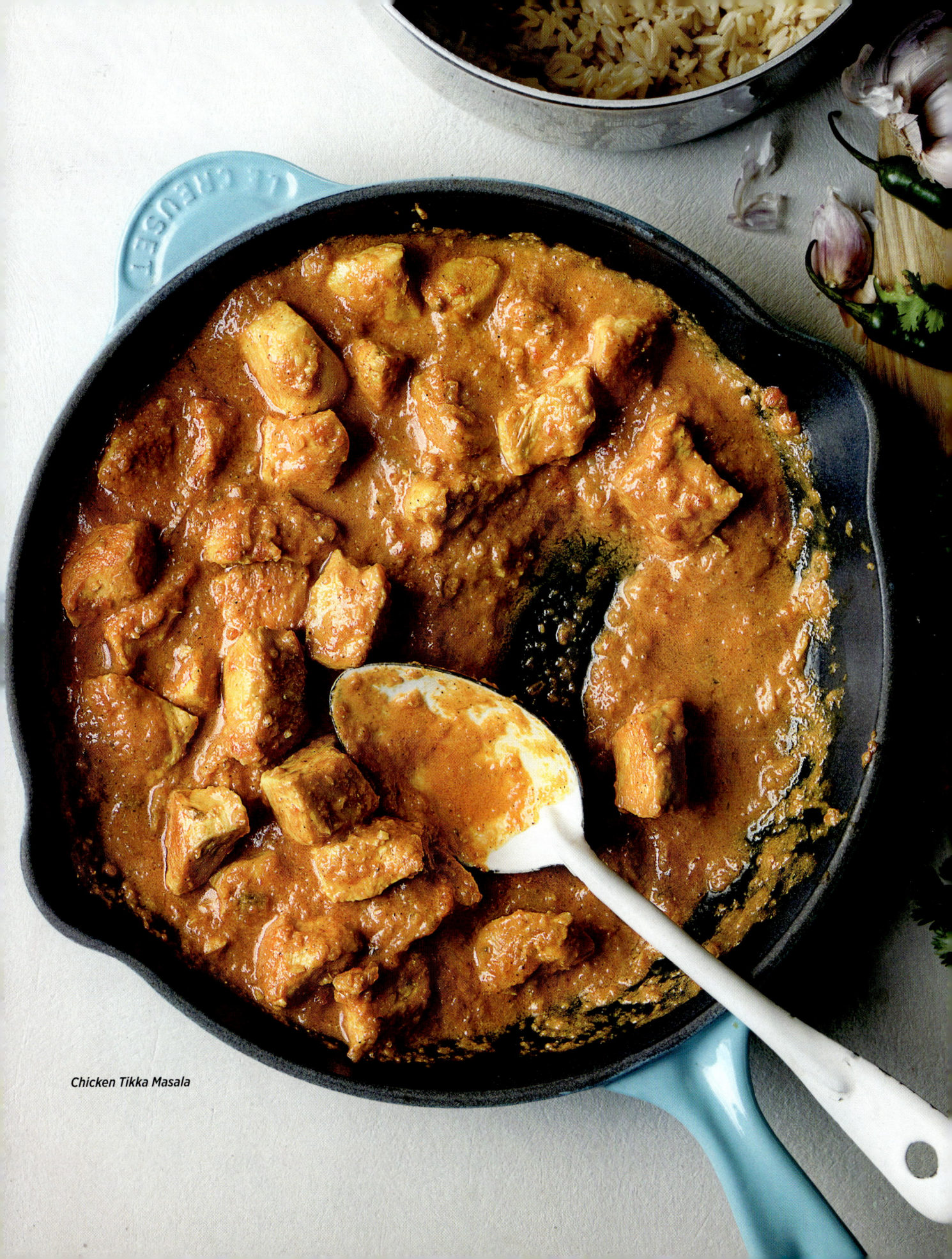

Chicken Tikka Masala

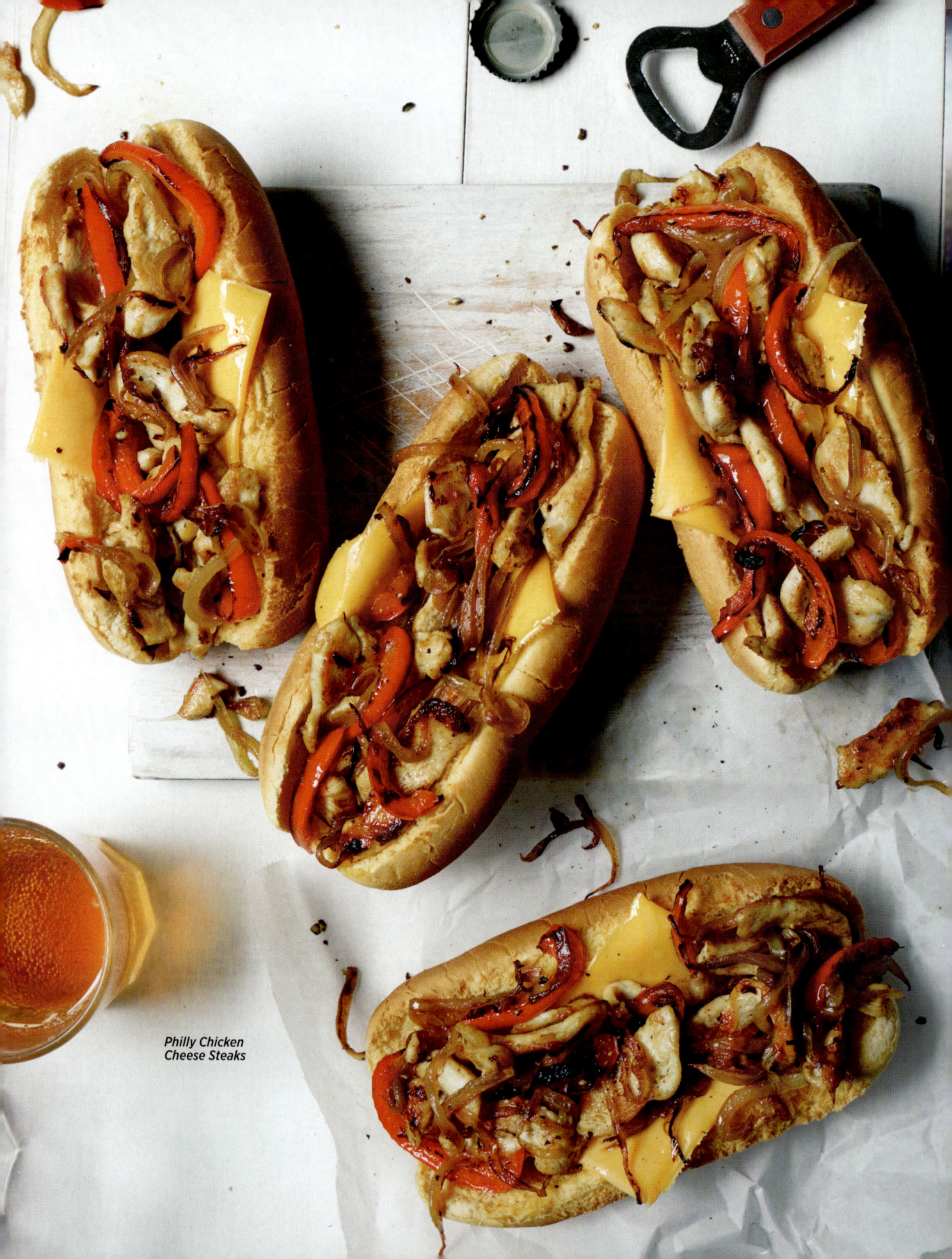

*Philly Chicken
Cheese Steaks*

PHILLY CHICKEN CHEESE STEAKS

SERVES 4 • UNDER 20 MINUTES

1 tablespoon canola oil

1 onion, thinly sliced

1 pound skinless boneless thin-sliced chicken breast, cut into strips

½ red bell pepper, thinly sliced

½ teaspoon salt

⅛ teaspoon black pepper

4 slices low-fat American cheese

4 reduced-calorie hot dog buns, toasted

1 Heat oil in medium skillet over medium-high heat. Add onion and cook, stirring frequently, until browned and very soft, about 10 minutes. Add chicken, bell pepper, salt, and black pepper; cook until chicken is golden brown and cooked through, 5–8 minutes.

2 Place 1 slice American cheese in each bun. Spoon chicken mixture down center of each bun. Close bun to help cheese melt slightly.

6 SmartPoints value

Per serving (1 cheese steak): 297 Cal, 9 g Total Fat, 2 g Sat Fat, 975 mg Sod, 22 g Total Carb, 4 g Sugar, 4 g Fib, 33 g Prot.

— COOK'S TIP —

This is a version of Philadelphia's favorite street food but with a twist: lean chicken breast instead of fatty beef. We used low-fat American cheese, but any low-fat cheese can be used.

GRILLED CHICKEN SANDWICHES WITH CHIPOTLE MAYONNAISE

SERVES 4 • UNDER 20 MINUTES

1 pound skinless boneless chicken breast, thinly sliced

1 teaspoon lime juice

⅛ teaspoon salt

⅛ teaspoon black pepper

2 tablespoons reduced-fat mayonnaise

1 tablespoon finely chopped canned chipotles en adobo, or to taste

1 cup mixed greens

8 slices reduced-calorie whole wheat bread, toasted

1 tomato, cut into 8 slices

1 Heat ridged grill pan over high heat. Sprinkle chicken with lime juice, salt, and pepper. Place chicken in pan and grill, turning once, until cooked through, about 5 minutes.

2 Stir mayonnaise and chipotles together in small cup.

3 Divide greens among 4 slices of toast. Top each with 2 tomato slices and one-quarter of chicken. Spread each remaining piece of toast with about 2 teaspoons chipotle mayonnaise and place on sandwiches.

5 SmartPoints value

Per serving (1 sandwich): 261 Cal, 7 g Total Fat, 1 g Sat Fat, 446 mg Sod, 21 g Total Carb, 3 g Sugar, 6 g Fib, 31 g Prot.

COOK'S TIP

This sandwich hits the spot when you're in the mood for smoky, spicy flavor. To turn the heat up or down a notch, simply adjust the amount of chipotles you add to the mayo.

MEXICAN-SPICED SHREDDED CHICKEN WITH HOMINY

SERVES 8 • GLUTEN FREE

2 teaspoons olive oil

1 large onion, chopped

1 teaspoon kosher salt, or to taste

2 garlic cloves, finely chopped

1½ teaspoons dried oregano

1 teaspoon ground coriander

1 teaspoon chili powder

1 teaspoon ground cumin

1 (15-ounce) can diced fire-roasted tomatoes with chiles

2 cups chicken broth

1½ pounds skinless boneless chicken breast

1 (30-ounce) can hominy, rinsed and drained

2 small zucchini, cut into chunks

¼ cup chopped fresh cilantro

1 Heat oil in large nonstick skillet over medium heat. Add onion and salt and cook, stirring frequently, until softened, about 7 minutes.

2 Add garlic, oregano, coriander, chili powder, and cumin to skillet; cook 1 minute, stirring.

3 Add tomatoes, broth, and chicken to skillet; bring to boil over high heat. Reduce heat to low and simmer, covered, until chicken is cooked through, about 7 minutes (if liquid in pan doesn't cover chicken, turn chicken halfway through cooking). When chicken is cooked through, transfer to plate.

4 Add hominy and zucchini to pan and increase heat to medium-high; cook until zucchini is tender and liquid is reduced, stirring occasionally, about 10 minutes.

5 Meanwhile, using 2 forks, finely shred chicken; add chicken back to pan and stir in cilantro.

4 SmartPoints value

Per serving (about 1 cup): 218 Cal, 5 g Total Fat, 1 g Sat Fat, 836 mg Sod, 21 g Total Carb, 3 g Sugar, 4 g Fib, 22 g Prot.

COOK'S TIP

This lightly spiced meal is fabulous on its own—it's packed with chicken, hominy, and vegetables. Or drain it slightly and use for soft tacos, or serve over rice.

HEARTY LEMON-CHICKEN SOUP WITH ORZO

SERVES 4

- 2 (10-ounce) bone-in chicken breasts, skin discarded
- 1 carrot, finely chopped
- 1 small celery stalk, finely chopped
- ½ onion, finely chopped
- ¾ teaspoon salt, or to taste
- ¼ teaspoon black pepper
- 4 cups reduced-sodium chicken broth
- ½ cup whole wheat orzo
- 2 large eggs
- 3 tablespoons lemon juice
- 2 tablespoons chopped fresh dill

1 Place chicken, carrot, celery, onion, ¼ teaspoon salt, and pepper in large saucepan. Add broth and bring to boil over high heat. Reduce heat; skim and discard any foam that rises to top. Lower heat and simmer, covered, until chicken is cooked through and vegetables are tender, about 20 minutes.

2 With slotted spoon, transfer chicken to plate to cool slightly. Add orzo to saucepan, adjust heat, and cook at bare simmer until tender, 6–8 minutes. Meanwhile, when chicken is cool enough to handle, shred meat and discard bones.

3 Whisk eggs, lemon juice, and remaining ½ teaspoon salt together in medium bowl until frothy. Stirring constantly, gradually add ½ cup hot liquid from soup into egg mixture. Stir egg mixture back into soup. Add chicken and cook, stirring constantly, just until heated through, about 1 minute (do not simmer). Stir in dill and ladle into bowls.

5 SmartPoints value

Per serving (about 1 cup): 240 Cal, 6 g Total Fat, 1 g Sat Fat, 950 mg Sod, 16 g Total Carb, 3 g Sugar, 2 g Fib, 29 g Prot.

COOK'S TIP

Make sure the soup doesn't simmer again once you've added the egg or it may curdle.

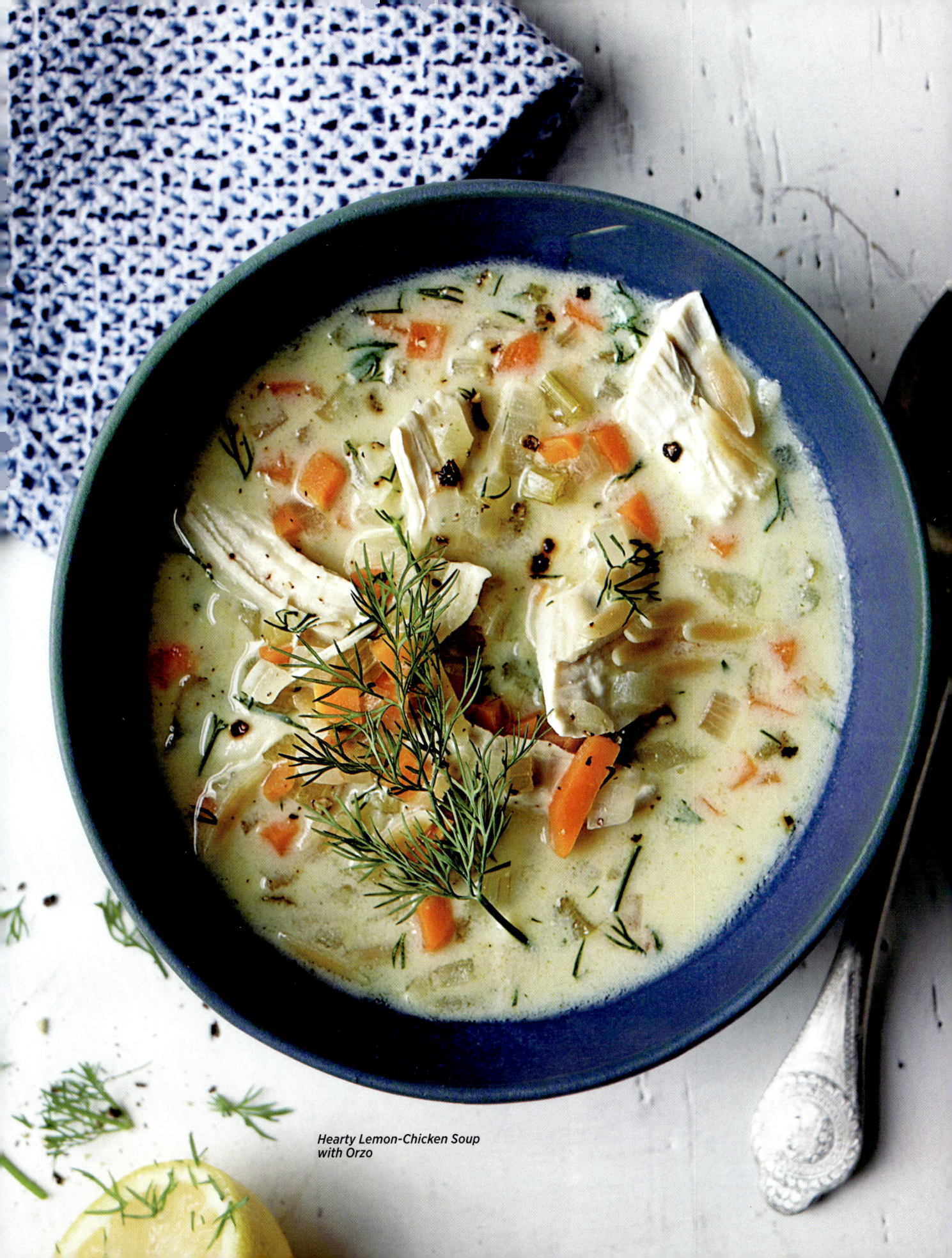

*Hearty Lemon-Chicken Soup
with Orzo*

TANGY SPINACH FLORENTINE SOUP WITH CHICKEN

SERVES 4 • UNDER 20 MINUTES

1 small onion, chopped

6 ounces baby spinach

3 cups chicken broth

½ cup whole wheat orzo or other small pasta shape, cooked according to package directions

2 cups cooked skinless boneless chicken breast, chopped

1 tablespoon lemon juice

¼ teaspoon salt, or to taste

¼ teaspoon black pepper

⅛ teaspoon ground nutmeg

1 Spray large saucepan with nonstick spray and place over medium heat. Add onion and spinach and cook, stirring frequently, until spinach is wilted, about 3 minutes. Remove from heat. Add broth and puree mixture with immersion blender or in batches in blender.

2 Return mixture to pan and add pasta, chicken, lemon juice, salt, pepper, and nutmeg. Cook over medium heat, stirring frequently, until hot, 4–5 minutes.

4 SmartPoints value

Per serving (about 1¼ cups): 213 Cal, 4 g Total Fat, 1 g Sat Fat, 791 mg Sod, 15 g Total Carb, 2 g Sugar, 3 g Fib, 29 g Prot.

UP THE PROTEIN

Top each serving of soup with a ¼-cup dollop of low-fat Greek yogurt for an additional 1 SmartPoints value.

EASY CHICKEN TORTILLA SOUP

SERVES 4 ● GLUTEN FREE

1 teaspoon olive oil

1½ cups chopped onion

¼ teaspoon salt, or to taste

2 garlic cloves, finely chopped

1 jalapeño pepper, seeded and minced

1 teaspoon chili powder

6 cups reduced-sodium chicken broth

1 (15-ounce) can diced fire-roasted tomatoes, drained

1¼ pounds skinless boneless chicken breast

1 cup lightly packed fresh cilantro leaves, chopped

⅓ cup lime juice

6 tablespoons shredded reduced-fat Mexican cheese blend

12 low-fat tortilla chips

1 Heat olive oil in large saucepan over medium heat. Add onion and salt and cook until onion softens, 5–6 minutes. Add garlic, jalapeño, and chili powder and cook 1 minute. Add broth, tomatoes, and chicken. Bring to simmer and cook, covered, until chicken is cooked through, about 20 minutes.

2 Remove chicken from soup and cool slightly. Using 2 forks, finely shred chicken. Return chicken to pan and add cilantro and lime juice. Serve soup garnished with cheese blend and crumbled tortilla chips.

5 SmartPoints value

Per serving (2 cups soup, 1½ tablespoons cheese, and 3 tortilla chips): 307 Cal, 8 g Total Fat, 2 g Sat Fat, 1,237 mg Sod, 21 g Total Carb, 8 g Sugar, 3 g Fib, 36 g Prot.

COOK'S TIP

You can use any reduced-fat shredded cheese in place of the Mexican cheese blend: Monterrey Jack or pepper Jack are classic.

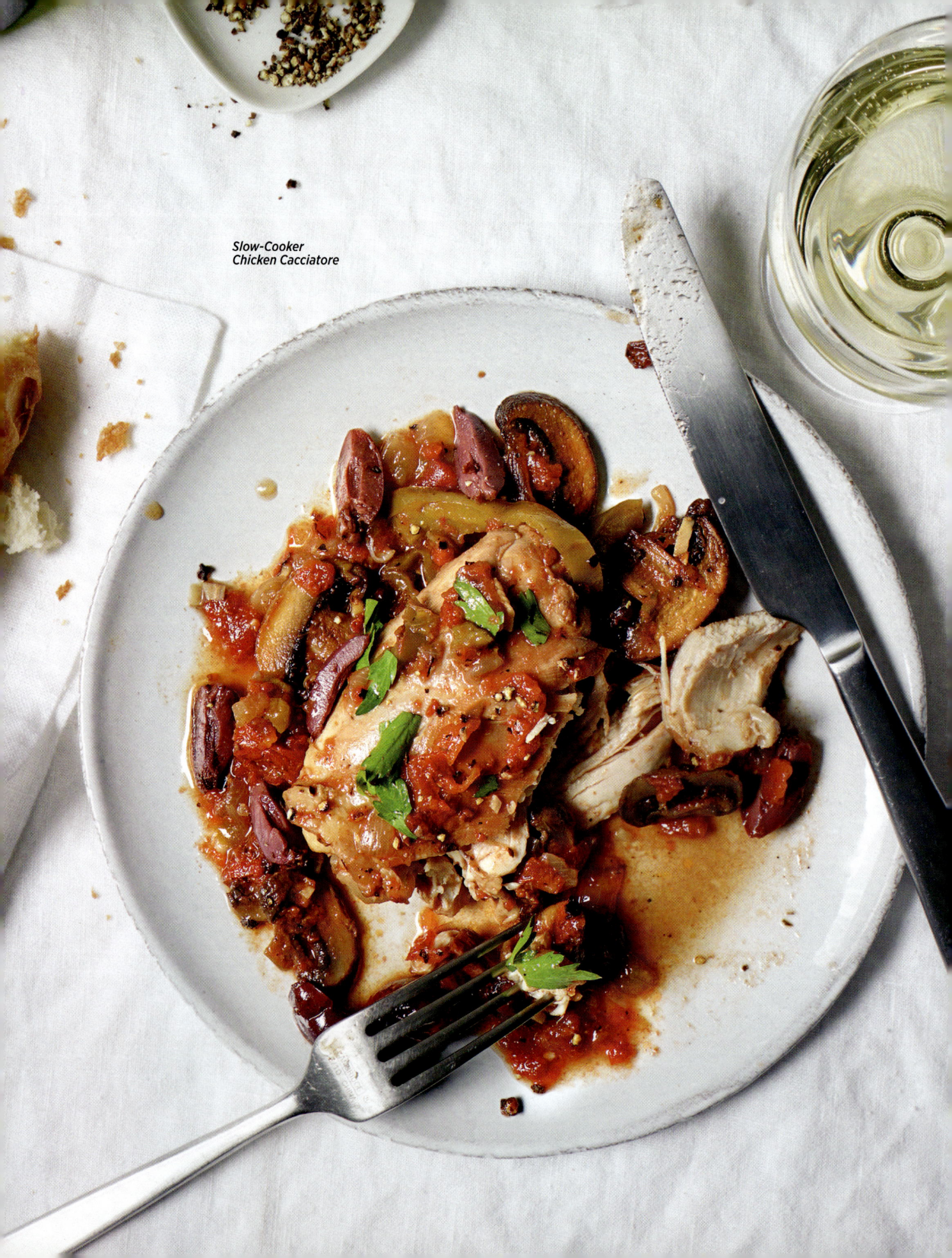

*Slow-Cooker
Chicken Cacciatore*

SLOW-COOKER CHICKEN CACCIATORE

SERVES 4 • GLUTEN FREE

1 (14½-ounce) can diced fire-roasted or crushed tomatoes

¼ cup red wine

1 tablespoon tomato paste

2 garlic cloves, finely chopped

¾ teaspoon dried oregano

¾ teaspoon salt, or to taste

¼ teaspoon black pepper

4 (5-ounce) skinless bone-in chicken thighs

2 cups sliced mushrooms

1 green bell pepper, thinly sliced

1 small onion, chopped

¼ cup sliced black olives

Chopped parsley for garnish

1 Whisk tomatoes, wine, tomato paste, garlic, oregano, salt, and black pepper together in 3- to 5-quart slow cooker. Add chicken, mushrooms, bell pepper, and onion. Cover and cook on Low 6–7 hours or on High 3–3½ hours.

2 Sprinkle with olives and parsley and serve.

5 SmartPoints value

Per serving (1 thigh and about ¾ cup vegetables): 300 Cal, 9 g Total Fat, 2 g Sat Fat, 862 mg Sod, 11 g Total Carb, 5 g Sugar, 3 g Fib, 41 g Prot.

COOK'S TIP

If you have a choice, use your slow cooker on the Low setting. Most dishes will be tastier when cooked longer, and most cookers heat more evenly on Low.

CHICKEN-AND-SPINACH PHYLLO PIE

SERVES 8

1 pound ground skinless chicken breast

1 onion, diced

1 garlic clove, minced

½ teaspoon curry powder

½ teaspoon cinnamon

¼ teaspoon ground allspice

¼ teaspoon salt

¼ teaspoon black pepper

½ cup tomato sauce

1 (10-ounce) package frozen chopped spinach, thawed and squeezed dry

1 cup crumbled reduced-fat feta

2 large egg whites, lightly beaten

8 (9 x 14-inch) sheets frozen phyllo, thawed

1 Place oven rack in bottom third of oven; preheat oven to 400°F. Spray 9-inch pie plate with nonstick spray.

2 To make filling, spray large skillet with nonstick spray and set over medium heat. Add chicken and onion; cook, breaking apart chicken with wooden spoon, until chicken is no longer pink, about 8 minutes. Add garlic, curry powder, cinnamon, allspice, salt, and pepper; cook, stirring frequently, until fragrant, about 1 minute. Stir in tomato sauce and simmer until mixture is thickened, about 5 minutes. Transfer filling to large bowl. Stir in spinach and feta; stir in egg whites.

3 Lay 1 phyllo sheet in pie plate; lightly spray with nonstick spray. Keep remaining phyllo covered with damp paper towel and plastic wrap to keep it from drying out. Repeat with 3 of the remaining phyllo sheets, placing corners at different angles and lightly spraying each sheet with nonstick spray. Spoon filling into crust.

4 Top filling with remaining 4 phyllo sheets, repeating layering and spraying with nonstick spray. Roll up edges of phyllo toward center to form 1½-inch-wide rim.

5 Bake on bottom rack of oven until phyllo is golden brown, 30–35 minutes. Let stand 5 minutes before serving. Cut into 8 wedges.

4 SmartPoints value

Per serving (1 wedge): 174 Cal, 4 g Total Fat, 2 g Sat Fat, 508 mg Sod, 15 g Total Carb, 1 g Sugar, 2 g Fib, 20 g Prot.

UP THE PROTEIN

Serve the pie with a protein-packed whole grain like quinoa. A ⅓-cup serving of cooked quinoa has a SmartPoints value of 2.

Chicken-and-Spinach
Phyllo Pie

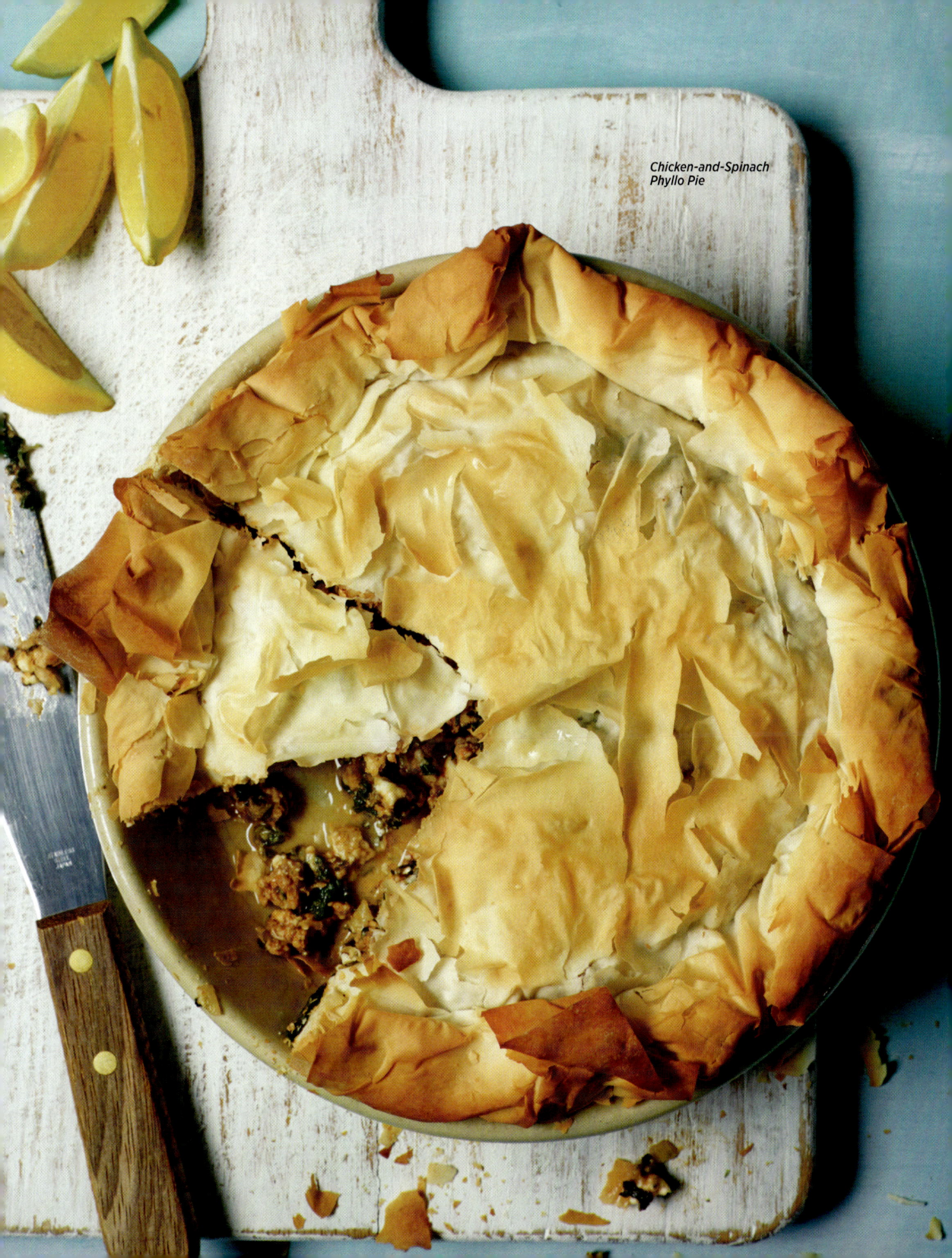

TANDOORI CHICKEN WITH CUCUMBER-SCALLION RAITA

SERVES 6 • GLUTEN FREE

1¾ cups plain fat-free yogurt

3 tablespoons lime juice

1½ tablespoons paprika

1 tablespoon grated peeled fresh ginger

2 garlic cloves, minced

2 teaspoons curry powder

½ teaspoon salt

6 (¼-pound) skinless bone-in chicken thighs

½ cucumber, peeled, seeded, and shredded

2 scallions, thinly sliced

¼ teaspoon ground cumin

1 Combine 1 cup yogurt, 2 tablespoons lime juice, paprika, ginger, garlic, curry powder, and ¼ teaspoon salt in zip-close plastic bag; add chicken. Squeeze out air and seal bag; turn to coat chicken. Refrigerate, turning bag occasionally, at least 1 hour or up to 8 hours.

2 Meanwhile, to make raita, stir remaining ¾ cup yogurt, remaining 1 tablespoon lime juice, remaining ¼ teaspoon salt, cucumber, scallions, and cumin together in small bowl. Cover and refrigerate until ready to serve.

3 Preheat oven to 450°F. Line large shallow baking pan with foil. Place wire rack in pan; spray rack with nonstick spray.

4 Remove chicken from marinade and place on rack. Discard marinade. Spray chicken with nonstick spray and bake until chicken is cooked through, about 25 minutes. Serve with raita.

3 SmartPoints value

Per serving (1 chicken thigh and 2 tablespoons raita): 153 Cal, 4 g Total Fat, 1 g Sat Fat, 328 mg Sod, 8 g Total Carb, 6 g Sugar, 1 g Fib, 21 g Prot.

COOK'S TIP

While the chicken bakes, you'll have time to prepare a quick-cooking side like couscous to serve with your meal; a ½-cup serving of cooked whole wheat couscous has a SmartPoints value of 3.

SAVORY SAUSAGE-APPLE CRUMBLES

SERVES 4

2 teaspoons canola oil

2 celery stalks, chopped

2 carrots, chopped

1 small onion, diced

1 small apple, cored and chopped

¾ teaspoon salt

1½ teaspoons garlic-herb seasoning

8 ounces cooked Italian-style chicken sausages, split and sliced into half-moons

1 cup chicken broth

2½ teaspoons cornstarch

1 cup quick-cooking rolled oats

3 tablespoons shredded Parmigiano-Reggiano

½ teaspoon paprika

2 tablespoons unsalted butter, softened

1 Preheat oven to 350°F. Set 4 (10-ounce) ramekins on rimmed baking sheet.

2 Heat oil in large skillet over medium-high heat. Add celery, carrots, onion, apple, salt, and 1 teaspoon garlic seasoning to skillet. Cook, stirring occasionally, until onions are translucent and soft, 6–8 minutes; stir in sausage.

3 Stir broth and cornstarch together in small cup; stir into skillet. Simmer, stirring occasionally, until reduced slightly and thickened, 5–6 minutes; remove from heat.

4 To make topping, combine oats, Parmigiano-Reggiano, paprika, and remaining ½ teaspoon garlic seasoning in medium bowl; add butter and incorporate with your fingers or with pastry cutter.

5 Spoon heaping ¾ cup sausage mixture into each ramekin; crumble ¼ cup topping over each and spray tops with nonstick spray. Bake until bubbling, 25–30 minutes.

8 SmartPoints value

Per serving (1 sausage crumble): 297 Cal, 15 g Total Fat, 6 g Sat Fat, 1,089 mg Sod, 27 g Total Carb, 8 g Sugar, 5 g Fib, 15 g Prot.

COOK'S TIP

These versatile mini casseroles are excellent for any meal—breakfast, lunch, or dinner.

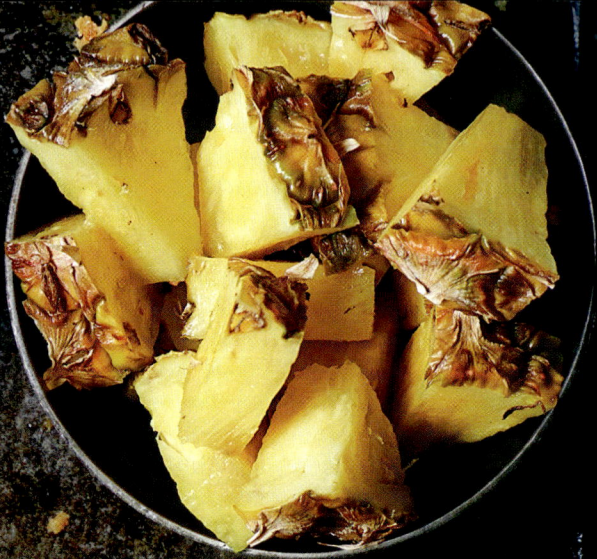

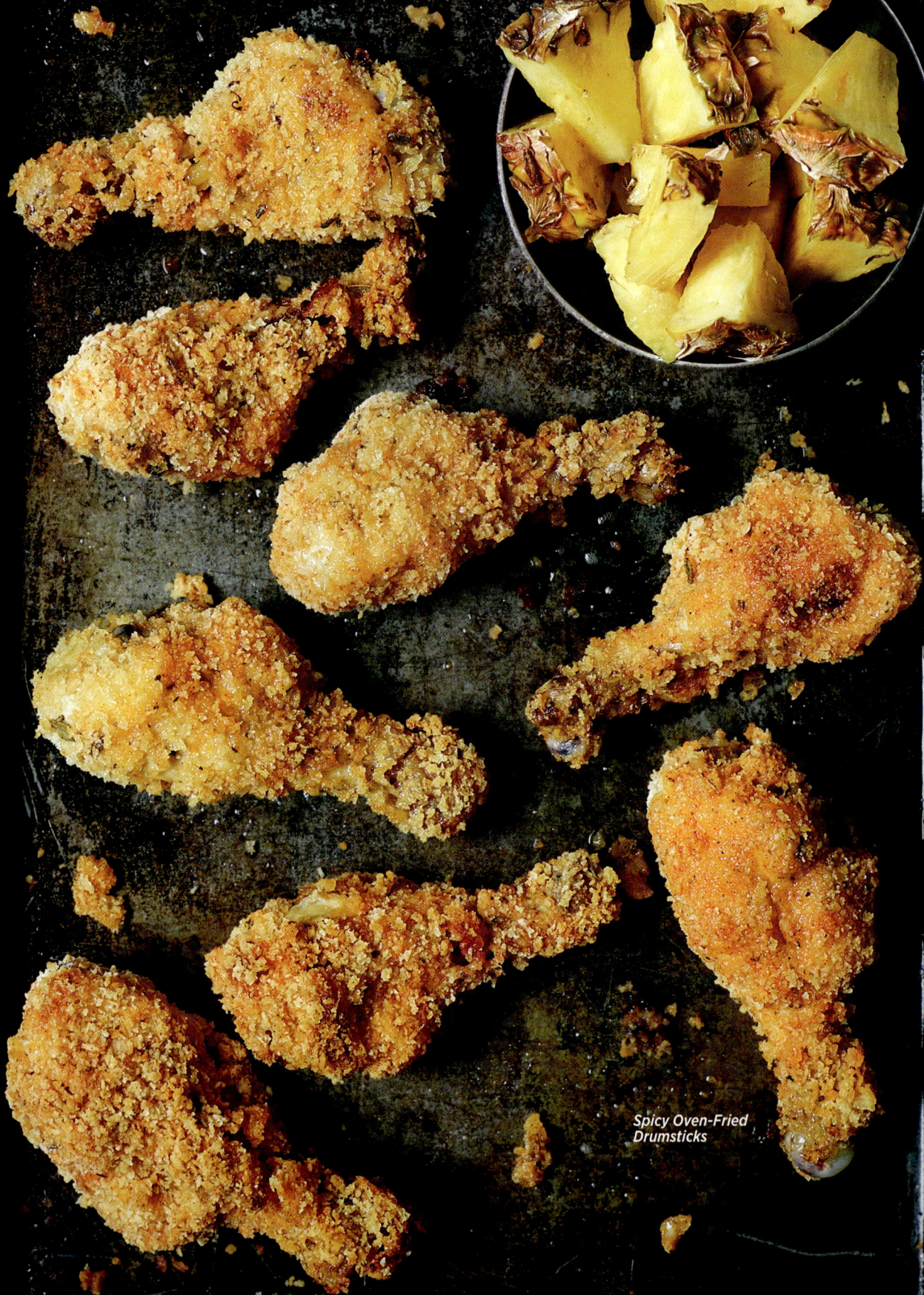

Spicy Oven-Fried Drumsticks

SPICY OVEN-FRIED DRUMSTICKS

SERVES 4

½ cup whole wheat panko (Japanese bread crumbs)

2 tablespoons all-purpose flour

1 teaspoon dried poultry seasoning or sage

¾ teaspoon salt

½ teaspoon black pepper

¼–½ teaspoon cayenne

¾ cup low-fat buttermilk

8 small skinless chicken drumsticks (about 1¾ pounds total)

1 Preheat oven to 450°F. Spray baking sheet with nonstick spray.

2 Mix panko, flour, poultry seasoning, salt, black pepper, and cayenne together in large shallow bowl. Pour buttermilk into another bowl. Dip drumsticks, one at a time, into buttermilk and roll in panko mixture to coat evenly.

3 Spray chicken lightly with nonstick spray and place in broiler pan. Bake until crispy and cooked through, about 25 minutes.

7 SmartPoints value

Per serving (2 drumsticks): 266 Cal, 12 g Total Fat, 3 g Sat Fat, 652 mg Sod, 15 g Total Carb, 2 g Sugar, 2 g Fib, 24 g Prot.

COOK'S TIP

A full ½ teaspoon of cayenne in this recipe will give you deliciously fiery drumsticks. Use a smaller amount if you prefer milder chicken, or serve the dish with a cooling side like raita or chopped pineapple.

LEMON-SAGE ROAST TURKEY BREAST

SERVES 8 • GLUTEN FREE

3 tablespoons unsalted butter, softened

3 tablespoons chopped fresh sage, plus extra for garnish (optional)

1 tablespoon chopped fresh thyme

½ teaspoon grated lemon zest, plus extra for garnish (optional)

½ teaspoon kosher salt

½ teaspoon black pepper

2 pounds skinless boneless turkey breast, in one piece

1½ cups chicken broth

6 garlic cloves, unpeeled

2 tablespoons lemon juice

1 Preheat oven to 400°F.

2 Combine 1½ tablespoons butter, sage, thyme, lemon zest, salt, and pepper in small bowl and mash with fork. Spread butter mixture all over turkey.

3 Place turkey in small roasting pan or large ovenproof skillet; pour ¾ cup broth around turkey and add garlic cloves to pan. Roast turkey, uncovered, basting turkey and turning garlic cloves twice, until turkey is cooked through and instant-read thermometer inserted into thickest part registers 165°F, about 45 minutes. Transfer turkey to cutting board, cover loosely with foil, and let rest 10–15 minutes.

4 Meanwhile, remove garlic from pan. Peel garlic cloves. Place roasting pan or skillet with turkey drippings on stovetop over high heat; add garlic cloves, remaining ¾ cup broth, and lemon juice. Bring mixture to boil, scraping bottom of skillet to incorporate drippings; continue boiling until sauce reduces and thickens slightly, mashing garlic to blend into sauce, 2–3 minutes. Remove from heat and strain sauce into small bowl; swirl in remaining 1½ tablespoons butter until melted.

5 Cut turkey into about 24 slices and arrange on serving platter; drizzle with any drippings from cutting board. Spoon sauce over turkey or serve on the side; garnish with more fresh lemon zest and chopped sage if desired.

3 SmartPoints value

Per serving (3 slices turkey and 1 tablespoon sauce): 183 Cal, 6 g Total Fat, 3 g Sat Fat, 391 mg Sod, 2 g Total Carb, 0 g Sugar, 0 g Fib, 28 g Prot.

COOK'S TIP

A roasted boneless turkey breast is a cook's secret weapon: It's perfect for small holiday tables that don't warrant a whole bird or for big ones that need even more white meat than one turkey offers.

TURKEY, ZUCCHINI, AND QUINOA MEAT LOAVES

SERVES 6 • GLUTEN FREE

½ cup quinoa, rinsed well

1 medium (7-ounce) zucchini, coarsely shredded

2 large egg whites, lightly beaten

½ cup chili sauce

½ onion, finely chopped

1 tablespoon chopped fresh sage

¾ teaspoon salt

½ teaspoon black pepper

1 pound ground skinless turkey

1 tablespoon spicy brown mustard

1 Cook quinoa according to package directions. Fluff with fork and let cool slightly.

2 Preheat oven to 425°F. Line large rimmed baking pan with foil; spray foil with nonstick spray.

3 Squeeze zucchini dry and place in large bowl with egg whites, ¼ cup chili sauce, onion, sage, salt, and pepper. Add turkey and quinoa and stir to mix well.

4 Shape into 6 (2½ x 4-inch) oval loaves. Place loaves on baking pan. Stir remaining ¼ cup chili sauce and mustard together in small bowl; spread mixture evenly over loaves.

5 Bake until instant-read thermometer inserted into side of each loaf registers 165°F, 30–35 minutes. Let stand 5 minutes before serving.

5 SmartPoints value

Per serving (1 meat loaf): 220 Cal, 8 g Total Fat, 2 g Sat Fat, 668 mg Sod, 17 g Total Carb, 3 g Sugar, 3 g Fib, 19 g Prot.

UP THE PROTEIN

Love cheese? Sprinkle 1 cup (about 4 ounces) shredded low-fat Cheddar or Colby cheese over the loaves during the last 5 minutes of baking for an additional 1 SmartPoints per serving.

TURKEY WITH APPLES, FENNEL, AND BARLEY

SERVES 4

1 tablespoon roasted garlic mustard or Dijon mustard

1 teaspoon packed brown sugar

½ teaspoon soy sauce

1 (1½-pound) boneless turkey breast

3 Golden Delicious apples, peeled, cored, and cut into ¾-inch-thick wedges

1 large fennel bulb, cut into ¾-inch wedges

1 red onion, sliced

¾ cup quick-cooking barley

¾ cup water

⅛ teaspoon salt

1 small head radicchio, thinly sliced

1 Preheat oven to 425°F. Line bottom of broiler pan with foil; spray foil with nonstick spray.

2 Mix mustard, sugar, and soy sauce together in small bowl. Place turkey on broiler pan; spread mustard mixture evenly over turkey. Scatter apples, fennel, and onion in pan. Roast until instant-read thermometer inserted into center of turkey registers 165°F and vegetables and apples are tender, 40–45 minutes.

3 Meanwhile, mix barley, water, and salt in large microwavable bowl. Cover with vented plastic wrap and microwave on High 8 minutes. Add radicchio, cover, and microwave until barley is tender, about 2 minutes.

4 Transfer turkey to cutting board and let rest 5 minutes. Cut into 12 slices. Serve with apples, vegetables, and barley.

3 SmartPoints value

Per serving (3 slices turkey, 1 cup vegetables and apples, and ½ cup barley): 349 Cal, 3 g Total Fat, 1 g Sat Fat, 391 mg Sod, 36 g Total Carb, 16 g Sugar, 7 g Fib, 43 g Prot.

COOK'S TIP

Got leftovers? Make an excellent soup for yourself by coarsley chopping the turkey and vegetables in a serving; mix it with 1 cup of chicken broth and the barley and heat it. The SmartPoints value will increase by 1.

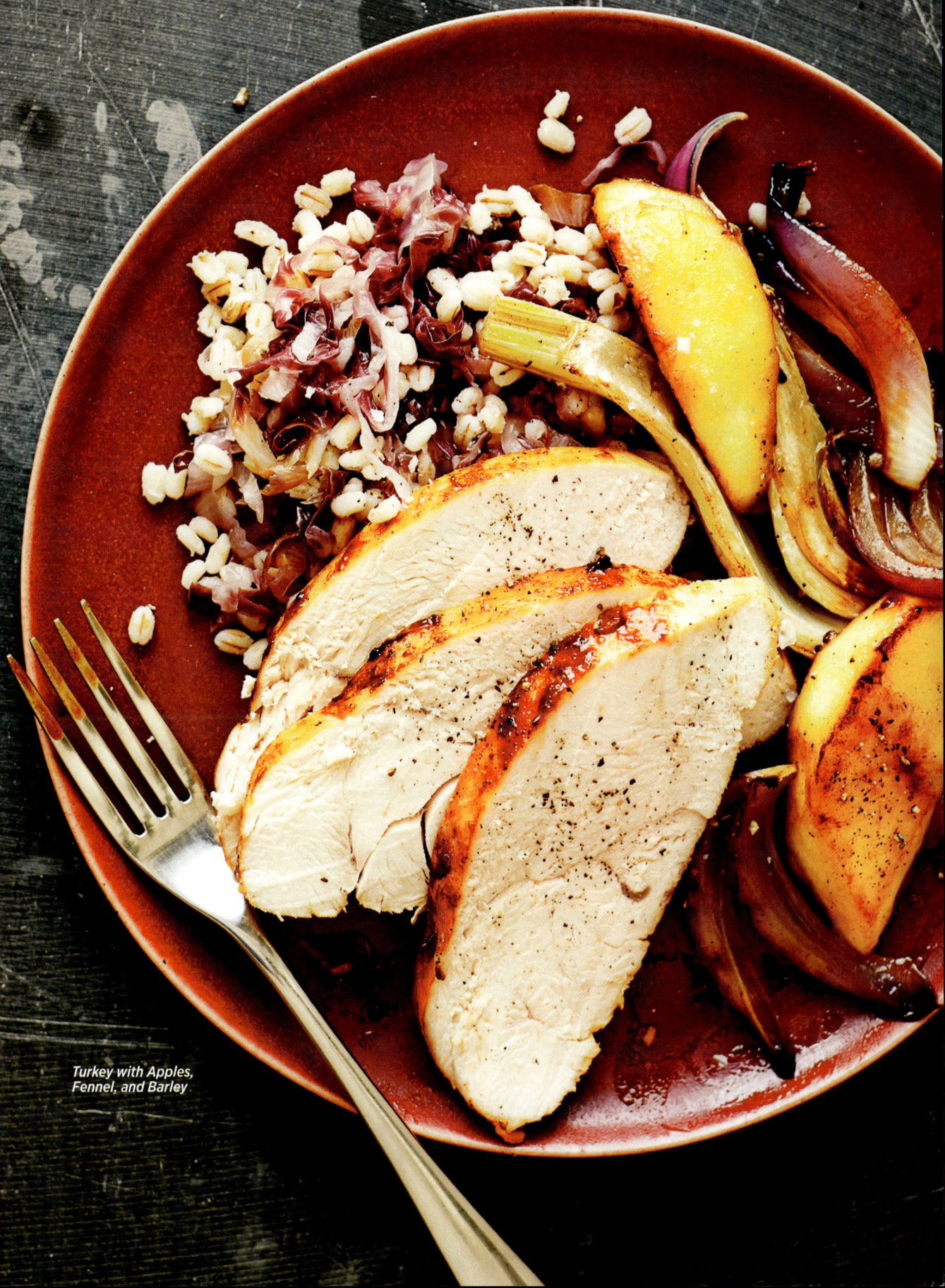

*Turkey with Apples,
Fennel, and Barley*

TURKEY-STUFFED CABBAGE LEAVES

SERVES 4 • GLUTEN FREE

8 outer leaves from large head green cabbage

¾ pound ground skinless turkey breast

1 onion, diced

½ cup cooked brown rice

1 large egg, lightly beaten

2 tablespoons finely chopped parsley

2 garlic cloves, minced

½ teaspoon cinnamon

⅛ teaspoon salt, or to taste

¼ teaspoon black pepper

1 (28-ounce) can diced tomatoes

1 cup chicken broth

1 Place cabbage leaves in large saucepan. Add enough water to cover leaves; set saucepan over high heat. Bring water to boil; boil until leaves are pliable and soft, about 10 minutes. Drain. When leaves are cool enough to handle, cut away thickest part of vein from bottom of leaves, making a V-shaped cut but leaving leaves intact.

2 Meanwhile, combine turkey, onion, rice, egg, parsley, garlic, cinnamon, salt, and pepper in large bowl; mix well.

3 Place about ¼ cup turkey mixture in center of each leaf. Fold in sides of leaves and roll up snuggly, burrito-style, fully covering filling.

4 Pour small amount of tomatoes into saucepan so thin layer covers bottom of pot. Place cabbage rolls in pot, packing them tightly to prevent opening during cooking; pour in remaining tomatoes and broth. Set pot over medium-high heat and bring to simmer; reduce heat to low and simmer, covered, 45 minutes.

4 SmartPoints value

Per serving (2 stuffed leaves and about ½ cup sauce): 267 Cal, 6 g Total Fat, 1 g Sat Fat, 1,184 mg Sod, 31 g Total Carb, 13 g Sugar, 7 g Fib, 27 g Prot.

COOK'S TIP

If the sauce is watery, you can reduce it slightly to make it thicker and concentrate the flavor: Transfer the stuffed cabbage leaves to a platter and keep them warm, return the saucepan to medium heat, and cook, uncovered, until the sauce is thickened.

SPICY TURKEY-CHEDDAR ENCHILADA PIE

SERVES 6

¾ pound ground skinless turkey

1 onion, chopped

1 teaspoon kosher salt

2 teaspoons chili powder

3 tablespoons all-purpose flour

1 cup fat-free milk

1 teaspoon ground cumin

12 corn tortillas

1 cup medium-hot prepared salsa

¾ cup shredded reduced-fat Cheddar

1 Preheat oven to 350°F. Spray large skillet with nonstick spray and place over medium-high heat. Add turkey, onion, salt, and chili powder to skillet; cook, breaking apart turkey with wooden spoon, until turkey is browned, 7–8 minutes. Remove turkey mixture from skillet and set aside.

2 Place skillet back over medium-high heat and add flour. Gradually whisk in milk. Bring to boil, then reduce heat to medium; simmer until thickened, about 2 minutes. Remove skillet from heat; stir in turkey mixture and cumin.

3 Wrap tortillas in damp paper towels and microwave on High until softened, about 15 seconds. Place 4 tortillas in bottom of 9-inch pie plate, overlapping slightly to cover bottom. Spread ⅓ of turkey mixture over tortillas. Spoon ⅓ cup salsa on top and sprinkle with ¼ cup Cheddar. Repeat layers with remaining ingredients.

4 Cover pie plate with foil and cook until cheese melts and filling is warmed through, about 20 minutes. Let stand, covered, 2 minutes before cutting into 6 wedges.

6 SmartPoints value

Per serving (1 wedge): 253 Cal, 5 g Total Fat, 1 g Sat Fat, 801 mg Sod, 32 g Total Carb, 5 g Sugar, 4 g Fib, 22 g Prot.

COOK'S TIP

Want more veggies in this delicious pie? Stir 1 cup chopped thawed frozen spinach, squeezed dry, into the turkey mixture after it cooks in Step 1.

*Warm Turkey
Taco Salad*

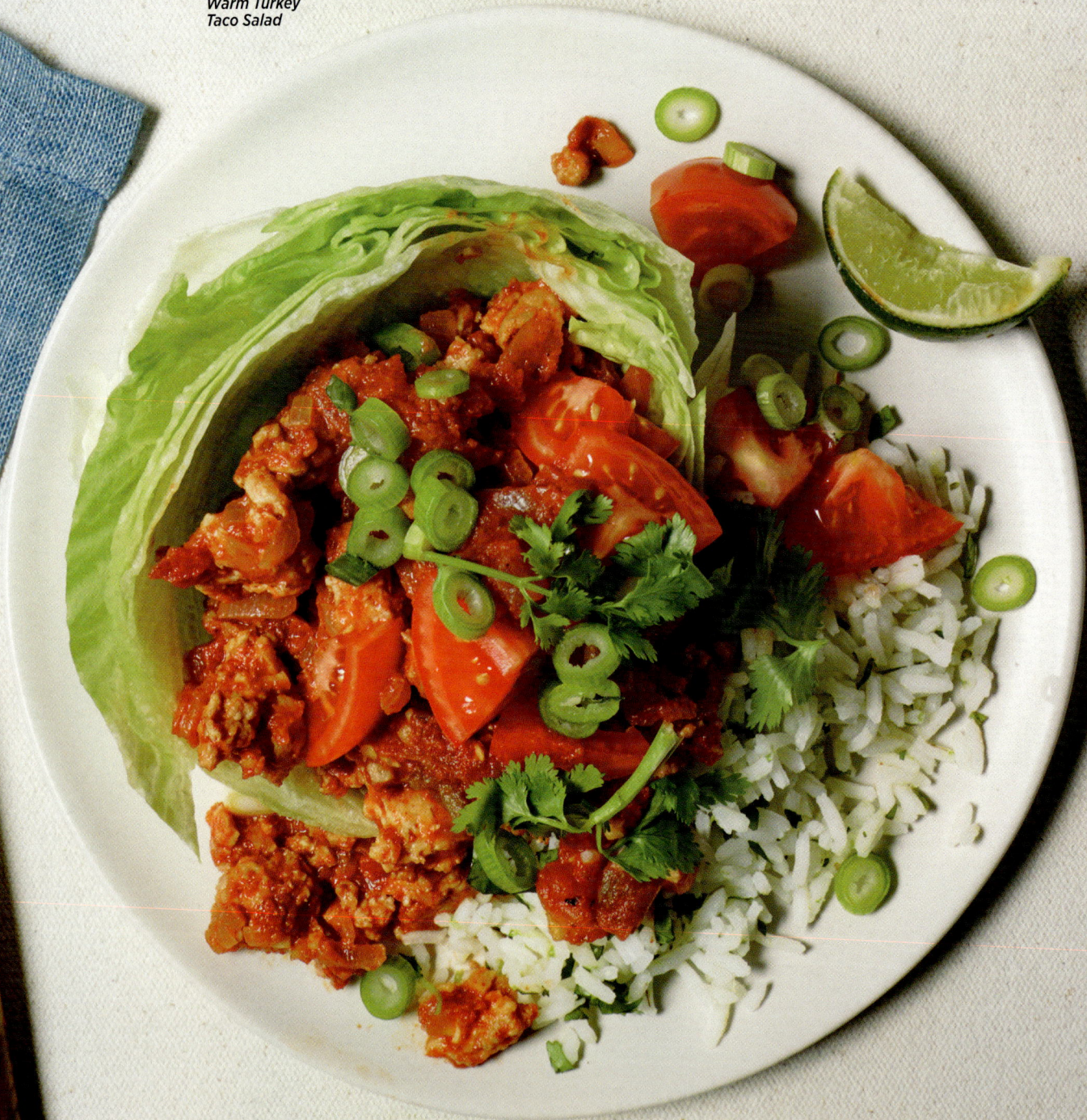

WARM TURKEY TACO SALAD

SERVES 4 • GLUTEN FREE

1 teaspoon olive oil

¾ pound ground skinless turkey

1 small onion, finely chopped

2 garlic cloves, minced

1 tablespoon chili powder

1 teaspoon ground cumin

½ teaspoon salt

1 canned chipotle en adobo, seeded and minced (leave seeds if you want more heat)

1 (14½-ounce) can crushed tomatoes

1½ tablespoons lime juice

1½ teaspoons brown sugar

1 cup cooked white rice, kept warm

2 teaspoons chopped fresh cilantro, plus extra for garnish

½ teaspoon grated lime zest

16 iceberg lettuce leaves

1 cup fresh chopped tomatoes

¼ cup prepared salsa

1 scallion, thinly sliced

1 Heat oil in large nonstick skillet over medium heat. Add turkey, onion, and garlic. Cook, breaking apart turkey with wooden spoon, until turkey is no longer pink and onion begins to soften, 3–5 minutes. Add chili powder, cumin, salt, chipotle, and crushed tomatoes; simmer, stirring occasionally, until turkey is fully cooked and sauce thickens, 8–10 minutes. Stir in 1 tablespoon lime juice and brown sugar; remove from heat.

2 Meanwhile, combine cooked rice, cilantro, lime zest, and remaining ½ tablespoon lime juice in small bowl.

3 To serve, make 4 lettuce cups by layering 4 lettuce leaves together for each serving. Place 1 lettuce cup on each of 4 plates and top each with ¾ cup turkey mixture, ¼ cup rice, ¼ cup chopped tomatoes, and 1 tablespoon salsa; garnish with scallion and cilantro.

5 SmartPoints value

Per serving (1 salad): 246 Cal, 8 g Total Fat, 2 g Sat Fat, 708 mg Sod, 25 g Total Carb, 8 g Sugar, 4 g Fib, 21 g Prot.

UP THE PROTEIN

Love cheese? Sprinkle each salad with ¼ cup (1 ounce) shredded low-fat Cheddar for an additional 1 SmartPoints.

ITALIAN WEDDING SOUP
WITH TURKEY MEATBALLS

SERVES 4

½ **pound ground skinless turkey**

1 **large egg white, lightly beaten**

2 **tablespoons plain dried bread crumbs**

1½ **tablespoons grated Parmesan**

1½ **teaspoons dried oregano**

½ **teaspoon garlic powder**

8 **cups low-sodium chicken broth**

2 **cups thinly sliced escarole**

½ **cup thinly sliced sweet onion**

⅓ **cup shredded carrot**

1 Combine turkey, egg white, bread crumbs, Parmesan, oregano, and garlic powder in medium bowl and mix gently. Shape into balls about ¾ inch in diameter.

2 Bring broth to boil in large saucepan. Stir in escarole, onion, carrot, and meatballs. Return soup to boil, then adjust heat so soup just simmers. Cook, uncovered, until meatballs are cooked through and float and escarole is tender, about 15 minutes.

4 SmartPoints value

Per serving (about 2¼ cups soup and about 8 meatballs): 151 Cal, 6 g Total Fat, 2 g Sat Fat, 978 mg Sod, 9 g Total Carb, 4 g Sugar, 2 g Fib, 14 g Prot.

COOK'S TIP

This Italian soup is full of great flavor. If you like, you can sprinkle it with some extra Parmesan: An additional 1½ tablespoons per serving will increase the SmartPoints value by 1.

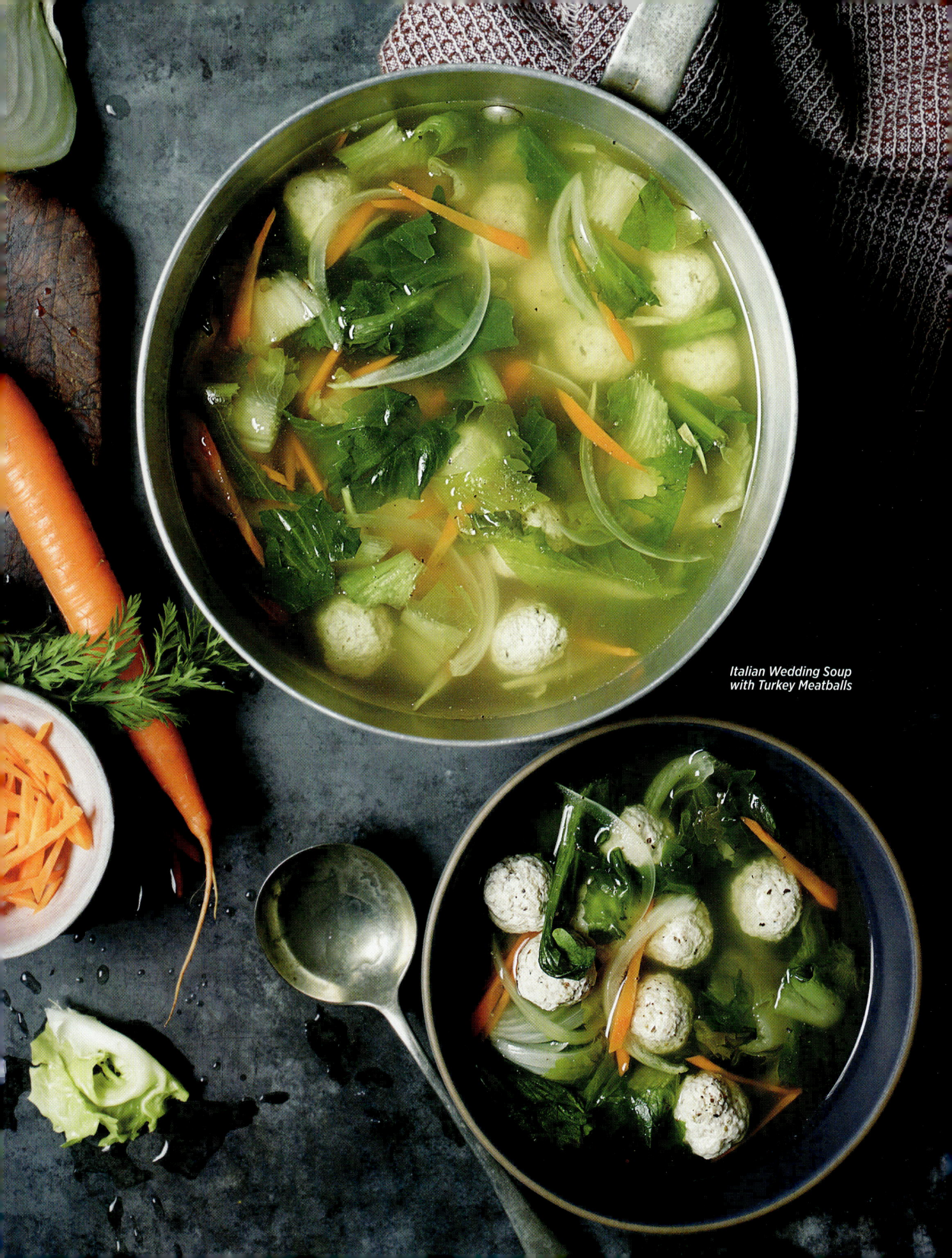
*Italian Wedding Soup
with Turkey Meatballs*

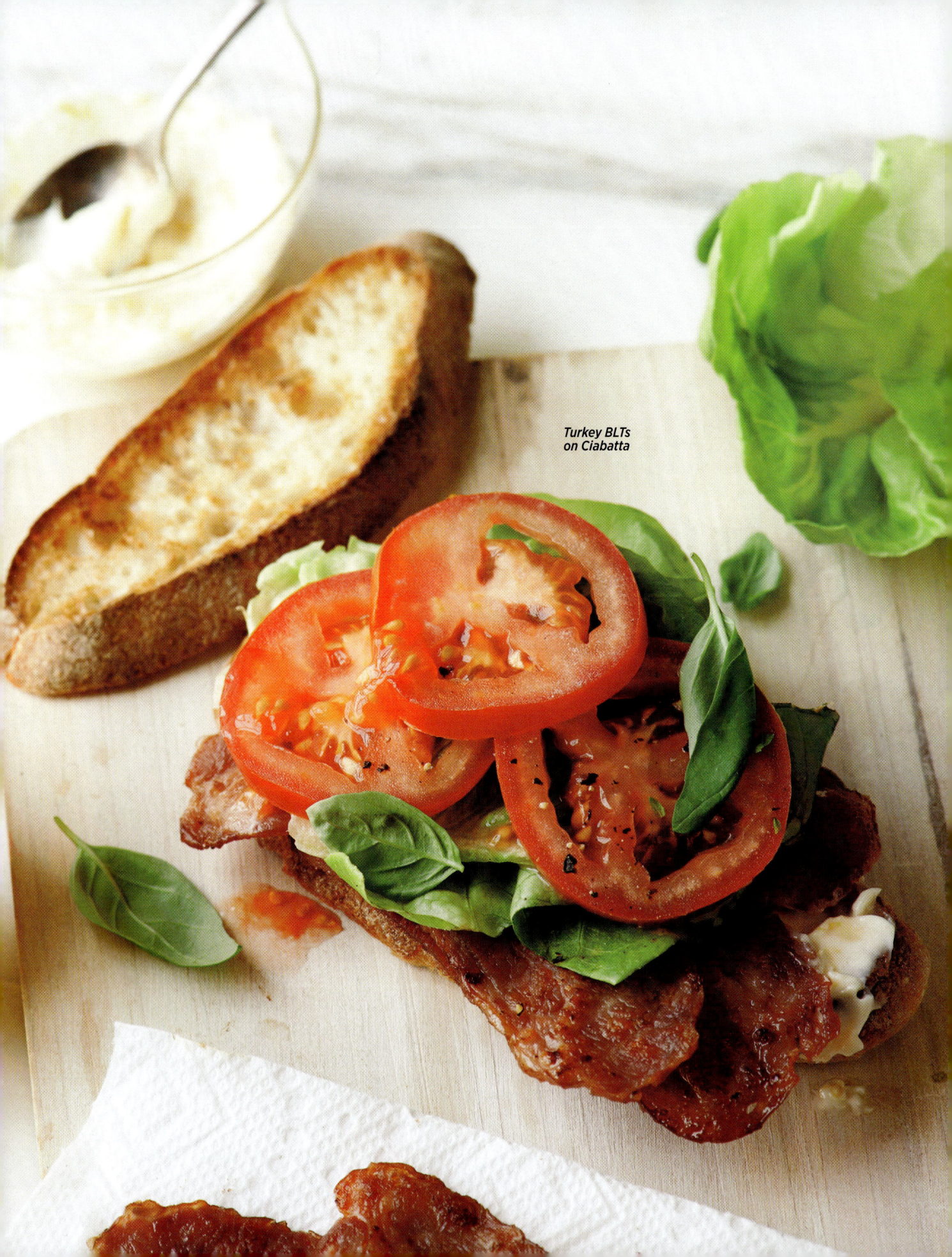

Turkey BLTs
on Ciabatta

TURKEY BLTS ON CIABATTA

SERVES 2 • UNDER 20 MINUTES

8 slices turkey bacon

3 tablespoons fat-free mayonnaise

1 teaspoon finely grated lemon zest

4 thin (½-ounce) slices ciabatta bread, toasted

1 tomato, sliced

3 leaves Boston or butter lettuce, sliced

⅛ teaspoon black pepper

6 basil leaves (optional)

1 Spray large heavy skillet with nonstick spray and set over medium-high heat. Add bacon and cook until browned, 2–3 minutes. Transfer to paper towel–lined plate; keep warm.

2 Stir mayonnaise and lemon zest together in small cup.

3 Spread lemon mayonnaise evenly on one side of each bread slice. Top 2 slices evenly with bacon, tomato, and lettuce. Sprinkle with pepper and top with basil, if using; cover sandwiches with remaining 2 slices ciabatta.

8 SmartPoints value

Per serving (1 sandwich): 254 Cal, 13 g Total Fat, 3 g Sat Fat, 1,040 mg Sod, 22 g Total Carb, 6 g Sugar, 2 g Fib, 14 g Prot.

UP THE PROTEIN

Thinly slice a shelled hard-cooked egg and divide the slices between the sandwiches, placing them under the bacon, for an additional 1 SmartPoints value per serving.

SWEDISH-STYLE TURKEY MEATBALLS WITH MUSHROOMS

SERVES 4

1 slice reduced-calorie wheat bread

¼ cup fat-free milk

1 pound ground skinless turkey

¾ teaspoon salt

¼ teaspoon black pepper

¼ teaspoon ground nutmeg

⅛ teaspoon ground allspice

1 teaspoon unsalted butter

¼ cup finely chopped onion

1 (10-ounce) container mushrooms, sliced

2 tablespoons all-purpose flour

1¼ cups reduced-sodium chicken broth

2 tablespoons light sour cream

2 tablespoons chopped fresh parsley

1 Place bread in shallow bowl. Add milk and let stand until bread softens, about 5 minutes. Squeeze bread dry; discard milk. Finely chop soaked bread.

2 Place turkey, bread, ½ teaspoon salt, pepper, nutmeg, and allspice in large bowl; mix gently just until combined. With damp hands, shape turkey mixture into 16 (1¼-inch) meatballs.

3 Spray large skillet with nonstick spray and set over medium heat. Add meatballs and cook, turning occasionally, until browned on all sides, about 8 minutes. Transfer meatballs to plate.

4 Melt butter in skillet. Add onion and cook, stirring to scrape up browned bits from bottom of pan, until tender, about 2 minutes. Add mushrooms and remaining ¼ teaspoon salt; increase heat and cook, stirring occasionally, until vegetables are browned and liquid evaporates, 5–6 minutes.

5 Whisk flour and broth together in medium bowl; stir into mushroom mixture. Stir in meatballs and bring to boil. Reduce heat and simmer, covered, stirring occasionally, until meatballs are cooked through, about 8 minutes. Remove skillet from heat; gently stir in sour cream and parsley until blended.

7 SmartPoints value

Per serving (4 meatballs and ½ cup sauce): 265 Cal, 13 g Total Fat, 4 g Sat Fat, 684 mg Sod, 10 g Total Carb, 2 g Sugar, 2 g Fib, 26 g Prot.

COOK'S TIP

For another taste of Scandinavia, place 1 tablespoon lingonberry preserves to the side of each serving for an additional 2 SmartPoints.

PAN-SEARED DUCK WITH BLUEBERRY SAUCE

SERVES 4 • GLUTEN FREE • UNDER 20 MINUTES

2 teaspoons olive oil

4 (5-ounce) skinless boneless duck breasts, trimmed

½ teaspoon salt

¼ teaspoon black pepper

1 small onion, finely chopped

⅓ cup dry red wine

⅓ cup no-sugar-added blueberry preserves

1½ teaspoons chopped fresh thyme or ½ teaspoon dried

1 Heat oil in large nonstick skillet over medium heat. Sprinkle duck with ¼ teaspoon of salt and the pepper. Add duck to skillet and cook until golden and instant-read thermometer inserted into center of breasts registers 165°F, about 5 minutes per side. Transfer to plate and keep warm.

2 Add onion to skillet and cook, stirring occasionally, until softened, about 4 minutes. Stir in wine, preserves, remaining ¼ teaspoon salt, and any accumulated duck juices. Increase heat to high and cook, stirring occasionally, until mixture is reduced to ½ cup, about 2 minutes. Stir in thyme.

3 Thinly slice each breast on diagonal and serve drizzled with sauce.

7 SmartPoints value

Per serving (1 duck breast and 2 tablespoons sauce): 242 Cal, 11 g Total Fat, 4 g Sat Fat, 549 mg Sod, 9 g Total Carb, 1 g Sugar, 1 g Fib, 16 g Prot.

COOK'S TIP

Try this recipe with other no-sugar-added preserves as well: Cherry and orange would also be excellent.

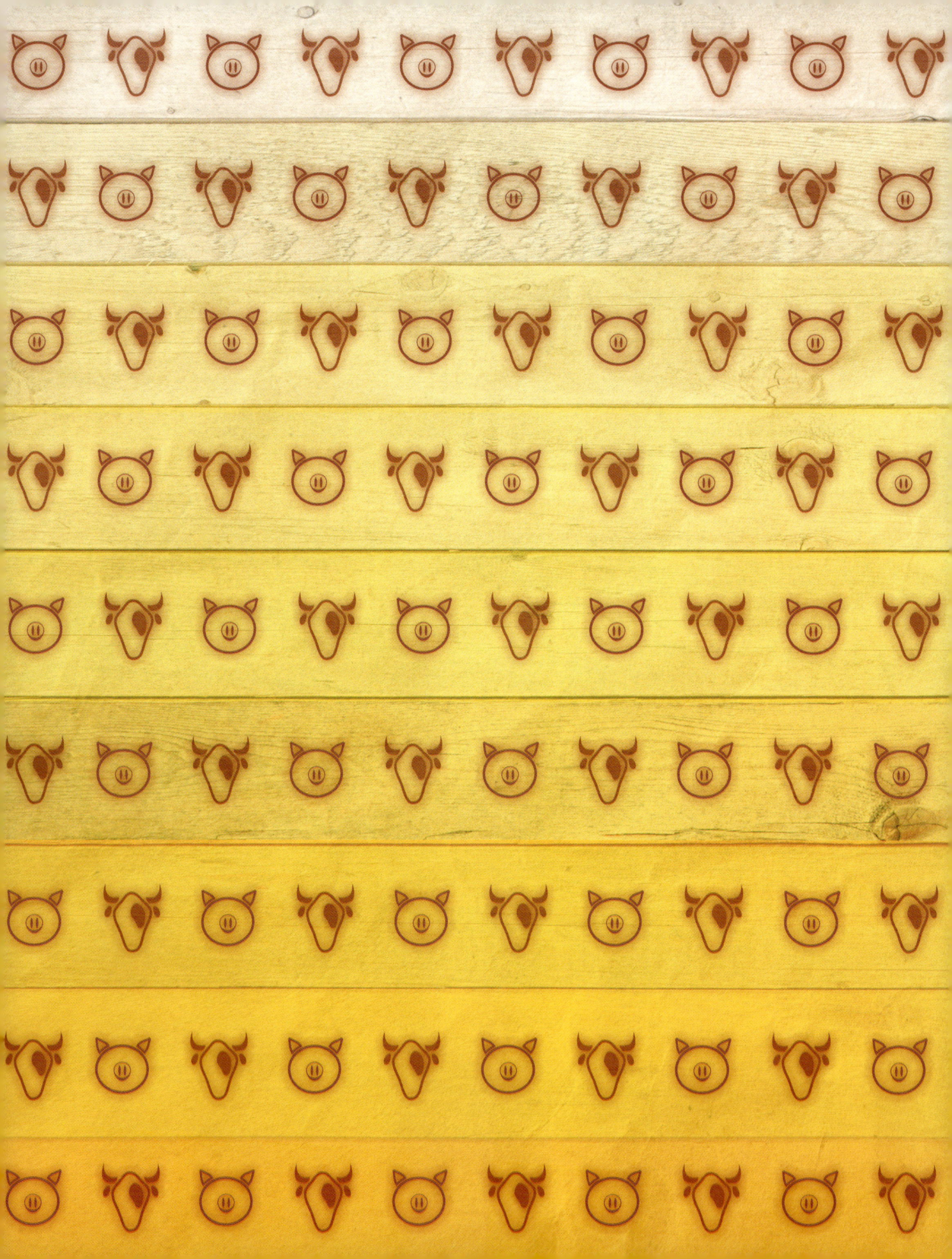

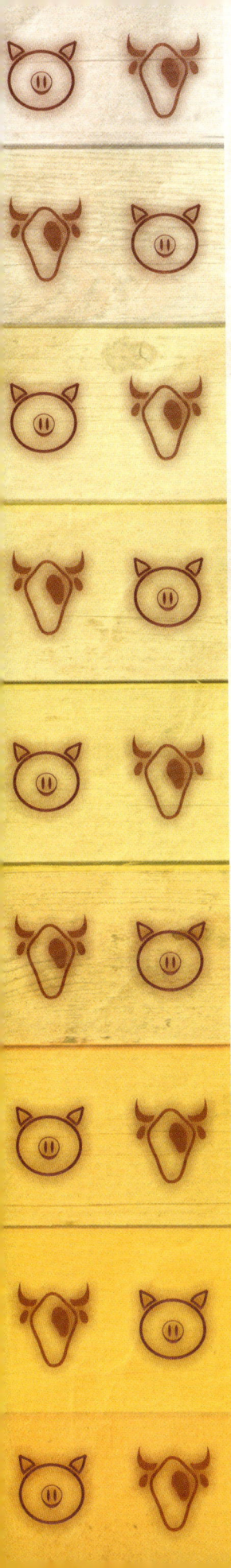

BEEF
PORK
LAMB
& BISON

BEEF TENDERLOIN WITH PARMESAN CRUST

SERVES 4 • GLUTEN FREE

1½ pounds lean beef tenderloin, in 1 piece, trimmed and tied

¼ teaspoon salt

¼ teaspoon black pepper

¾ teaspoon canola oil

¼ cup grated Parmesan

¼ cup finely chopped fresh parsley

1 tablespoon reduced-fat mayonnaise

1½ teaspoons Dijon mustard

3 garlic cloves, minced

1 Preheat oven to 450°F. Position rack in top third of oven.

2 Sprinkle beef with salt and pepper. Heat oil in large ovenproof skillet over medium-high heat. Add beef and cook until browned on all sides, about 10 minutes. Remove beef from pan and set on cutting board.

3 Combine Parmesan, parsley, mayonnaise, mustard, and garlic in small bowl. Remove and discard string from tenderloin. Spread Parmesan mixture over top and sides of tenderloin; return to skillet. Transfer skillet to oven and roast until instant-read thermometer inserted into center of beef registers 145°F for medium, about 25 minutes. Transfer beef to cutting board and let stand 10 minutes. Cut into 8 slices.

7 SmartPoints value

Per serving (2 slices beef): 302 Cal, 14 g Total Fat, 5 g Sat Fat, 396 mg Sod, 1 g Total Carb, 0 g Sugar, 0 g Fib, 40 g Prot.

COOK'S TIP

Steamed asparagus sprinkled with lemon and dill makes a simple but elegant side to this superb roast.

SIRLOIN SPOON ROAST WITH GRAVY AND THYME POTATOES

SERVES 12

1 (3-pound) lean boneless top sirloin roast, trimmed and tied

¾ teaspoon black pepper

1¼ teaspoons salt

4 shallots, chopped

2 pounds small new potatoes, cut into wedges

1½ teaspoons olive oil

1¼ cups beef broth

3 garlic cloves, finely chopped

1 tablespoon chopped fresh thyme

2 teaspoons all-purpose flour

1 Preheat oven to 450°F.

2 Sprinkle roast with pepper and 1 teaspoon salt. Scatter shallots evenly over bottom of large metal roasting pan. Place roast on top of shallots. Toss potatoes, oil, and remaining ¼ teaspoon salt on large rimmed baking sheet. Spread potatoes in single layer. Transfer beef and potatoes to oven and roast 20 minutes. Reduce oven temperature to 325°F. Pour ½ cup broth around beef. Continue to roast beef and potatoes, turning potatoes once or twice, until instant-read thermometer inserted into center of beef registers 145°F for medium, about 30 minutes more. Transfer beef to cutting board and cover loosely with foil; let stand 15 minutes.

3 Sprinkle potatoes with garlic and thyme. Return to oven and roast, turning potatoes once or twice, until potatoes are very tender, about 10 minutes longer.

4 Meanwhile, to make gravy, set roasting pan with shallots over medium heat on stovetop. Stir in flour and cook, stirring, 1 minute. Whisk in remaining ¾ cup broth and bring to simmer. Simmer until sauce bubbles and thickens, about 3 minutes. Cut beef across grain into 12 slices and serve with potatoes and gravy.

4 SmartPoints value

Per serving (1 slice beef, about 4 potato wedges, and 2 tablespoons gravy): 221 Cal, 5 g Total Fat, 2 g Sat Fat, 406 mg Sod, 14 g Total Carb, 1 g Sugar, 1 g Fib, 28 g Prot.

COOK'S TIP

Got leftovers? This beef is superb for sandwiches or diced for salads or for making a luxurious breakfast of steak and eggs.

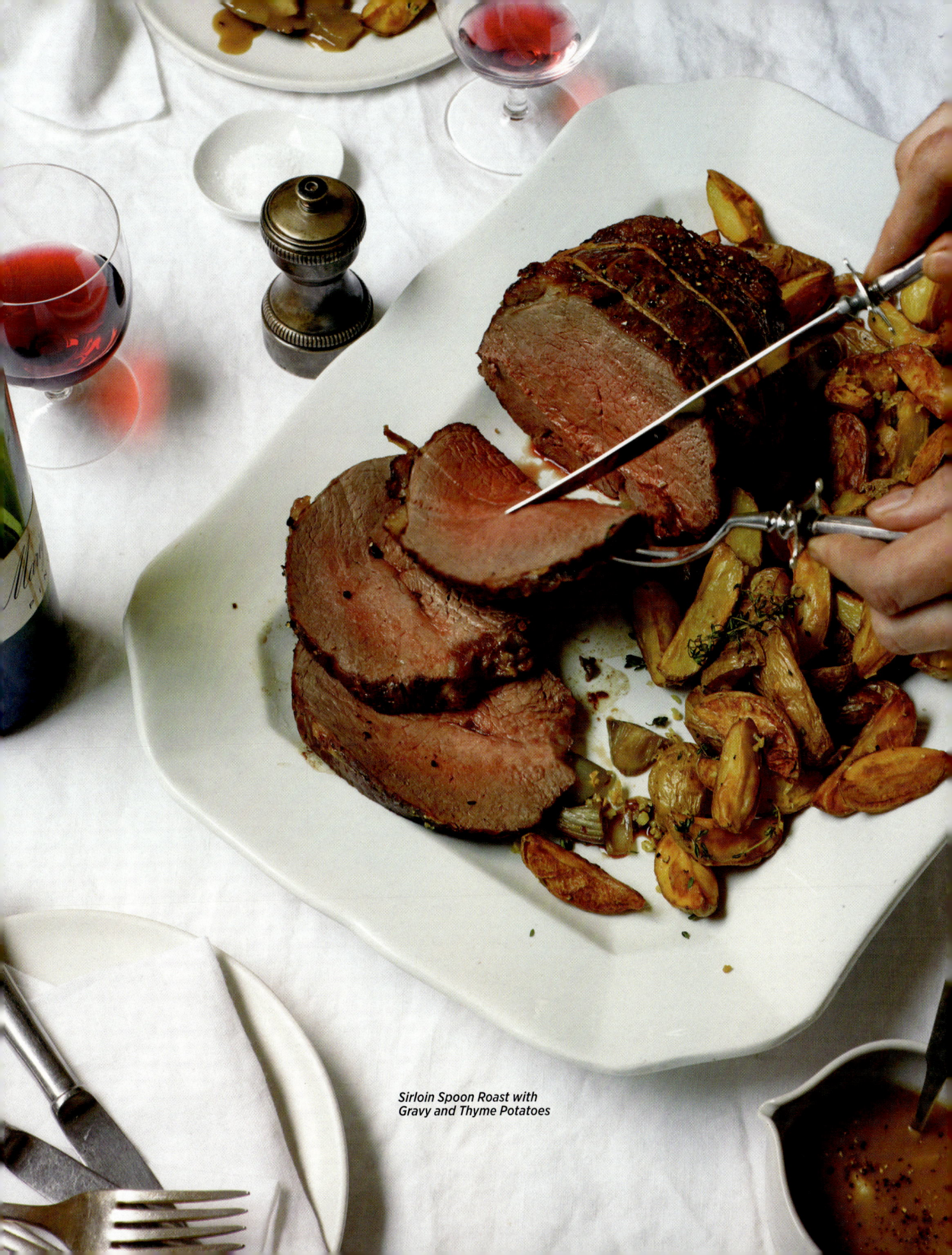

*Sirloin Spoon Roast with
Gravy and Thyme Potatoes*

Easy Oven-Barbecued Brisket

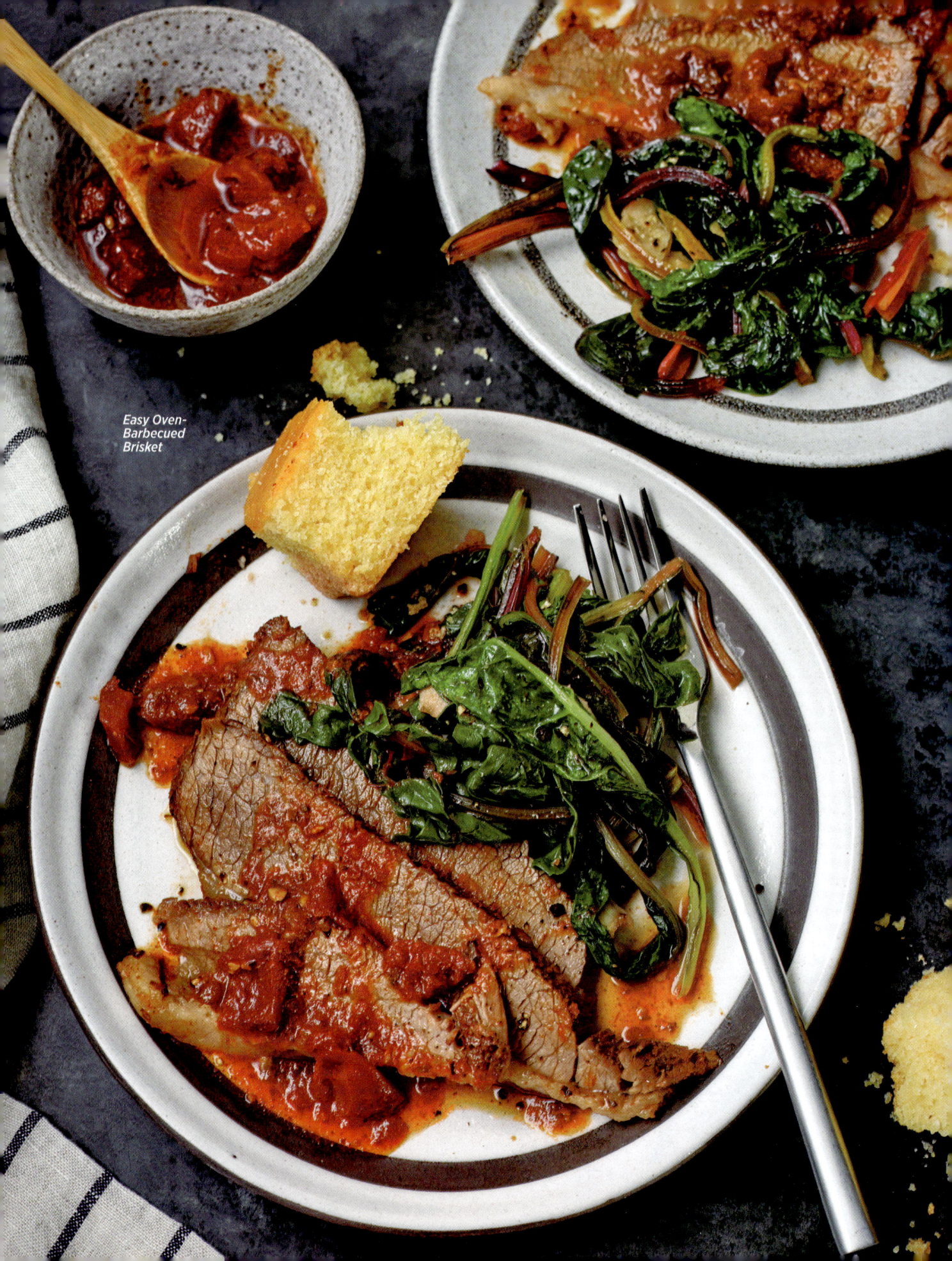

EASY OVEN-BARBECUED BRISKET

SERVES 8 ● GLUTEN FREE

2 large garlic cloves, crushed through garlic press

1 tablespoon chili powder

2 teaspoons ground cumin

1 teaspoon dried oregano

1 (2¼-pound) lean beef brisket, trimmed

¾ teaspoon kosher salt

1 (14½-ounce) can diced tomatoes with green peppers and onions

1½ cups water

½ cup chili sauce

1 teaspoon finely chopped canned chipotle en adobo

1 Combine garlic, chili powder, cumin, and oregano in cup. Rub beef with spice mixture. Wrap beef in plastic wrap and refrigerate at least 3 hours or overnight.

2 Preheat oven to 350°F. Unwrap beef; sprinkle both sides with salt and spray with nonstick spray. Place beef in large Dutch oven. Cover and bake 1½ hours.

3 Stir tomatoes, water, chili sauce, and chipotle together in medium bowl. Pour tomato mixture over beef; turn beef to coat. Cover and bake until beef is fork-tender, about 1½ hours longer.

4 Transfer brisket to cutting board. With spoon, skim and discard any fat from sauce. Cut brisket across grain into 24 slices. Serve with sauce.

5 SmartPoints value

Per serving (3 slices brisket and about ⅓ cup sauce): 231 Cal, 10 g Total Fat, 3 g Sat Fat, 571 mg Sod, 7 g Total Carb, 3 g Sugar, 2 g Fib, 28 g Prot.

COOK'S TIP

For an even tastier brisket, refrigerate the beef and sauce in an airtight container overnight, then gently reheat. This will allow the flavors to meld and more fully develop.

FILET MIGNON WITH RED WINE SAUCE

SERVES 4 • GLUTEN FREE • UNDER 20 MINUTES

4 (¼-pound) lean filets mignons, trimmed and patted dry

¾ teaspoon coarse sea salt

½ teaspoon black pepper

¾ cup red wine, such as Burgundy or Bordeaux

2 teaspoons unsalted butter

1 tablespoon chopped fresh chives or parsley

1 Spray large cast-iron skillet with nonstick spray and set over medium-high heat.

2 Rub filets all over with salt and pepper. When skillet is hot, cook filets for about 4 minutes without turning. Turn filets and cook until instant-read thermometer inserted into side registers 145°F for medium, about 4 minutes more. Place filets on cutting board and cover loosely with aluminum foil; let rest while you make sauce.

3 Meanwhile, to make sauce, pour wine into skillet and increase heat to high. Reduce liquid by about three-quarters, scraping bottom and sides of pan, about 3 minutes. If any juice has seeped out of steak while it's resting, add it to skillet. Remove skillet from heat and swirl in butter just until melted.

4 Thinly slice filets against grain and place on plates; drizzle with sauce. Garnish with chives or parsley.

5 SmartPoints value

Per serving (1 filet and 1 tablespoon sauce): 224 Cal, 9 g Total Fat, 4 g Sat Fat, 415 mg Sod, 2 g Total Carb, 0 g Sugar, 0 g Fib, 25 g Prot.

COOK'S TIP

Try serving these luscious steaks with steamed sugar snap peas drizzled with lemon juice.

STEAK PIZZAIOLA WITH GARLIC BREAD

SERVES 4

3 teaspoons olive oil

1 small onion, thinly sliced

4 garlic cloves, minced

¼ teaspoon red pepper flakes

1 (28-ounce) can whole peeled tomatoes

1 teaspoon dried oregano

½ teaspoon salt

3 tablespoons coarsely chopped fresh parsley

1 (1-pound) lean flank steak, trimmed

½ small (8-ounce) whole wheat baguette

1 Heat 2 teaspoons oil in medium saucepan over medium-high heat. Add onion, 3 garlic cloves, and red pepper flakes. Cook, stirring occasionally, until onion softens, about 5 minutes. Add tomatoes, ½ teaspoon oregano, and ¼ teaspoon salt; bring to boil. Reduce heat and simmer, stirring occasionally with wooden spoon to break up tomatoes, until sauce thickens slightly, about 8 minutes. Remove saucepan from heat and stir in parsley.

2 Spray broiler pan with nonstick spray and preheat broiler. Sprinkle steak with remaining ¼ teaspoon salt. Place steak on broiler pan and broil 5 inches from heat, turning once, until instant-read thermometer inserted into center of steak registers 145°F for medium, about 5 minutes per side. Transfer steak to cutting board; let stand 5 minutes.

3 Split baguette lengthwise, then cut each piece in half again, making 4 equal pieces. Mix remaining 1 teaspoon oil, remaining garlic clove, and remaining ½ teaspoon oregano in small bowl. Brush mixture on cut sides of bread. Place bread, cut side up, on broiler rack and broil until lightly browned, about 2 minutes.

4 Cut steak into 12 slices. Serve with sauce and bread.

6 SmartPoints value

Per serving (3 slices steak, ¾ cup sauce, and 1 piece garlic bread): 322 Cal, 10 g Total Fat, 3 g Sat Fat, 954 mg Sod, 29 g Total Carb, 9 g Sugar, 4 g Fib, 30 g Prot.

UP THE PROTEIN

Want heftier portions of steak? For 2 extra SmartPoints, use 1¾ pounds of flank steak, cut it into 20 slices, and serve 5 slices for each serving.

GRILLED FLANK STEAK WITH MARJORAM SALSA VERDE

SERVES 8 • GLUTEN FREE

2 teaspoons black pepper

2 teaspoons ground allspice

1¼ teaspoons salt

1 teaspoon sugar

2 pounds lean flank steak, trimmed

1 garlic clove, minced

1 tablespoon finely grated lemon zest

2 tablespoons lemon juice

¼ teaspoon ground nutmeg

⅓ cup finely chopped fresh parsley

2 tablespoons finely chopped fresh marjoram

2 tablespoons plus 1 teaspoon olive oil

1 Mix pepper, allspice, 1 teaspoon salt, and sugar together in small bowl; sprinkle over both sides of steak, patting so mixture adheres. Place steak on plate; cover with plastic wrap.

2 Combine garlic, lemon zest, lemon juice, remaining ¼ teaspoon salt, nutmeg, parsley, marjoram, and 2 tablespoons oil in small bowl; let stand, unrefrigerated, to allow flavors to blend.

3 Heat ridged grill pan over high heat. Brush steak with remaining 1 teaspoon oil. When pan is very hot, place steak on pan and let sear without moving for 3–4 minutes. Turn steak, reduce heat to medium, and cook until instant-read thermometer inserted into side of steak registers 145°F for medium, about 4 minutes longer. Transfer steak to cutting board and let stand 5 minutes.

4 Slice steak thinly against grain into 24 slices; arrange on warmed serving platter and spoon salsa over steak.

5 SmartPoints value

Per serving (3 slices steak and scant 1 tablespoon salsa): 205 Cal, 10 g Total Fat, 3 g Sat Fat, 430 mg Sod, 2 g Total Carb, 1 g Fib, 25 g Prot.

COOK'S TIP

If you're making this recipe for company, you can prepare the salsa and the steak the day before and refrigerate them. Just remember to take both out of the refrigerator about 20 minutes before cooking so they can come to room temperature.

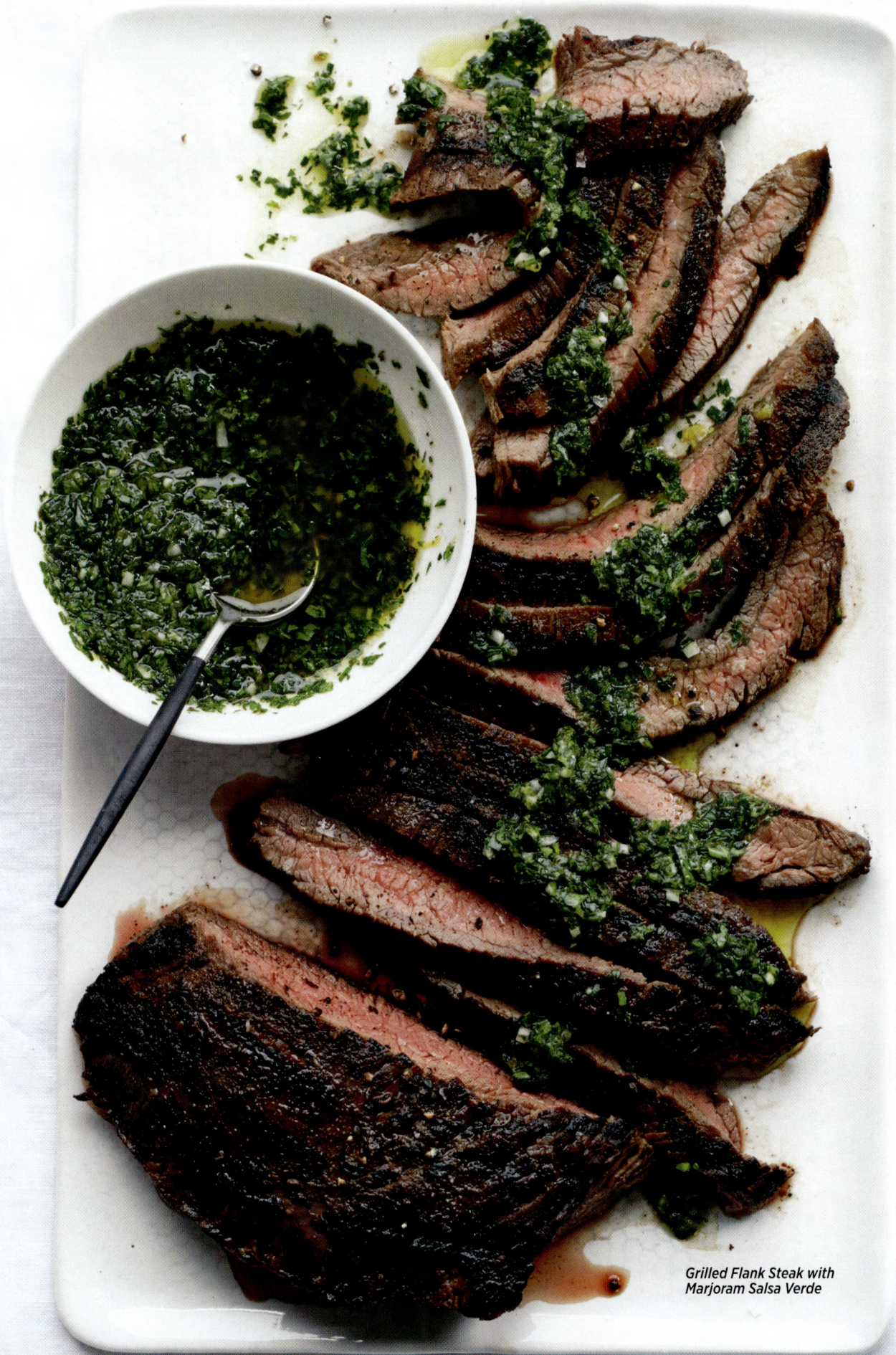

Grilled Flank Steak with Marjoram Salsa Verde

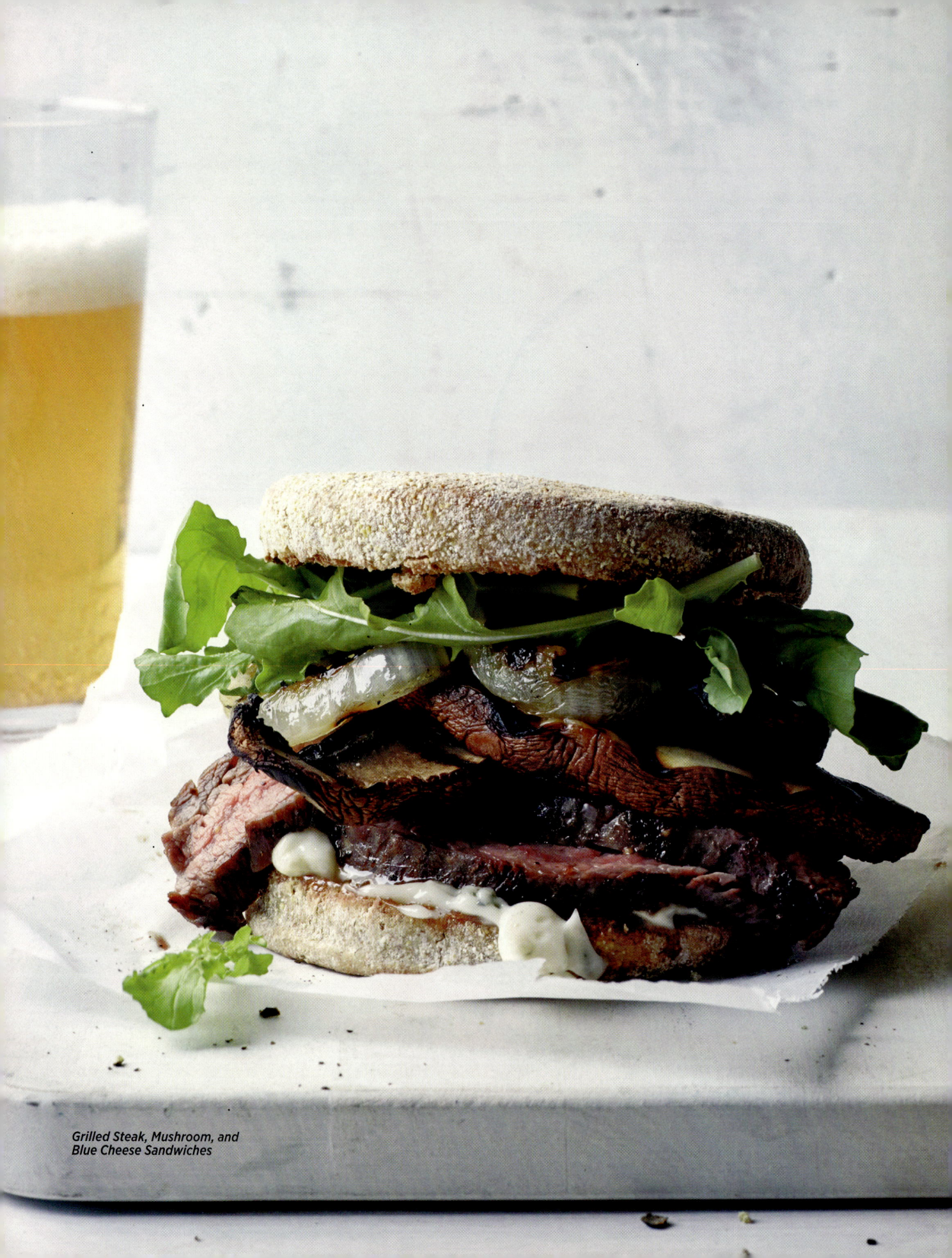

*Grilled Steak, Mushroom, and
Blue Cheese Sandwiches*

GRILLED STEAK, MUSHROOM, AND BLUE CHEESE SANDWICHES

SERVES 4

¾ **pound lean flank steak, trimmed**

2 portobello mushroom caps, cut into eight ½-inch-thick slices

1 small onion, cut into 4 slices

½ **teaspoon salt**

¼ **teaspoon black pepper**

3 tablespoons reduced-calorie mayonnaise

3 tablespoons crumbled blue cheese

1⅓ **cups baby arugula**

4 light whole wheat English muffins, toasted

1 Prepare outdoor grill for medium-high heat cooking or place ridged grill pan over medium-high heat.

2 Lightly spray steak, mushrooms, and onion with nonstick spray; sprinkle with salt and pepper. Grill, turning once, until vegetables are lightly charred and tender and instant-read thermometer inserted into center of steak registers 145°F for medium, about 10 minutes. Transfer steak to cutting board and let stand 5 minutes before slicing thinly against the grain.

3 Meanwhile, stir mayonnaise and blue cheese together in small cup.

4 To assemble sandwiches, spread each muffin bottom with about 1½ tablespoons mayonnaise mixture. Top each with one-quarter of sliced steak, mushrooms, onions, and arugula and cover with muffin tops.

7 SmartPoints value

Per serving (1 sandwich): 301 Cal, 11 g Total Fat, 4 g Sat Fat, 731 mg Sod, 25 g Total Carb, 4 g Sugar, 5 g Fib, 26 g Prot.

COOK'S TIP

Arugula is a natural with steak and meaty mushrooms, but you can also use any crisp green in these sandwiches.

HANGER STEAK WITH POLENTA "FRIES"

SERVES 4 ● GLUTEN FREE ● UNDER 20 MINUTES

1 (16-ounce) package plain fat-free polenta

¾ teaspoon salt

1 tablespoon chopped fresh rosemary

1 teaspoon finely grated lemon zest

1 (1-pound) lean hanger steak, trimmed

¼ teaspoon black pepper

1 Preheat broiler.

2 Cut polenta crosswise in half; then, working with one piece at a time, set polenta on flat (cut) end and cut lengthwise into ½-inch-thick slices. Cut slices into ½-inch-thick strips that look like French fries. Spread fries in single layer on large baking sheet. Spray fries with nonstick spray and sprinkle with ¼ teaspoon salt. Broil 6 inches from heat until crisp and browned in spots, about 10 minutes (no need to turn them). While still hot, sprinkle with ½ tablespoon rosemary and lemon zest.

3 Meanwhile, heat grill pan over medium-high heat. Sprinkle steak with remaining ½ teaspoon salt and pepper. Place steak on grill pan and cook until browned and instant-read thermometer inserted into center of steak registers 145°F, about 4 minutes per side. Let steak rest on cutting board 5 minutes. Cut diagonally against grain into 20 (½-inch-thick) slices. Sprinkle steak with remaining ½ tablespoon rosemary and serve with polenta fries.

6 SmartPoints value

Per serving (5 slices steak and about 10 polenta fries): 242 Cal, 6 g Total Fat, 2 g Sat Fat, 829 mg Sod, 17 g Total Carb, 0 g Sugar, 1 g Fib, 27 g Prot.

COOK'S TIP

Serve the steak with fresh baby arugula or other greens drizzled with lemon juice and sprinkled with salt and pepper to taste.

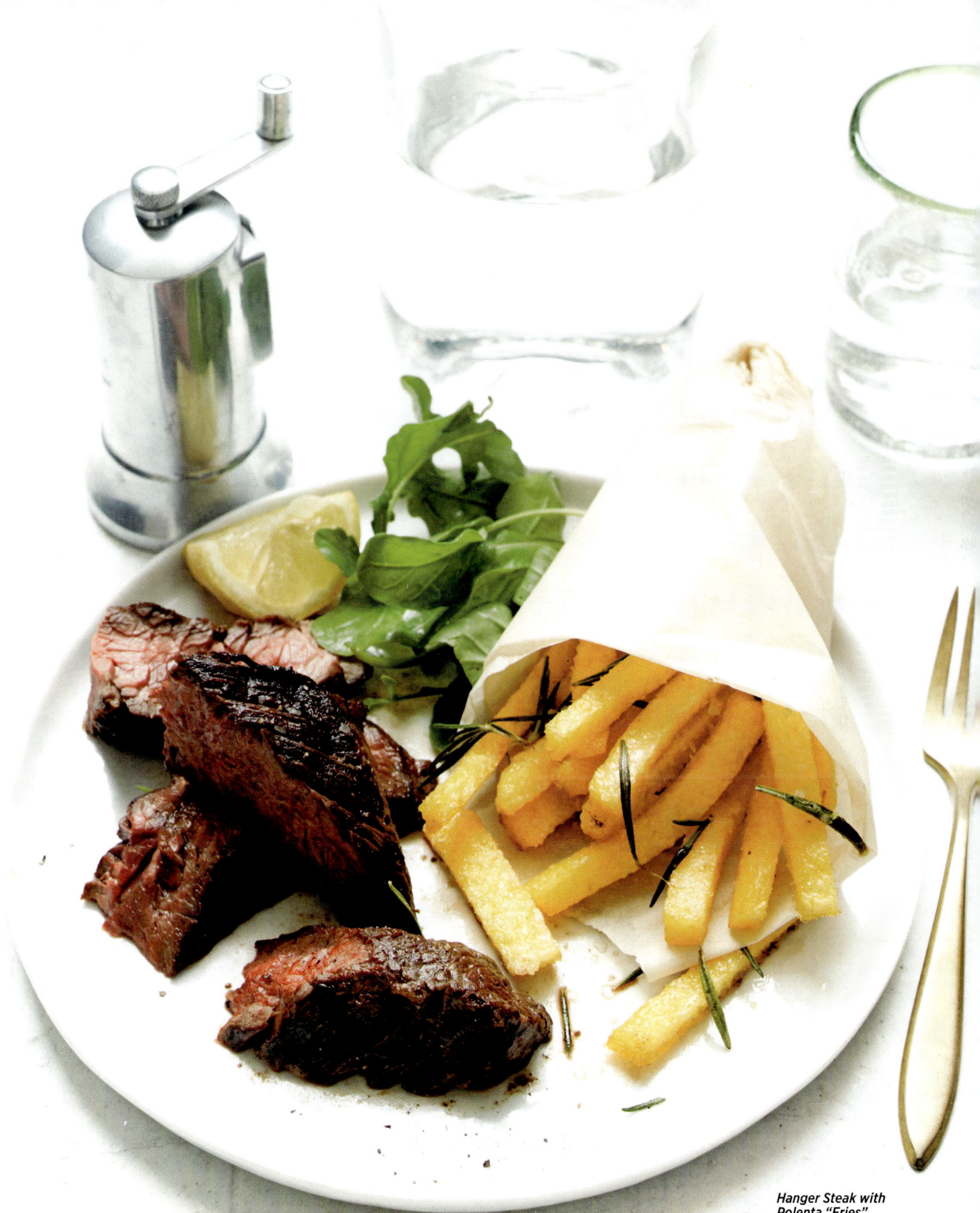

Hanger Steak with Polenta "Fries"

Vietnamese Beef Pho

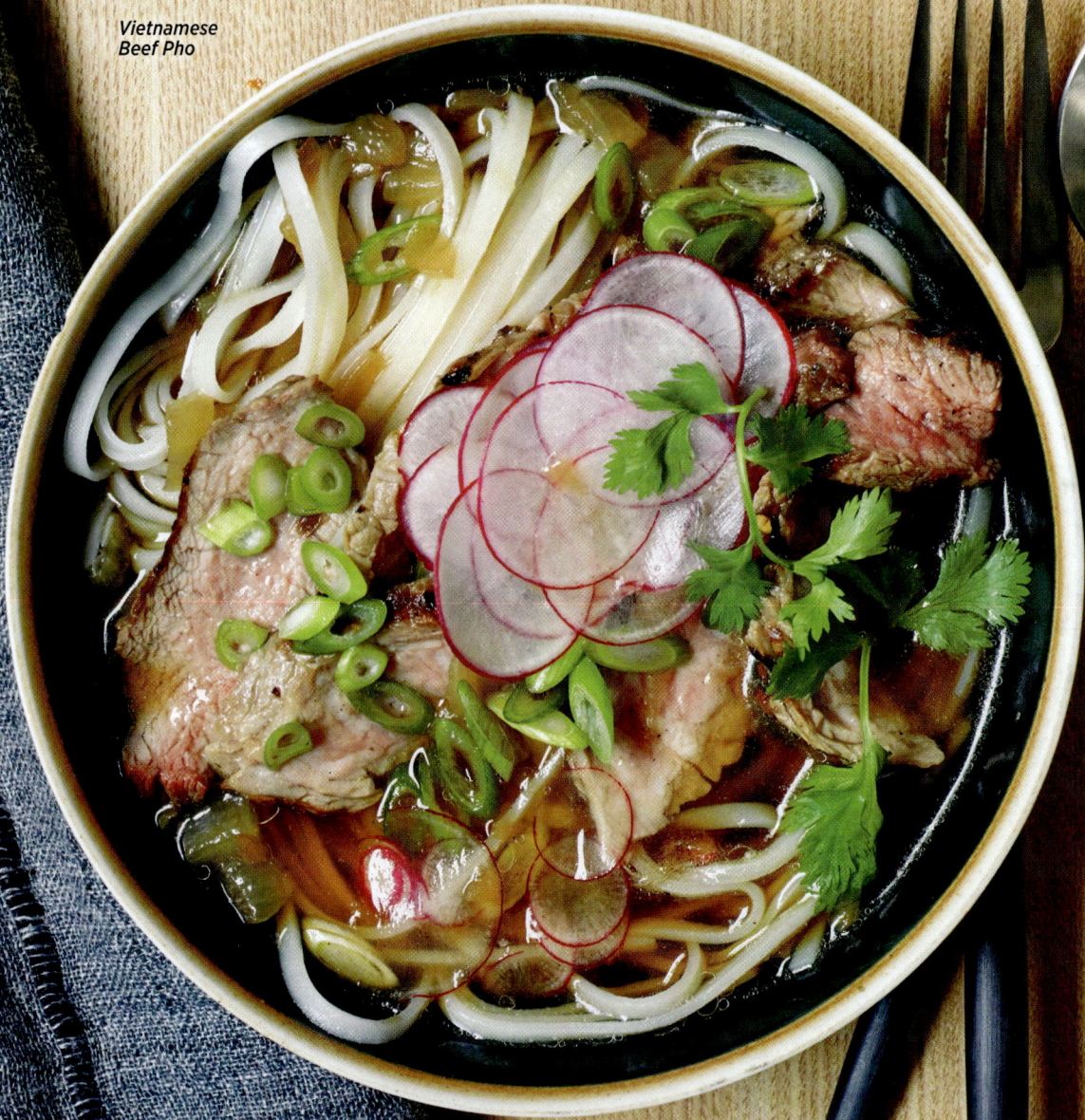

VIETNAMESE BEEF PHO

SERVES 4 • GLUTEN FREE

¾ **pound lean sirloin beef, trimmed**

¼ **teaspoon salt, or to taste**

¼ **teaspoon black pepper**

2 **teaspoons canola oil**

1 **cup chopped onion**

4 **cups low-sodium beef broth**

2 **cinnamon sticks**

2 **star anise pods**

10 **black peppercorns**

1½ **tablespoons Asian fish sauce**

4 **ounces dried flat rice noodles**

3 **scallions, white and light green parts, thinly sliced**

4 **radishes, thinly sliced**

¼ **cup fresh cilantro leaves**

4 **lime wedges**

1 Heat ridged grill pan over medium-high heat. Sprinkle steak with ⅛ teaspoon salt and the pepper. Place steak on grill pan and cook until browned and instant-read thermometer inserted into center of steak registers 145°F for medium, 6–8 minutes per side. Transfer steak to cutting board and let stand 5 minutes.

2 Meanwhile, heat oil in large saucepan over medium heat. Add onion and cook, covered, stirring occasionally, until golden, about 8 minutes. Add broth, cinnamon sticks, star anise, peppercorns, and remaining ⅛ teaspoon salt and bring to boil. Reduce heat to low, and simmer, covered, 5 minutes. Stir in fish sauce.

3 Cook rice noodles according to package directions. Drain and divide among 4 shallow bowls.

4 Remove cinnamon sticks, star anise, and peppercorns from broth mixture. Slice beef very thinly against the grain into about 20 slices. Layer beef over noodles. Top beef with scallions, radishes, and cilantro. Ladle broth over beef and serve with lime wedges.

6 SmartPoints value

Per serving (1 bowl): 280 Cal, 6 g Total Fat, 1 g Sat Fat, 1,134 mg Sod, 33 g Total Carb, 4 g Sugar, 3 g Fib, 24 g Prot.

UP THE PROTEIN

Sliced hard-cooked egg is a classic ingredient in Vietnamese pho. If you like, top each bowl with ½ of a thinly sliced hard-cooked egg and increase the per-serving SmartPoints by 1.

SKILLET BEEF-AND-BEER STEW WITH POTATOES

SERVES 4

1 pound lean beef round, trimmed and cut into ½-inch cubes

1 teaspoon salt, or to taste

1 onion, chopped

1 green bell pepper, chopped

3 garlic cloves, finely chopped

2 potatoes, peeled and diced

½ pound baby-cut carrots

1 (12-ounce) bottle light beer

½ cup beef broth

2 bay leaves

2 teaspoons fresh thyme or ¾ teaspoon dried

2 tablespoons cornstarch

1 Spray large skillet with nonstick spray and heat over medium-high heat. Add beef, sprinkle with salt, and cook, stirring frequently, until browned, about 8 minutes. Transfer beef to plate and set aside. Add onion, bell pepper, and garlic to skillet and cook, stirring, until softened, about 3 minutes. Stir in potatoes, carrots, beer, broth, bay leaves, and thyme; bring to boil. Return beef to skillet. Reduce heat, and simmer, covered, until meat is tender, 45 minutes–1 hour.

2 Stir cornstarch and ½ cup broth from skillet together in small cup; add back to skillet and stir to combine. Cook until slightly thickened and bubbling, about 5 minutes; cook, stirring occasionally, 2 minutes more. Discard bay leaves.

7 SmartPoints value

Per serving (about 2 cups): 326 Cal, 6 g Total Fat, 2 g Sat Fat, 795 mg Sod, 33 g Total Carb, 6 g Sugar, 5 g Fib, 29 g Prot.

COOK'S TIP

If you like, add ½ pound trimmed sugar snap peas to the stew along with the cornstarch mixture in Step 2.

ITALIAN BEEF AND LENTIL SLOW-COOKER STEW

SERVES 6 • GLUTEN FREE

1 small onion, chopped

1 garlic clove, finely chopped

1 large zucchini, diced

1 pound lean beef round, trimmed and cut into 1-inch chunks

½ teaspoon dried oregano, crushed

1 (14½-ounce) can diced tomatoes, with juice

1 tablespoon canned tomato paste

¾ cup dry lentils

4 cups beef broth

1 teaspoon salt

¼ teaspoon black pepper

¼ cup lightly packed fresh basil leaves, cut into strips

1 Place all ingredients except basil in 5- to 6-quart slow cooker; stir well. Cook on Low until beef is very tender, 6–7 hours.

2 Stir in basil and cook 5 minutes longer.

4 SmartPoints value

Per serving (1½ cups): 229 Cal, 5 g Total Fat, 2 g Sat Fat, 1,153 mg Sod, 21 g Total Carb, 4 g Sugar, 9 g Fib, 26 g Prot.

COOK'S TIP

You can substitute 2 cups of fresh green beans, cut into 2-inch lengths, for the zucchini, and 2 tablespoons of chopped fresh parsley for the basil.

MINI SHEPHERD'S PIES

SERVES 6 • GLUTEN FREE

1¼ pounds Yukon Gold potatoes, cut into 1-inch pieces

1 teaspoon salt

1 scallion, finely chopped

⅔ cup fat-free milk

Pinch black pepper

¾ pound ground lean beef (7% fat or less)

1 small onion, finely chopped

2 carrots, finely chopped

1 garlic clove, finely chopped

2½ teaspoons garlic-herb seasoning

1 cup canned tomato sauce

1¼ cups frozen cut green beans, thawed

6 tablespoons low-fat shredded Cheddar

1 Preheat oven to 400°F. Place 6 (6-ounce) ramekins on rimmed baking sheet; set aside.

2 Place potatoes in medium saucepan; add enough water to cover and stir in ¼ teaspoon salt. Bring to boil over high heat; reduce heat to medium-low and simmer, covered, until tender, 12–15 minutes. Drain potatoes and return to saucepan; stir in scallion, milk, pepper, and ¼ teaspoon salt. Mash with potato masher until somewhat smooth; set aside.

3 Meanwhile, spray large skillet with nonstick spray; set over medium-high heat. Add beef, onion, carrot, garlic, garlic seasoning, and remaining ½ teaspoon salt; sauté, breaking apart beef with spoon, until onions are translucent and carrots are just tender, about 10 minutes. Stir in tomato sauce; remove from heat.

4 Divide beef mixture evenly among ramekins. Top each with layer of green beans and layer of mashed potatoes; sprinkle each with 1 tablespoon Cheddar. Bake until heated through, about 20 minutes.

4 SmartPoints value

Per serving (1 pie): 200 Cal, 4 g Total Fat, 2 g Sat Fat, 575 mg Sod, 24 g Total Carb, 7 g Sugar, 4 g Fib, 18 g Prot.

COOK'S TIP

If you like, you can freeze these pies right in the ramekins after baking. If frozen, thaw in the refrigerator, and then bake until heated through, about 35 to 40 minutes.

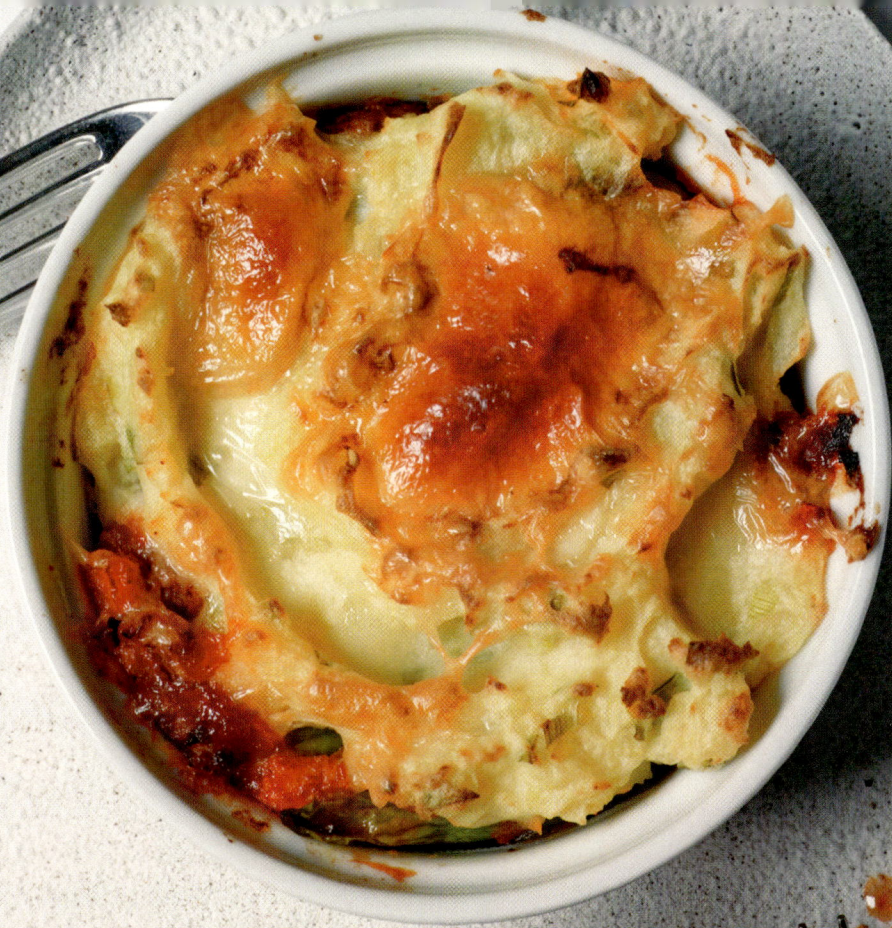

Mini Shepherd's Pies

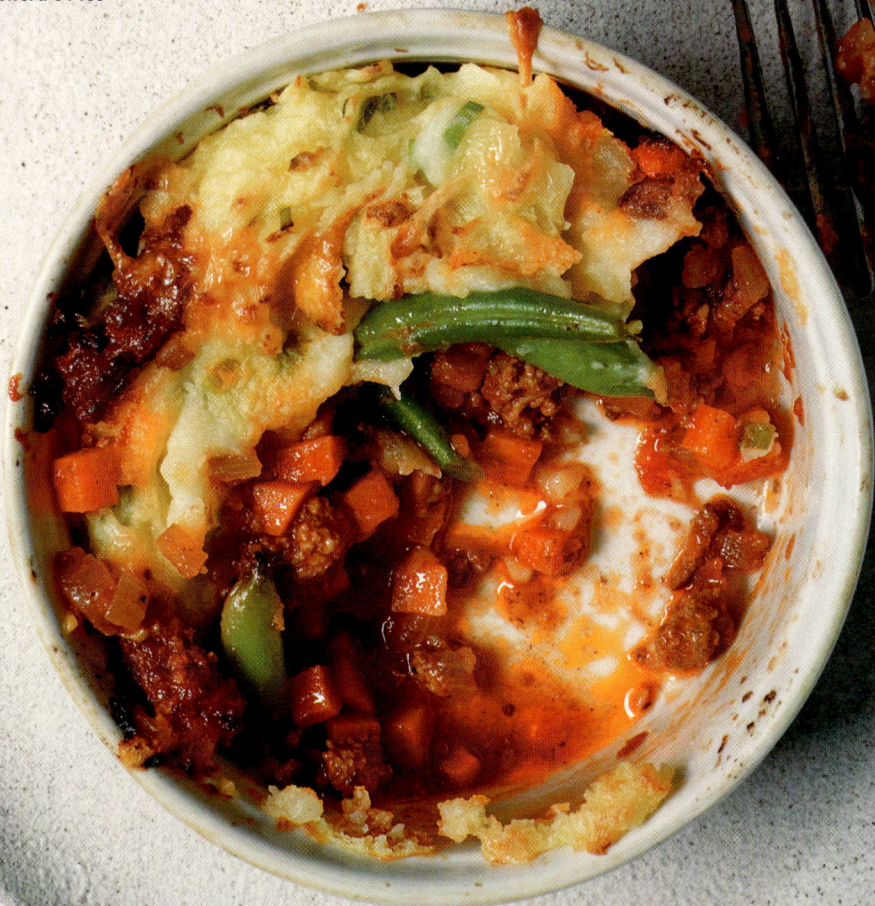

BAKED PENNE WITH BEEF AND CAULIFLOWER

SERVES 6

1¼ pounds ground lean beef (7% fat or less)

¼ teaspoon salt

1 (8-ounce) container sliced cremini mushrooms

1 (24-ounce) jar fat-free marinara sauce

¼ teaspoon red pepper flakes, or to taste

4 ounces (about 1¼ cups) whole wheat penne

½ head cauliflower, cut into small florets (about 4 cups)

½ cup part-skim ricotta

¾ cup shredded reduced-fat Italian cheese blend

1 Spray large skillet with nonstick spray and set over medium-high heat. Add beef and salt; cook, breaking apart beef with wooden spoon, until browned, about 5 minutes. With slotted spoon, transfer beef to medium bowl. Return skillet to medium-high heat. Add mushrooms and cook, stirring frequently, until mushrooms have released their liquid, about 5 minutes. Remove skillet from heat and stir in marinara, red pepper flakes, and reserved beef.

2 Preheat oven to 375°F. Spray 2-quart shallow baking dish lightly with nonstick spray.

3 Cook pasta according to package directions just until al dente, adding cauliflower during last 3 minutes of cooking time. Drain well.

4 Stir pasta mixture into skillet with beef mixture. Transfer to prepared baking dish and spread evenly. Spoon ricotta by small teaspoonfuls over pasta. Bake until bubbling at edges, about 25 minutes. Sprinkle with cheese blend and bake until cheese melts, 8–10 minutes longer.

8 SmartPoints value

Per serving (1½ cups): 331 Cal, 9 g Total Fat, 5 g Sat Fat, 512 mg Sod, 29 g Total Carb, 7 g Sugar, 4 g Fib, 33 g Prot.

UP THE PROTEIN

Love cheese? Sprinkle each serving of this casserole with 1 tablespoon of grated Parmesan for an additional 1 SmartPoints per serving.

TERIYAKI BURGERS WITH CHILI KETCHUP

SERVES 4

1 pound ground lean beef (7% fat or less)

¼ cup finely chopped red onion

2 tablespoons teriyaki sauce

¼ teaspoon salt

¼ teaspoon black pepper

½ cup ketchup

1 teaspoon sun-dried hot chile pepper or red pepper flakes, or to taste

4 romaine lettuce leaves

1 large tomato, cut into 8 slices

1 Combine beef, onion, teriyaki sauce, salt, and black pepper in large bowl. Mix well and shape mixture into 4 patties, each about 1 inch thick.

2 Spray ridged grill pan with nonstick spray and set over medium-high heat. When pan is hot, add burgers and grill until cooked through and instant-read thermometer inserted into side of each patty registers 160°F, 4–5 minutes per side.

3 Mix ketchup and chile together in small bowl. Serve each burger on lettuce leaf with 2 tomato slices and 2 tablespoons ketchup.

5 SmartPoints value

Per serving (1 burger): 205 Cal, 6 g Total Fat, 3 g Sat Fat, 840 mg Sod, 12 g Total Carb, 9 g Sugar, 1 g Fib, 26 g Prot.

COOK'S TIP

You can also cook these phenomenally tasty burgers on an outdoor grill—just be sure to adjust the cooking time.

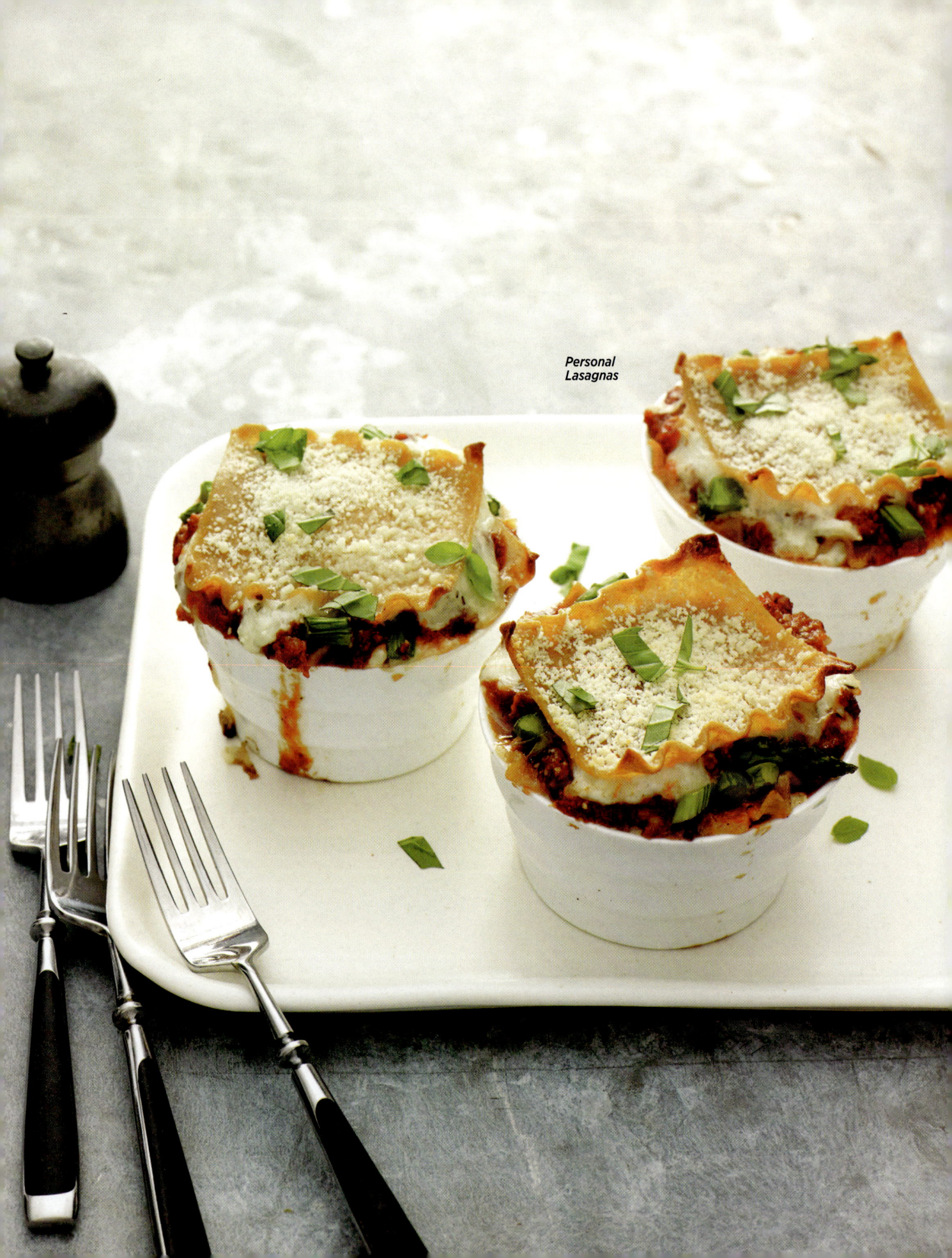

Personal Lasagnas

PERSONAL LASAGNAS

SERVES 12

9 ounces whole wheat lasagna noodles

1½ cups shredded part-skim mozzarella

¾ cup part-skim ricotta

2 large egg whites

¾ teaspoon dried oregano

1¼ pounds ground lean beef (5% fat or less)

1½ cups finely chopped asparagus

¼ teaspoon kosher salt, or to taste

¼ teaspoon black pepper, or to taste

1 (28-ounce) can crushed tomatoes with onion and garlic

¼ cup grated Parmesan

2 tablespoons chopped fresh basil

1 Preheat oven to 375°F.

2 Cook pasta according to package directions for al dente; drain.

3 Meanwhile, combine mozzarella, ricotta, egg whites, and oregano in medium bowl; set aside. Cook beef over medium-high heat in medium nonstick skillet, breaking apart with wooden spoon, until no longer pink, about 6 minutes. Add asparagus, salt, and pepper; cook, stirring occasionally, until asparagus is bright green, about 2 minutes. Add tomatoes and stir to combine; set aside.

4 Slice noodles in half widthwise, and then cut each half into 2 pieces so you have 4 equal-size pieces from each noodle.

5 Generously spray 12 (6-ounce) ramekins with nonstick spray. Sprinkle ½ teaspoon Parmesan in bottom of each ramekin and tilt to evenly cover bottoms. Place 1 noodle piece on bottom of each ramekin; top with about 1½ tablespoons beef mixture and then about 1 tablespoon cheese mixture. Repeat layering 2 more times to form 3 layers of noodles, beef, and cheese in each cup. Place final noodle square on each lasagna; sprinkle each with ½ teaspoon remaining Parmesan.

6 Cover lasagnas tightly with foil and bake 20 minutes; uncover and cook until browned on top, about 5 minutes more. Remove from oven; let cool 3 minutes. Sprinkle with basil just before serving.

5 SmartPoints value

Per serving (1 lasagna): 216 Cal, 7 g Total Fat, 4 g Sat Fat, 313 mg Sod, 19 g Total Carb, 3 g Sugar, 3 g Fib, 21 g Prot.

COOK'S TIP

Wrap and freeze these mini lasagnas for a fabulous dinner anytime. Just thaw and reheat when you're ready for supper.

SPAGHETTI SQUASH BOLOGNESE WITH MUSHROOMS

SERVES 6 • GLUTEN FREE

1 teaspoon olive oil

1 onion, chopped

1 red bell pepper, chopped

3 garlic cloves, finely chopped

½ pound cremini mushrooms, chopped

1 pound ground lean beef (7% fat or less)

¾ teaspoon salt

¼ teaspoon black pepper

1 (28-ounce) can crushed tomatoes

1 (3-pound) spaghetti squash

3 tablespoons grated pecorino

¼ cup loosely packed fresh basil leaves, whole or thinly sliced

1 Heat oil in large nonstick skillet over medium-high heat. Add onion and bell pepper; cook, covered, stirring occasionally, until vegetables are tender, about 3 minutes. Add garlic and cook, stirring constantly, until fragrant, about 30 seconds. Add mushrooms and cook, uncovered, stirring occasionally, until tender, about 3 minutes. Add beef, ½ teaspoon salt, and black pepper; cook, breaking apart beef with spoon, just until no longer pink, about 3 minutes.

2 Stir in tomatoes; bring to boil. Reduce heat and simmer until flavors are blended, about 8 minutes.

3 Meanwhile, pierce squash all over with tip of small sharp knife; place on double layer of paper towels in microwave. Microwave on High until tender, about 14 minutes, turning once halfway through microwaving time. Let stand 5 minutes; then split squash lengthwise and use a spoon to scoop out and discard seeds.

4 With fork, scrape out squash pulp into medium bowl; toss with remaining ¼ teaspoon salt. Divide squash evenly among 6 bowls. Top with sauce; sprinkle evenly with pecorino and basil.

3 SmartPoints value

Per serving (generous ¾ cup sauce and ⅔ cup squash): 233 Cal, 7 g Total Fat, 3 g Sat Fat, 619 mg Sod, 25 g Total Carb, 6 g Sugar, 3 g Fib, 21 g Prot.

COOK'S TIP

The cooked squash will be very hot after microwaving, so protect your hands with mitts if necessary when splitting it in Step 3.

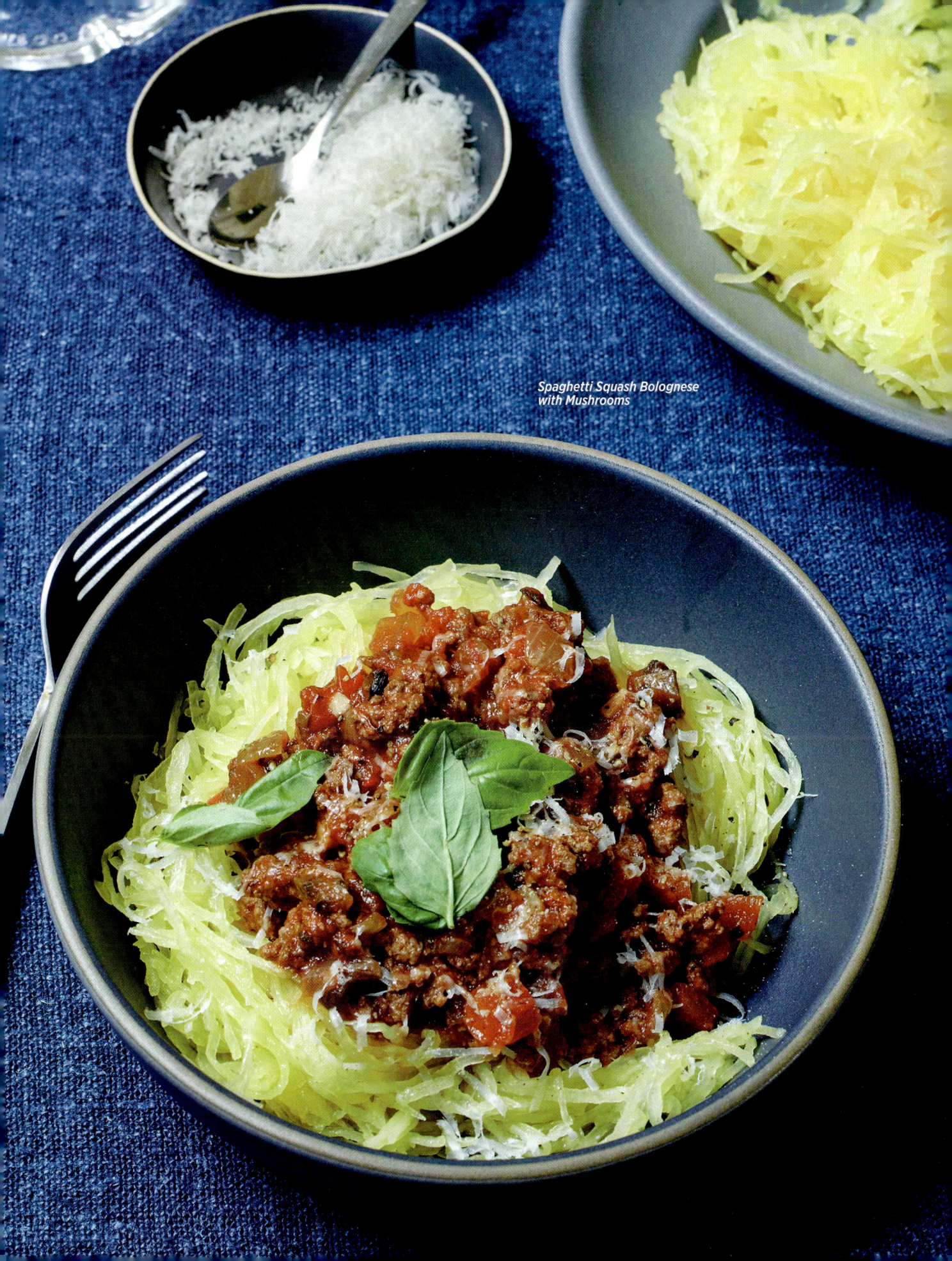

Spaghetti Squash Bolognese with Mushrooms

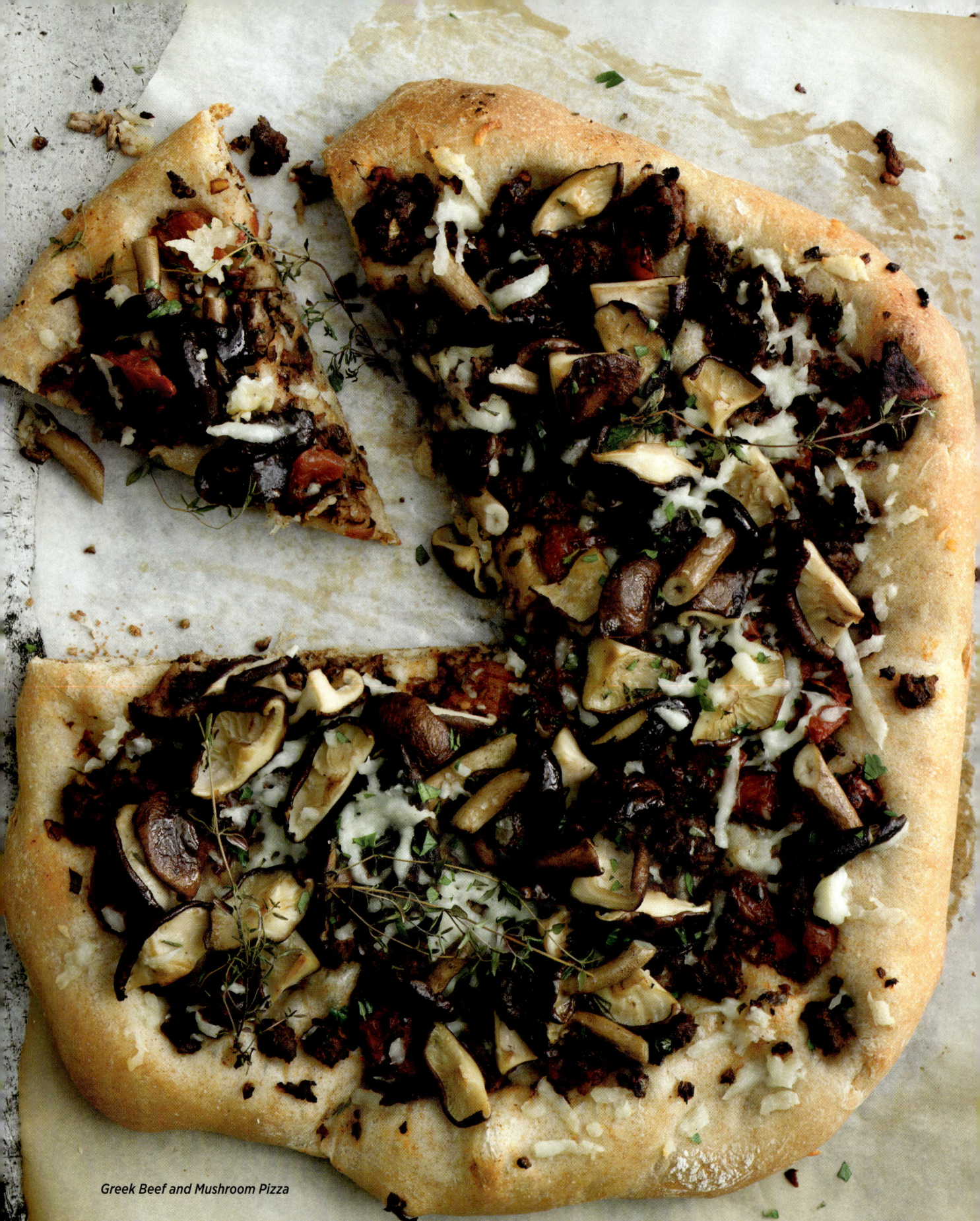

Greek Beef and Mushroom Pizza

GREEK BEEF AND MUSHROOM PIZZA

SERVES 6

2 teaspoons olive oil

1 small onion, finely chopped

½ pound ground lean beef
(7% fat or less)

4 ounces shiitake mushrooms,
stems removed and caps
thinly sliced

1 tomato, chopped

2 tablespoons chopped
fresh parsley

1 tablespoon fresh thyme leaves

1 tablespoon chopped
fresh oregano

1 teaspoon cinnamon

½–1 teaspoon ancho
chile powder

½ teaspoon salt

¼ teaspoon black pepper

1 (10-ounce) prebaked thin
whole wheat pizza crust

2 ounces haloumi cheese,
shredded (about ½ cup)

1 Preheat oven to 400°F; adjust oven rack to lower third of oven. Spray large baking sheet with nonstick spray.

2 Heat oil in large nonstick skillet over medium heat. Add onion and cook, stirring frequently, until softened, about 3 minutes. Add beef and mushrooms and cook, breaking apart beef with wooden spoon, until beef is browned, about 5 minutes. Stir in tomato, parsley, thyme, oregano, cinnamon, chile powder, salt, and pepper; cook, stirring occasionally, until thickened, about 2 minutes.

3 Place pizza crust on baking sheet. Top crust evenly with beef mixture, then with haloumi. Bake until cheese melts and crust is crisp, 15–20 minutes. Let stand 5 minutes before serving. Cut into 6 wedges.

6 SmartPoints value

Per serving (1 wedge): 223 Cal, 7 g Total Fat, 3 g Sat Fat, 495 mg Sod, 24 g Total Carb, 2 g Sugar, 5 g Fib, 15 g Prot.

COOK'S TIP

Haloumi, a firm creamy cheese from Cyprus, is made from a combination of sheep's and goat's milk. If you can't find it, you can use ¼ cup crumbled feta and ¼ cup shredded mozzarella.

ROASTED PORK TENDERLOIN

SERVES 6 • GLUTEN FREE

2 tablespoons chopped fresh thyme or 2 teaspoons dried thyme

2 tablespoons chopped fresh oregano or 2 teaspoons dried oregano

1 teaspoon garlic powder

1 teaspoon onion powder

1 teaspoon salt

1 teaspoon black pepper

2 teaspoons olive oil

2 pounds lean pork tenderloin, trimmed

1 Preheat oven to 400°F. Spray shallow roasting pan with nonstick spray.

2 Combine thyme, oregano, garlic powder, onion powder, salt, and pepper in small bowl; set aside. Rub oil over pork. Sprinkle spice mixture all over pork and transfer to prepared pan.

3 Roast until instant-read thermometer inserted into center of pork reads 145°F, 25–30 minutes. Let roast stand 3 minutes before slicing crosswise into 24 slices.

3 SmartPoints value

Per serving (4 slices pork): 187 Cal, 5 g Total Fat, 1 g Sat Fat, 470 mg Sod, 2 g Total Carb, 0 g Sugar, 1 g Fib, 32 g Prot.

COOK'S TIP

For variety, try seasoned oils (such as roasted red pepper olive oil or garlic olive oil) and different herbs and spices (such as parsley, rosemary, onion powder, and cumin), and this can be a healthy go-to meal at least once a week: Leftovers are great in salads.

SLOW-ROASTED PORK IN MOLE SAUCE

SERVES 12 • GLUTEN FREE

3 pounds lean pork tenderloin, trimmed

1 tablespoon paprika

1 teaspoon salt

3 poblano peppers, seeded, deveined, and sliced

2 onions, thinly sliced

¼ cup water

2 teaspoons olive oil

4 garlic cloves, finely chopped

3 tablespoons chopped canned chipotles en adobo, or to taste

1½ tablespoons ground cumin

½ cup fresh cilantro leaves, finely chopped

2 tablespoons unsweetened cocoa powder

3 cups chopped fresh tomatoes

½ cup raisins

3 tablespoons peanut butter

1 Preheat oven to 450°F.

2 Rinse and dry pork tenderloin; rub paprika and salt all over.

3 Spray large, heavy ovenproof pot with nonstick spray; set over high heat. Place pork in pot and sear on all sides, about 4 minutes.

4 Remove pot from heat and nestle 1 whole sliced poblano and 1 whole sliced onion under pork; add water to pot and cover tightly. Bake 20 minutes; reduce heat to 200°F and continue to bake until pork is very tender, about 2 hours. When pork has cooked for 1½ hours, start mole sauce.

5 To make mole sauce, heat oil in large skillet over medium heat. When oil begins to shimmer, add garlic and chipotles. Cook, stirring, until garlic is fragrant, about 1 minute. Add remaining onion and poblano slices; cook, stirring frequently, until onion starts to turn golden brown, about 10 minutes. Stir in cumin, ¼ cup cilantro, and cocoa; stir until well mixed. Stir in tomatoes and simmer 10–15 minutes.

6 When pork is done, remove pot from oven but leave oven on. Transfer pork to cutting board; remove vegetables and juices and add to mole sauce with raisins and peanut butter. Mix well and simmer 5 minutes more. Working in small batches, puree mole sauce in blender.

7 Thinly slice pork and return to pot. Cover pork with mole sauce and cook 1 hour longer. Serve garnished with remaining ¼ cup cilantro.

4 SmartPoints value

Per serving (1⅓ cups meat and sauce): 208 Cal, 6 g Total Fat, 1 g Sat Fat, 302 mg Sod, 13 g Total Carb, 7 g Sugar, 3 g Fib, 27 g Prot.

COOK'S TIP

Preparing a batch of this utterly delicious pork will really pay off. Turn leftovers into burritos if you like.

BARBECUE PORK
WITH FRESH KIMCHI

SERVES 4

½ head Napa cabbage, shredded (about 4 cups)

1 cup shredded carrot

3 scallions, thinly sliced

2 tablespoons rice vinegar

1 tablespoon finely chopped pickled ginger

1 tablespoon liquid from jar of pickled ginger

2 tablespoons Sriracha or other hot sauce

¼ teaspoon salt

1 tablespoon soy sauce

1 tablespoon hoisin sauce

1 (1¼-pound) lean pork tenderloin, trimmed

1 To make kimchi, combine cabbage, carrot, scallions, vinegar, ginger, ginger juice, 1 tablespoon Sriracha, and salt in large bowl and toss. Let stand at least 10 minutes for flavors to blend.

2 Preheat oven to 425°F. Spray small shallow roasting pan with nonstick spray.

3 Whisk soy sauce, hoisin sauce, and remaining 1 tablespoon Sriracha together in small bowl. Brush mixture over pork. Place pork in pan and roast until instant-read thermometer inserted into center of pork registers 145°F for medium, 20–25 minutes. Transfer pork to cutting board and let stand 10 minutes. Cut pork into 12 slices and serve with kimchi.

3 SmartPoints value

Per serving (3 slices pork and ¾ cup kimchi): 215 Cal, 3 g Total Fat, 1 g Sat Fat, 747 mg Sod, 13 g Total Carb, 7 g Sugar, 3 g Fib, 31 g Prot.

COOK'S TIP

Serve this spicy dish with a side of nutty quinoa garnished with cilantro; a ½-cup portion of cooked quinoa per serving will increase the SmartPoints value by 3.

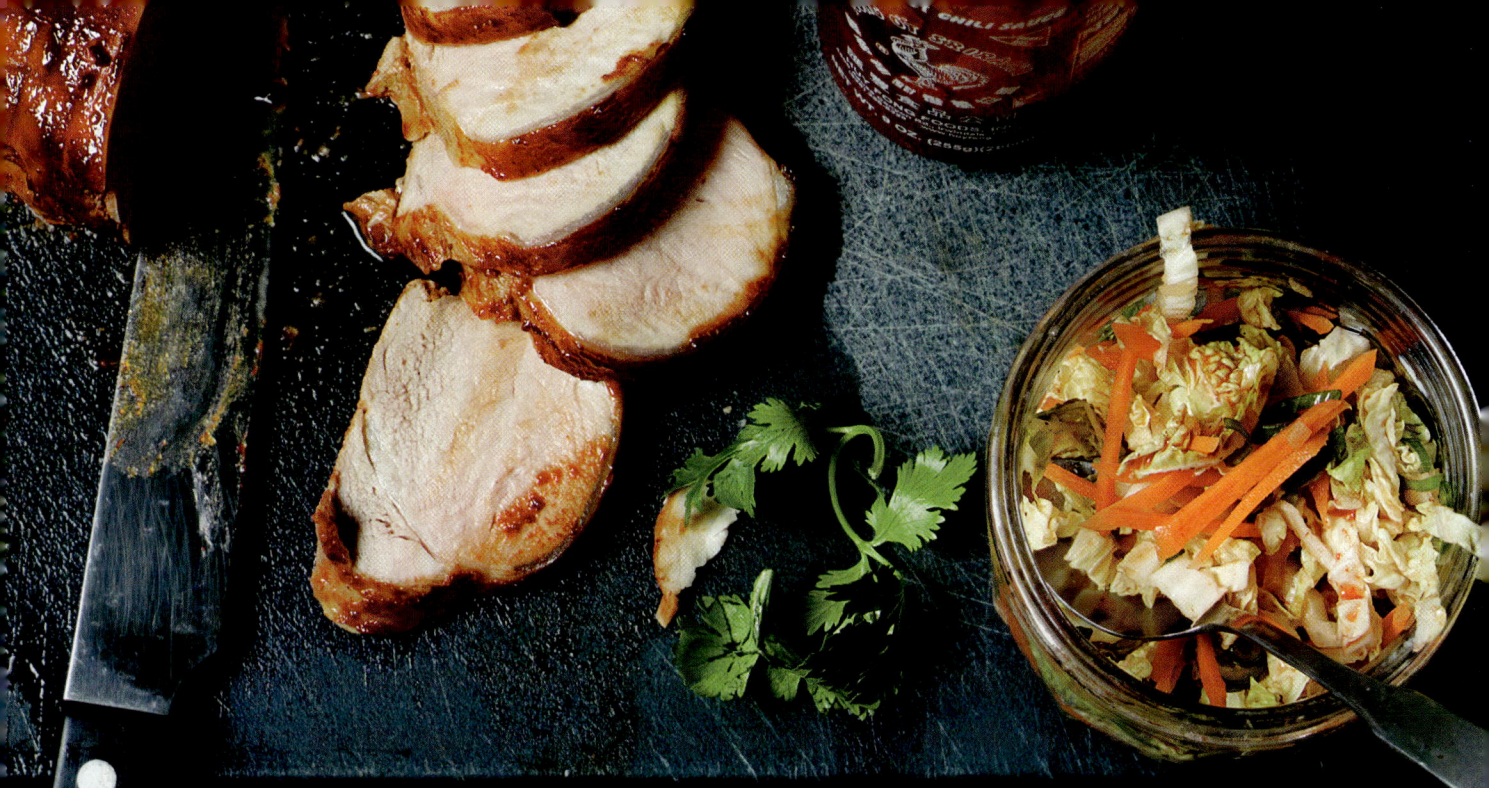

*Barbecue Pork
with Fresh Kimchi*

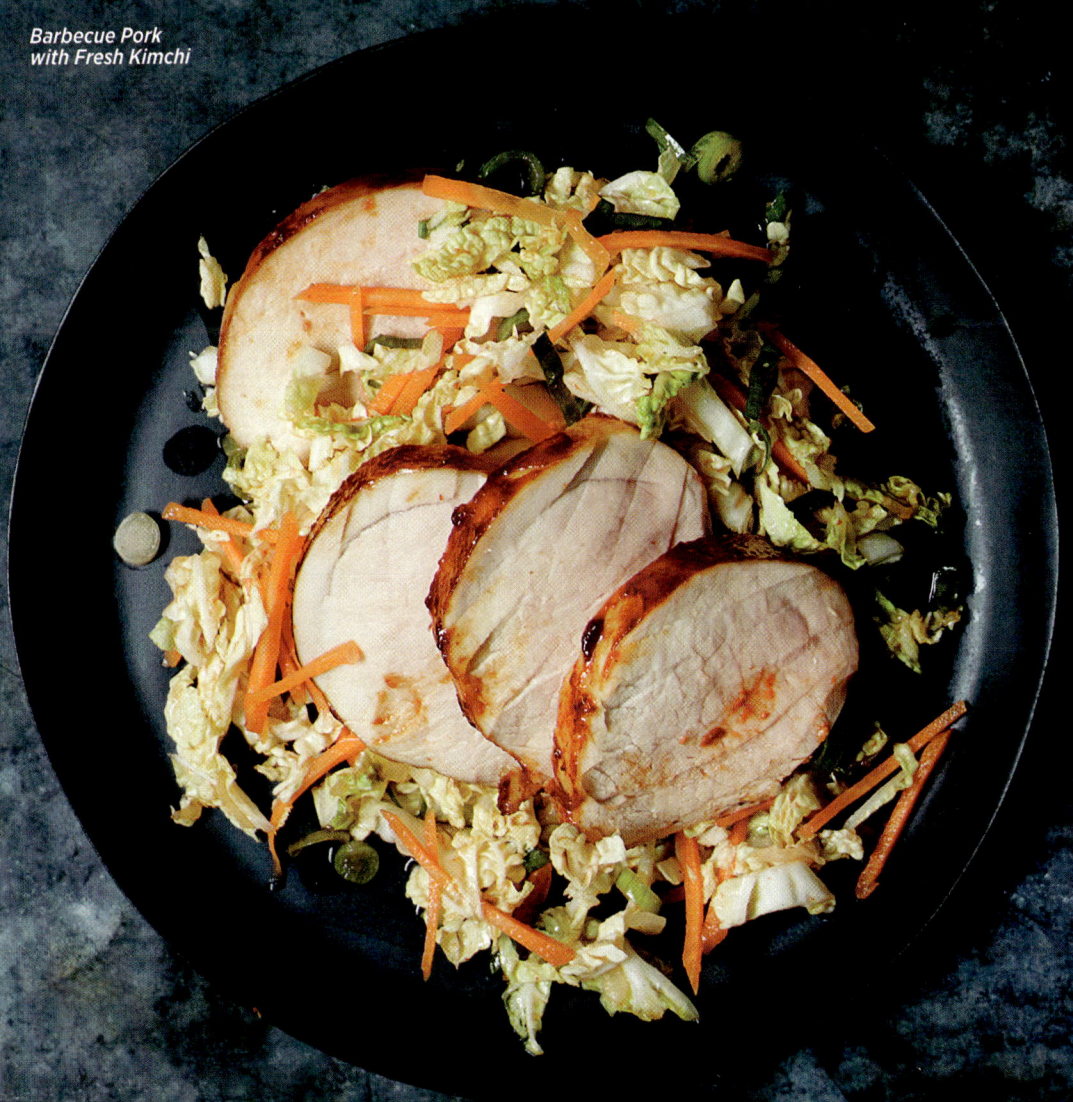

PORK PICCATA WITH GARLICKY SPINACH

SERVES 4

3 tablespoons all-purpose flour

1 teaspoon salt

½ teaspoon black pepper, or to taste

1 pound lean pork tenderloin, trimmed and cut into 16 thin slices

2½ teaspoons olive oil

¾ cup chicken broth

¼ cup lemon juice

2 teaspoons cornstarch

2 teaspoons salted butter

1 tablespoon capers, drained

2 garlic cloves, finely chopped

12 ounces baby spinach

1 Combine flour, ½ teaspoon salt, and ¼ teaspoon pepper on plate; dredge pork in flour, coating both sides and shaking off excess.

2 Heat 2 teaspoons oil in large nonstick skillet over medium-high heat. Add pork (in 2 batches if necessary) and cook just until cooked through and golden, about 1½ minutes per side; set aside on platter and cover to keep warm.

3 Whisk broth, lemon juice, cornstarch, ¼ teaspoon salt, and ⅛ teaspoon pepper together in cup until blended. Pour into same skillet and stir with wooden spoon to scrape up browned bits from bottom of skillet. Simmer until slightly thickened, about 1 minute. Remove skillet from heat; stir in butter until melted. Stir in capers and spoon mixture over pork; cover to keep warm.

4 Heat remaining ½ teaspoon oil in same skillet over medium-high heat. Add garlic and cook, stirring, until fragrant, about 30 seconds. Add spinach to skillet in batches, tossing mixture and adding more spinach as it cooks down; add remaining ¼ teaspoon salt and remaining ⅛ teaspoon pepper. Cook, tossing, until wilted and tender, about 2 minutes more. Serve spinach with pork.

5 SmartPoints value

Per serving (4 slices pork, about 3 tablespoons sauce, and ½ cup spinach): 227 Cal, 8 g Total Fat, 3 g Sat Fat, 930 mg Sod, 11 g Total Carb, 1 g Sugar, 2 g Fib, 28 g Prot.

COOK'S TIP

For some Italian spice with your spinach, add ¼ teaspoon red pepper flakes to the skillet along with the garlic in Step 4.

GRILLED PORK WRAPS WITH PINEAPPLE SLAW

SERVES 4

3 tablespoons lime juice

2 teaspoons olive oil

1 teaspoon dried oregano

½ teaspoon garlic powder

½ teaspoon ground cumin

¾ teaspoon salt

¾ pound lean pork tenderloin, trimmed and cut into ½-inch-thick slices

2 cups packaged coleslaw mix

½ cup diced pineapple

½ cup lightly packed fresh cilantro leaves, coarsely chopped

1 scallion, thinly sliced

4 large whole wheat tortillas

1 Combine 1 tablespoon lime juice, 1 teaspoon oil, oregano, garlic powder, cumin, and ½ teaspoon salt in medium bowl; add pork and toss to coat. Let marinate 15 minutes, or cover and refrigerate up to 2 hours.

2 Meanwhile, combine coleslaw mix, pineapple, cilantro, scallion, remaining 2 tablespoons lime juice, remaining 1 teaspoon oil, and remaining ¼ teaspoon salt in another medium bowl.

3 Spray ridged grill pan with nonstick spray and place over medium-high heat.

4 Place pork in pan; brush with any remaining marinade. Cook pork, turning once, until instant-read thermometer inserted into pork registers 145°F, 6–8 minutes; let stand 3 minutes. Divide pork evenly among tortillas and top each with ½ cup slaw.

6 SmartPoints value

Per serving (1 wrap): 261 Cal, 5 g Total Fat, 1 g Sat Fat, 771 mg Sod, 40 g Total Carb, 5 g Sugar, 5 g Fib, 24 g Prot.

— COOK'S TIP —

If you like, while the pork rests you can grill the tortillas on the hot grill pan until lightly browned on both sides.

Cider-Brined Pork Chops
with Greens and Peas

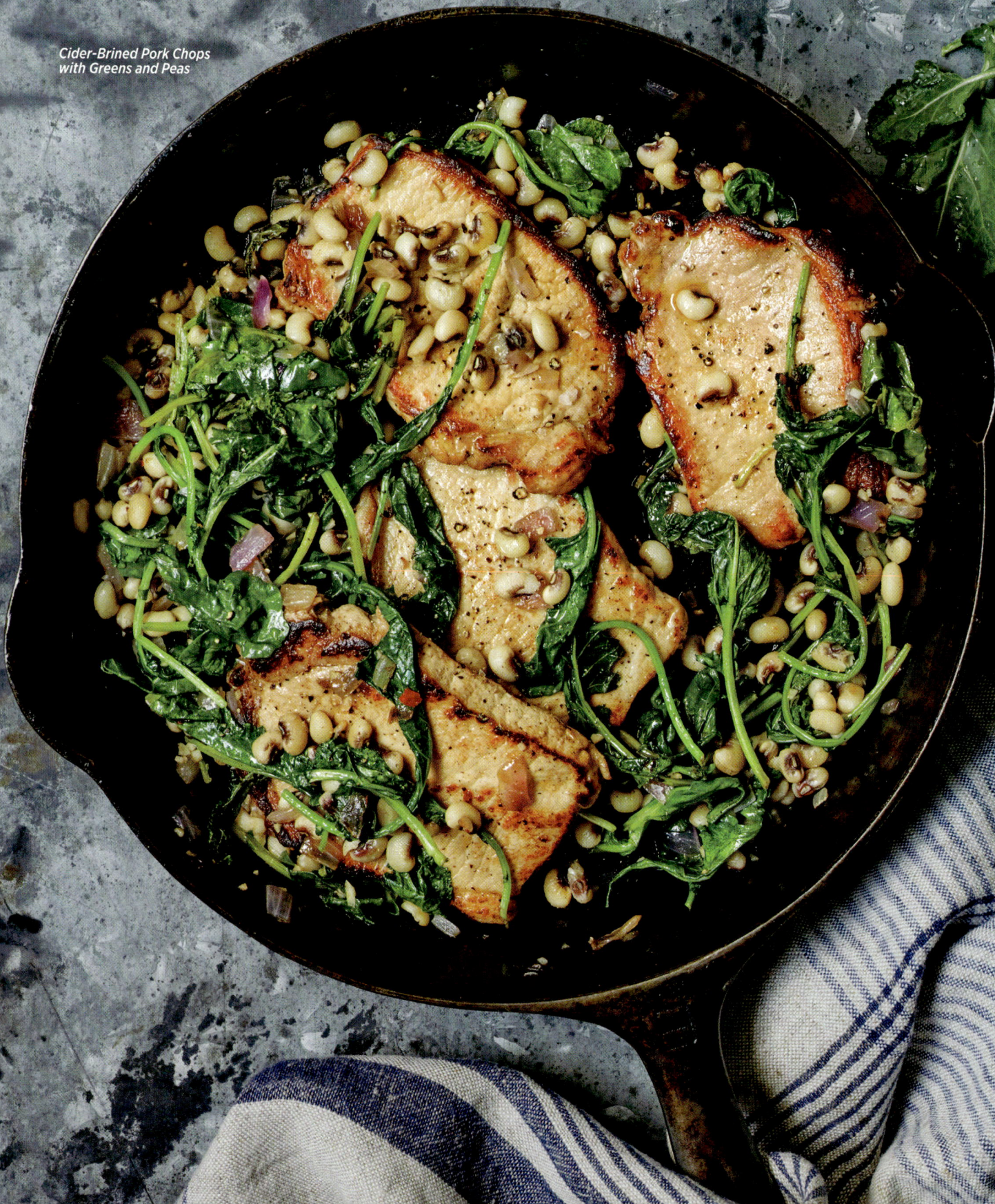

CIDER-BRINED PORK CHOPS WITH GREENS AND PEAS

SERVES 4 ● GLUTEN FREE

1½ cups apple cider

⅔ cup plus 2 tablespoons water

2½ teaspoons kosher salt

3 whole cloves

4 (¼-pound) lean boneless pork loin chops, trimmed

¼ teaspoon black pepper

2 teaspoons canola oil

1 red onion, chopped

1½ cups frozen black-eyed peas, thawed

2 garlic cloves, finely chopped

¼ teaspoon red pepper flakes

1 (5-ounce) container baby kale

1 teaspoon apple cider vinegar

1 Stir cider, ⅔ cup water, 2 teaspoons salt, and cloves together in medium bowl until salt dissolves; add pork chops. Cover and refrigerate 3 hours.

2 Remove pork from brine; pat dry with paper towels and sprinkle with black pepper. Discard brine. Heat 1 teaspoon oil in large skillet over medium-high heat. Add pork and cook until instant-read thermometer inserted into sides of chops registers 145°F, 3–4 minutes per side. Transfer to plate and keep warm.

3 Heat remaining 1 teaspoon oil in skillet over medium-high heat. Add onion and cook, covered, stirring occasionally, until golden, about 2 minutes. Add black-eyed peas, garlic, and red pepper flakes; cook, stirring constantly, until fragrant, about 1 minute. Add kale, remaining 2 tablespoons water, and remaining ½ teaspoon salt; cook, covered, stirring occasionally, just until greens wilt, about 2 minutes. Stir vinegar into greens and serve with pork.

6 SmartPoints value

Per serving (1 pork chop and ½ cup greens mixture): 269 Cal, 9 g Total Fat, 2 g Sat Fat, 561 mg Sod, 19 g Total Carb, 4 g Sugar, 4 g Fib, 26 g Prot.

COOK'S TIP

To thaw the black-eyed peas quickly, rinse them in a colander under hot running water about 1 minute. You can also use canned black-eyed peas in this recipe; they will have a slightly softer texture but will be delicious as well.

THREE-BEAN AND PORK SLOW-COOKER CHILI

SERVES 10 • GLUTEN FREE

1 onion, chopped

2 garlic cloves, finely chopped

1 cup chopped carrots

1 tablespoon chili powder

1 teaspoon dried oregano, crushed

1 small jalapeño pepper, seeded and chopped

½ teaspoon salt

½ teaspoon black pepper

2 pounds lean pork loin, trimmed and cut into 1-inch chunks

1 (15-ounce) can black beans, rinsed and drained

1 (15-ounce) can kidney beans, rinsed and drained

1 (15-ounce) can pinto beans, rinsed and drained

1 cup canned tomato puree

2 (14½-ounce) cans diced tomatoes with green pepper, celery, and onion

1 (6-ounce) can tomato paste

Combine onion, garlic, carrots, chili powder, oregano, jalapeño, salt, and black pepper in 5- to 6-quart slow cooker and stir. Add remaining ingredients and stir again. Cover and cook until pork is very tender, 6–8 hours on Low or 3–4 hours on High.

5 SmartPoints value

Per serving (1 cup): 259 Cal, 3 g Total Fat, 1 g Sat Fat, 929 mg Sod, 31 g Total Carb, 8 g Sugar, 10 g Fib, 28 g Prot.

COOK'S TIP

Serve your chili with a variety of 0 SmartPoints toppings so everyone can customize their own bowl: Chopped cilantro, sliced scallions, sliced radishes, diced tomato, pickled jalapeños, and lime wedges are all excellent.

SPICY SOUTHWEST PORK-AND-LENTIL BURGERS

SERVES 4

¼ cup dry green (French) lentils, picked over and rinsed

¾ pound lean ground pork

1 roasted red pepper (water-packed), drained and minced

1 teaspoon ancho chile powder

2 teaspoons ground cumin

2 teaspoons dried oregano

¾ teaspoon salt, or to taste

4 reduced-calorie sandwich thins

2 tablespoons tomatillo salsa

2 tablespoons light sour cream

1 Cook lentils according to package directions; drain and transfer to large bowl. Coarsely mash with potato masher or fork. Let stand until cool, about 10 minutes.

2 Meanwhile, line bottom of broiler pan with foil. Spray broiler rack with nonstick spray. Preheat broiler.

3 Add pork, roasted pepper, chile powder, cumin, oregano, and salt to lentils; stir until combined. Form mixture into 4 (½-inch-thick) patties. Place patties on broiler pan. Broil 4 inches from heat until instant-read thermometer inserted into side of each burger registers 160°F, about 4 minutes on each side.

4 Place burgers on bottom of sandwich thins, top each with ½ tablespoon salsa and ½ tablespoon sour cream, and cover with tops.

6 SmartPoints value

Per serving (1 burger): 247 Cal, 5 g Total Fat, 2 g Sat Fat, 703 mg Sod, 22 g Total Carb, 1 g Sugar, 8 g Fib, 24 g Prot.

COOK'S TIP

Instead of cooking just a ¼ cup of dry lentils, consider preparing a whole cup for about 3 cups of cooked lentils. You can use ¾ cup in this recipe, then refrigerate the remainder up to 3 days to use in soups and salads.

GARLIC-STUDDED ROAST LEG OF LAMB WITH NEW POTATOES

SERVES 8 • GLUTEN FREE

1 (3-pound) lean boneless leg of lamb, trimmed, rolled, and tied

3 large garlic cloves, thinly sliced crosswise

1½ teaspoons salt

½ teaspoon black pepper

1½ pounds very small new potatoes, halved

1 large red bell pepper, cut into 1-inch strips

1 large yellow bell pepper, cut into 1-inch strips

1 large onion, cut into ¾-inch-thick wedges through root end

1 tablespoon chopped fresh thyme

½ cup dry white wine

1 lemon, cut into wedges

1 Preheat oven to 400°F. Spray rimmed baking sheet with nonstick spray.

2 Make about 20 slits in lamb with tip of long thin knife, each slit about 1 inch deep and ½ inch wide. Insert garlic slices into slits. Rub lamb with ¾ teaspoon salt and ¼ teaspoon black pepper.

3 Toss potatoes, bell peppers, onion, thyme, remaining ¾ teaspoon salt, and remaining ¼ teaspoon black pepper in roasting pan. Spread vegetables out and place lamb in center. Pour wine over vegetables. Roast, stirring vegetables once, until instant-read thermometer inserted into center of lamb registers 145°F for medium and potatoes and vegetables are tender, 1 hour–1 hour 10 minutes. Transfer lamb to cutting board and let stand 10 minutes.

4 Meanwhile, pour off and reserve pan juices. Skim and discard any fat. Cut lamb into 24 slices. Serve lamb with vegetables, pan juices, and lemon wedges.

5 SmartPoints value

Per serving (3 slices lamb, 1 cup vegetables, and ½ tablespoon pan juices): 267 Cal, 5 g Total Fat, 2 g Sat Fat, 553 mg Sod, 18 g Total Carb, 3 g Sugar, 3 g Fib, 32 g Prot.

COOK'S TIP

Steamed asparagus sprinkled with lemon juice and fresh chopped dill is a perfect side dish for this lamb.

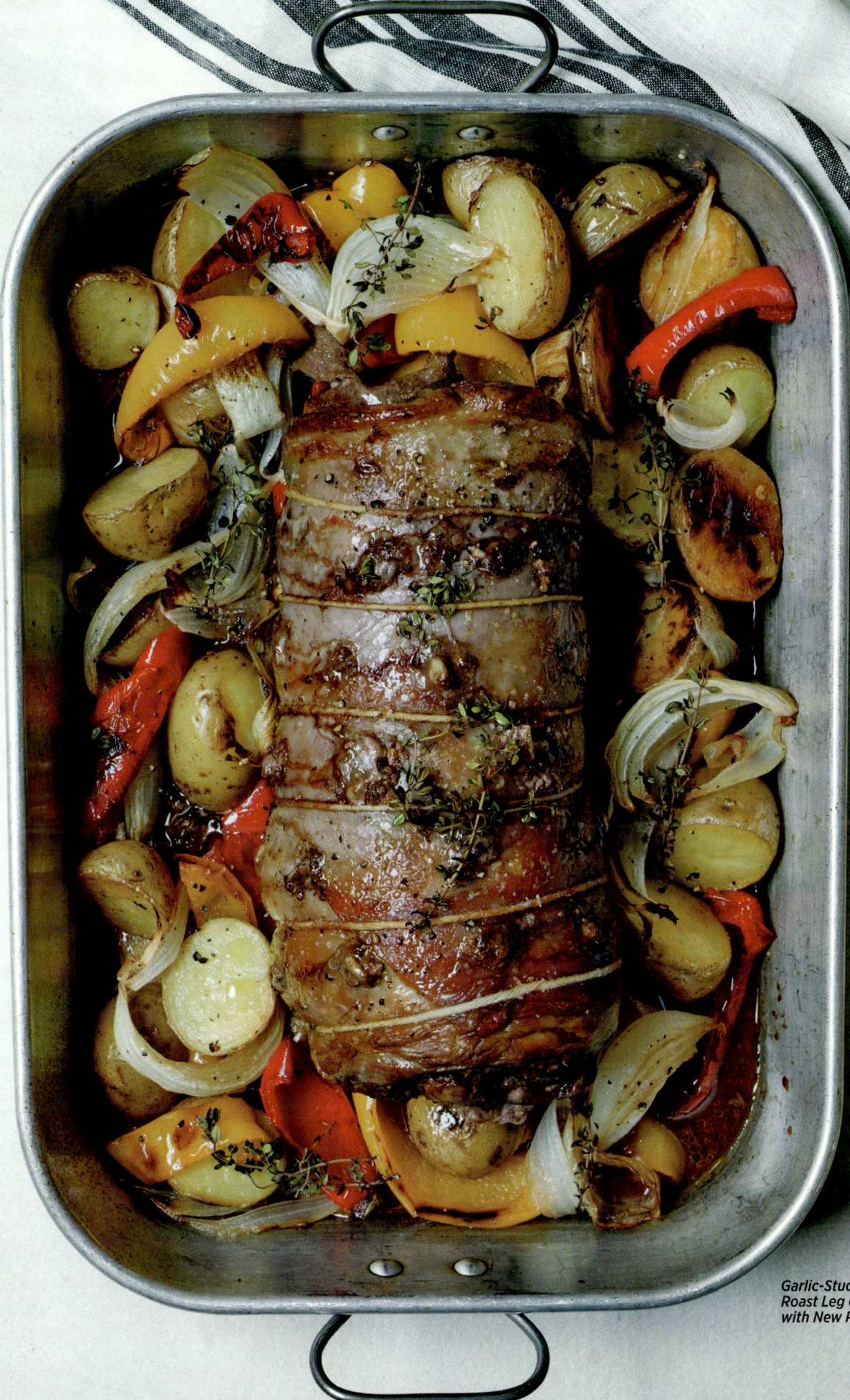

Garlic-Studded Roast Leg of Lamb with New Potatoes

ROSEMARY LAMB CHOPS WITH BALSAMIC SAUCE

SERVES 4 • GLUTEN FREE • UNDER 20 MINUTES

4 (4-ounce) lean bone-in lamb loin chops, about ¾ inch thick, trimmed

1½ teaspoons chopped fresh rosemary

½ teaspoon salt

¼ teaspoon black pepper

1 teaspoon olive oil

2 teaspoons unsalted butter

1 shallot, finely chopped

¾ cup beef broth

2 tablespoons balsamic vinegar

2 teaspoons honey

1 Sprinkle lamb with rosemary, salt, and pepper. Heat oil in large heavy skillet over medium-high heat. Add lamb and cook until browned and instant-read thermometer inserted into center of each chop registers 145°F for medium, 3–4 minutes on each side. Transfer to plate.

2 Melt butter in same skillet over low heat. Add shallot and cook, stirring occasionally, until it begins to soften, about 1 minute. Add broth, vinegar, and honey, scraping up browned bits from bottom of skillet. Bring to boil and cook until slightly thickened, 4–5 minutes. Add lamb and cook, turning once, until heated through, about 1 minute.

5 SmartPoints value®

Per serving (1 lamb chop and 2 teaspoons sauce): 211 Cal, 10 g Total Fat, 4 g Sat Fat, 537 mg Sod, 5 g Total Carb, 4 g Sugar, 0 g Fib, 24 g Prot.

UP THE PROTEIN

White beans are a classic to serve with lamb. A ⅓ cup of small white beans has a SmartPoints value of 2. Mix them with diced red onion and diced bell pepper and sprinkle with red-wine vinegar.

SLOW-COOKER LAMB STEW
WITH LEEKS AND CARROTS

SERVES 6

**2 pounds lean leg of lamb,
trimmed into 1-inch cubes**

¼ cup all-purpose flour

**1½ teaspoons kosher salt,
or to taste**

½ teaspoon black pepper

2 teaspoons olive oil

**3 leeks, halved lengthwise and
cut into 1½-inch pieces,
rinsed well**

1 pound baby-cut carrots, halved

1 cup chicken broth

3 tablespoons Dijon mustard

**2 tablespoons fresh
minced rosemary**

2 garlic cloves, finely chopped

1 Toss lamb with flour, 1 teaspoon salt, and ¼ teaspoon pepper in large bowl. Heat oil in large skillet over medium-high heat. Working in batches, add lamb to skillet and brown on all sides; add to slow cooker.

2 Add leeks and carrots to slow cooker; stir to combine. Whisk broth, mustard, rosemary, and garlic together in medium bowl. Pour over lamb and vegetables; cover and cook on Low until lamb shreds easily with fork, about 6 hours. Stir in remaining ½ teaspoon salt and ¼ teaspoon pepper.

4 SmartPoints value

Per serving (1 cup): 287 Cal, 7 g Total Fat, 2 g Sat Fat, 924 mg Sod, 18 g Total Carb, 5 g Sugar, 3 g Fib, 35 g Prot.

COOK'S TIP

Most slow cookers heat more evenly on Low, and most foods will be tastier with longer cooking. That's why we recommend cooking this stew on Low, but if you're pressed for time you can use the High setting and the stew should be done in 3 to 3½ hours.

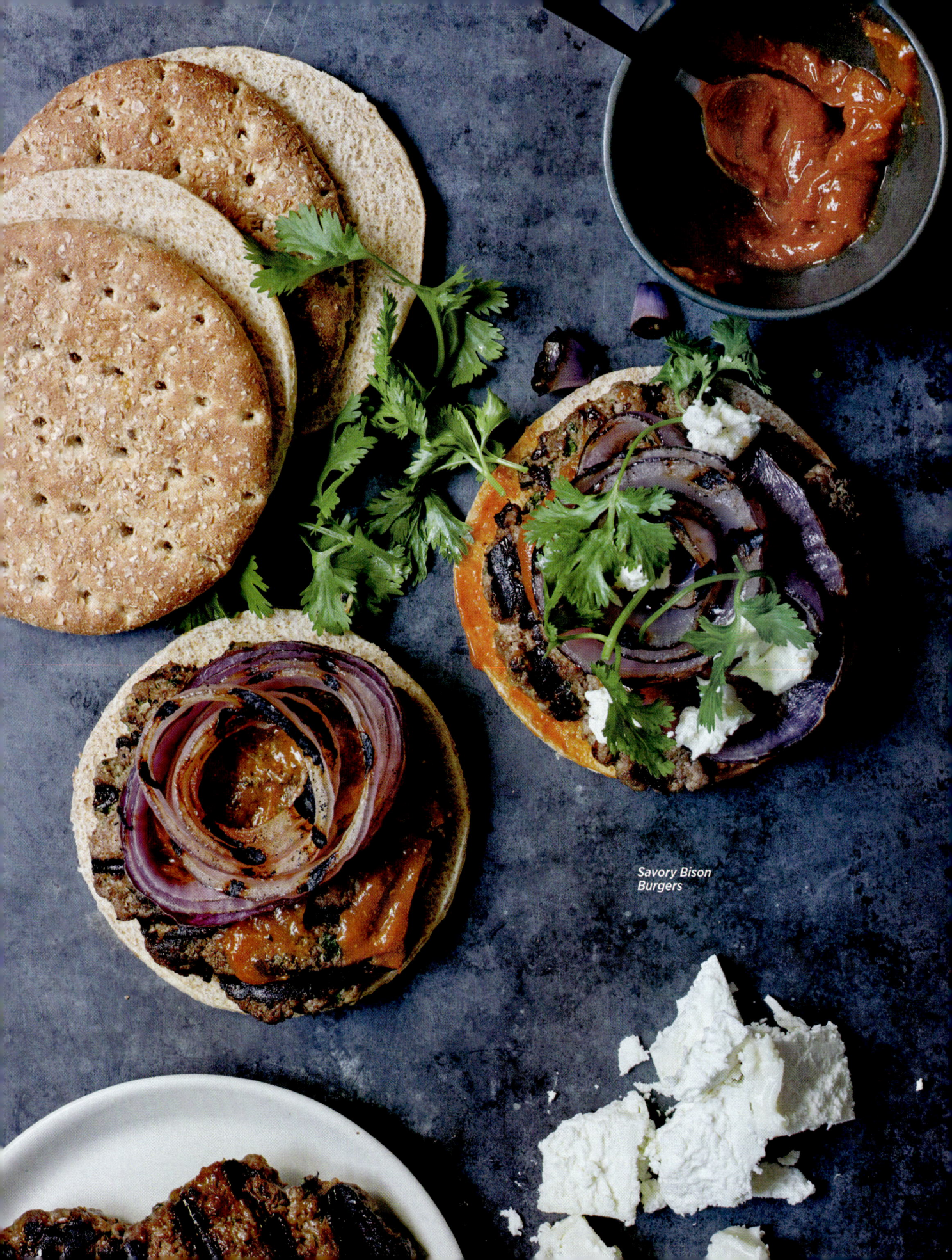

*Savory Bison
Burgers*

SAVORY BISON BURGERS

SERVES 4

1 pound ground lean bison (buffalo) meat

¼ cup finely chopped fresh cilantro

2 garlic cloves, crushed through garlic press

1 teaspoon ground cumin

¼ teaspoon black pepper

½ teaspoon salt

1 red onion, cut into ½-inch rounds

¼ cup ketchup

1 teaspoon curry powder

4 whole wheat sandwich thins, split

4 tablespoons crumbled low-fat goat cheese

Fresh cilantro sprigs

1 Preheat grill to medium-high or prepare medium-high fire, or heat grill pan over medium-high heat.

2 Place bison, cilantro, garlic, cumin, and pepper in large bowl; mix gently just until combined. With damp hands, shape bison mixture into 4 (½-inch-thick) patties. Sprinkle salt on both sides of patties and spray both sides with nonstick spray.

3 Place patties and onion on grill rack; grill until instant-read thermometer inserted into side of patties registers 160°F and onions are browned and tender, 3–4 minutes per side.

4 Stir ketchup and curry powder together in small bowl. Layer bottom of each sandwich thin with 1 burger, curry-ketchup, onion, goat cheese, and cilantro sprigs. Top with remaining bread.

5 SmartPoints value

Per serving (1 burger): 225 Cal, 5 g Total Fat, 2 g Sat Fat, 566 mg Sod, 17 g Total Carb, 5 g Sugar, 3 g Fib, 29 g Prot.

COOK'S TIP

If you prefer toasted sandwich thins, place the split thins cut side down on the grill rack about 1 minute before burgers are done, or toast them under the broiler.

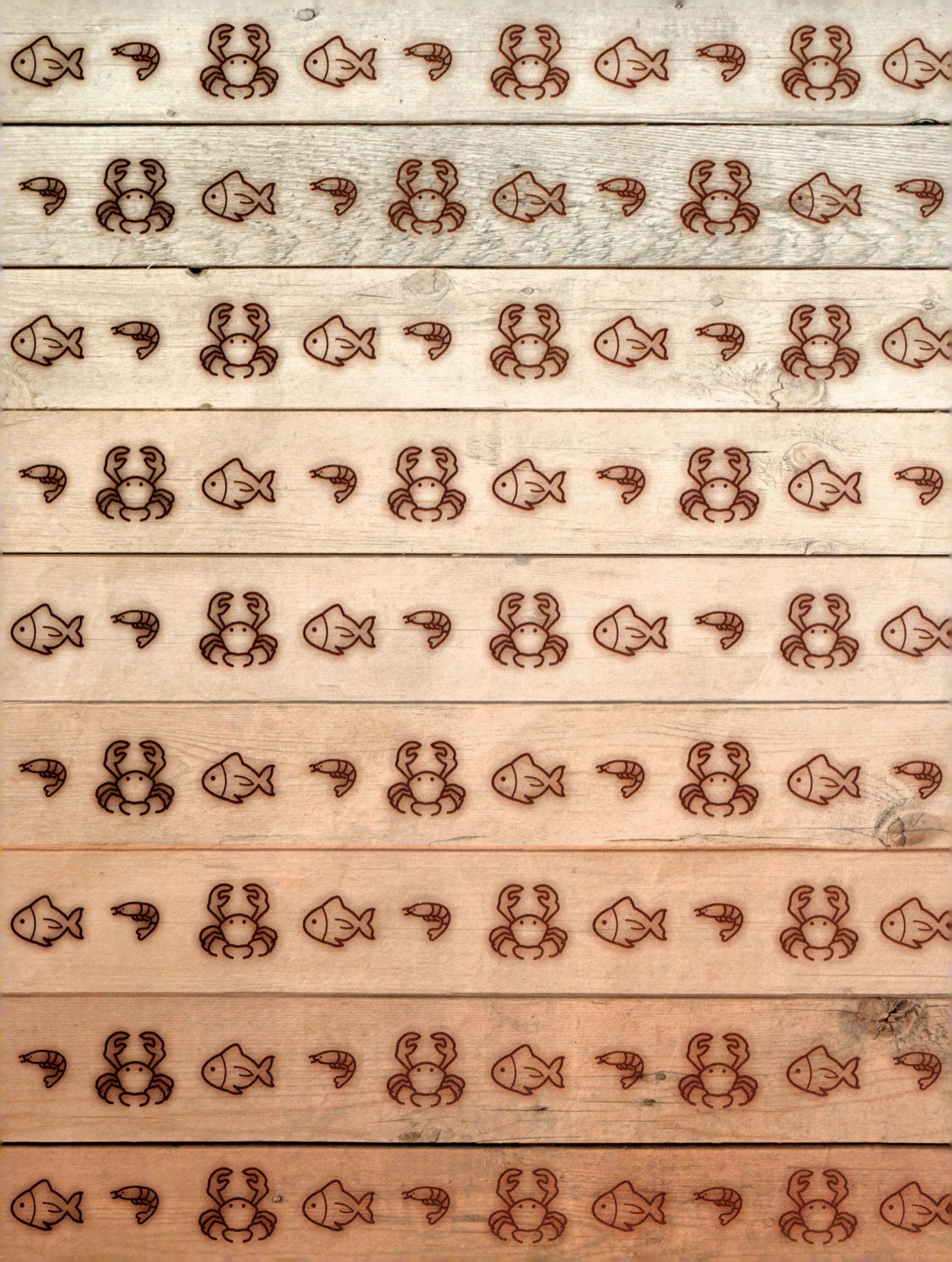

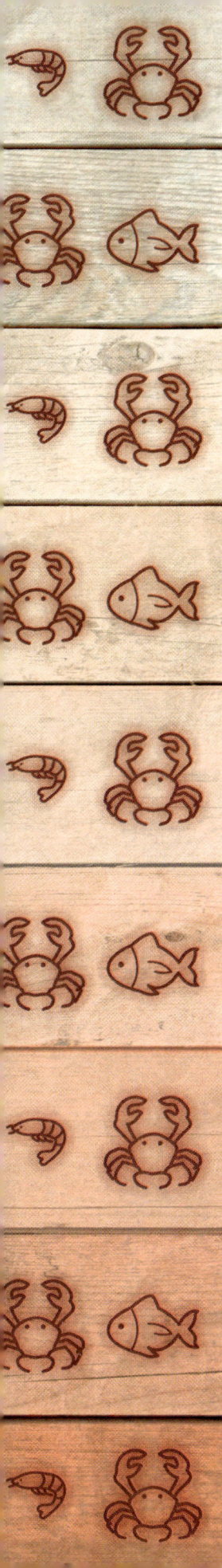

CHAPTER 4

FISH
SHRIMP
SCALLOPS
CRAB
MUSSELS
CLAMS
& LOBSTER

PHYLLO-WRAPPED SALMON FILLET

SERVES 8

1 tablespoon olive oil

2 shallots, minced

2 onions, chopped

1 pound mushrooms, sliced

2 teaspoons salt

½ teaspoon black pepper

2 teaspoons finely grated lemon zest

1 tablespoon lemon juice

6 sheets phyllo, thawed if frozen

2 pounds skinless salmon fillet, in one piece, any pin bones removed

1 Preheat oven to 425°F.

2 Heat oil in large nonstick skillet over medium heat. Add shallots and onions. Cook, stirring occasionally, until golden, about 5 minutes. Add mushrooms, 1 teaspoon salt, and ¼ teaspoon pepper. Cook until almost dry, stirring occasionally, about 10 minutes. Stir in lemon zest and lemon juice.

3 Line baking sheet with parchment paper or spray with nonstick spray. Lightly spray one sheet phyllo with nonstick spray and place on baking sheet. Cover with second sheet and spray with nonstick spray. Repeat with third sheet. Place salmon on phyllo and sprinkle with remaining 1 teaspoon salt and ¼ teaspoon pepper. Place mushroom mixture on top of fish. Wrap phyllo over fish, envelope-style. Repeat spraying and layering with 3 more sheets of phyllo. Wrap around fish to cover completely.

4 Bake fish until phyllo crisps and browns and fish inside is cooked through but still slightly pink at center, about 20 minutes. Slice into 8 equal pieces.

7 SmartPoints value

Per serving (1 slice): 294 Cal, 15 g Total Fat, 3 g Sat Fat, 722 mg Sod, 13 g Total Carb, 3 g Sugar, 2 g Fib, 26 g Prot.

COOK'S TIP

To remove pin bones from a salmon fillet, use clean needlenose pliers or clean tweezers.

COCONUT-CURRY SALMON STIR-FRY

SERVES 4 • UNDER 20 MINUTES

2 teaspoons coconut oil

2 garlic cloves, finely chopped

2 teaspoons minced peeled fresh ginger

2 jalapeño peppers, seeded and finely chopped, or to taste

¼ cup green curry paste

¾ pound skinless wild salmon fillet, cut into ¾-inch cubes

2 red bell peppers, thinly sliced

2 yellow bell peppers, thinly sliced

3 cups sugar snap peas, trimmed

½ cup light (low-fat) coconut milk

½ cup chicken broth

1 teaspoon salt

⅓ cup chopped fresh cilantro

⅓ cup chopped scallions

2 tablespoons lime juice

¼ cup toasted coconut chips

1 Heat coconut oil in large skillet or wok over medium heat. Add garlic, ginger, and jalapeño and stir-fry until fragrant, 2–3 minutes.

2 Add curry paste, salmon, bell peppers, and snap peas to pan and cook, stirring frequently, until salmon browns, about 5 minutes. Stir in coconut milk, broth, and salt and bring to boil. Simmer until salmon is cooked through and vegetables are crisp-tender, about 5 minutes.

3 Stir in cilantro, scallions, and lime juice. Sprinkle with coconut chips.

8 SmartPoints value

Per serving (2 cups stir-fry and 1 tablespoon coconut chips): 319 Cal, 15 g Total Fat, 10 g Sat Fat, 764 mg Sod, 26 g Total Carb, 6 g Sugar, 6 g Fib, 23 g Prot.

UP THE PROTEIN

Love seafood? Add ½ pound of either medium peeled and deveined shrimp or bay scallops along with the coconut in Step 2 and increase the per-serving SmartPoints value by 1.

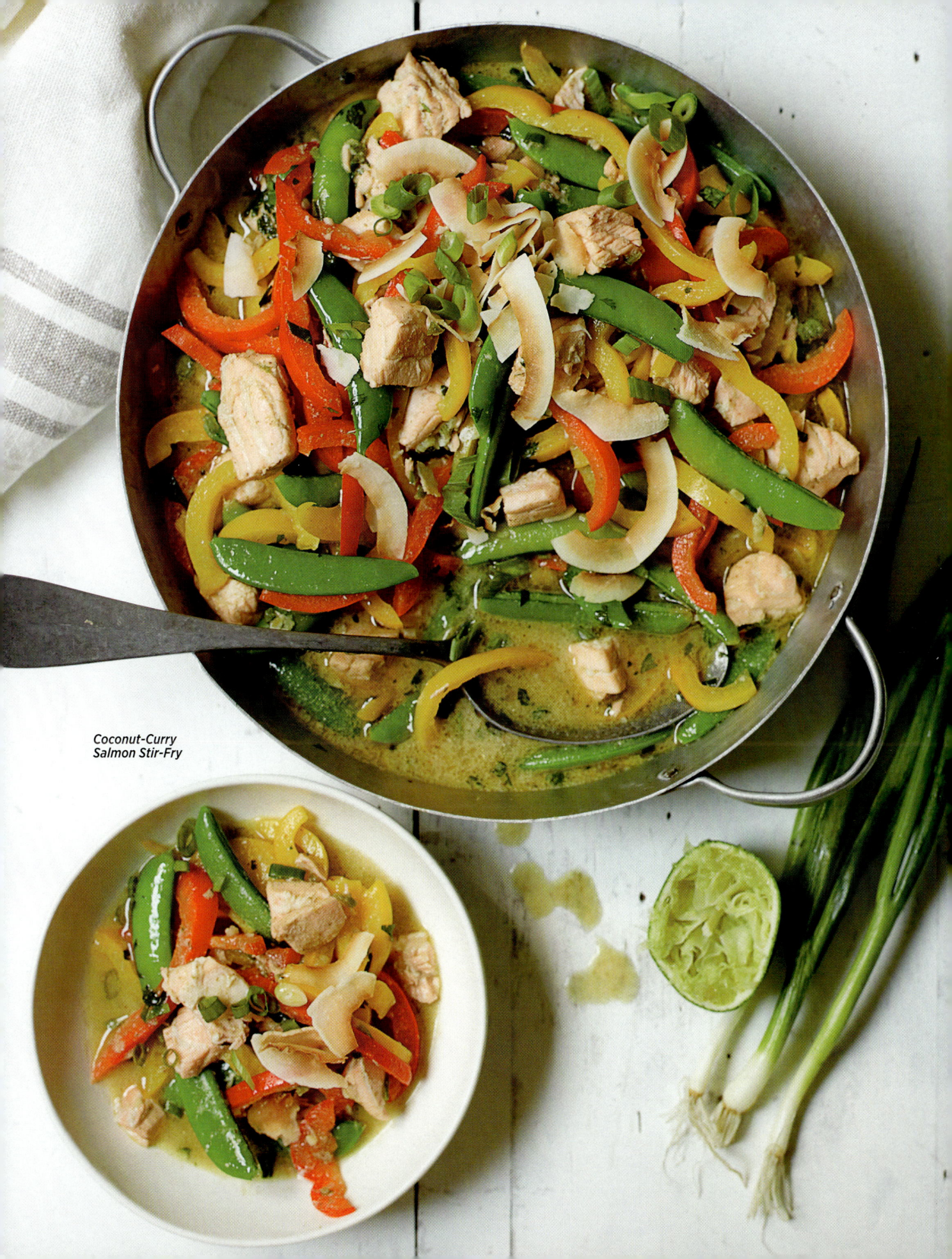

Coconut-Curry Salmon Stir-Fry

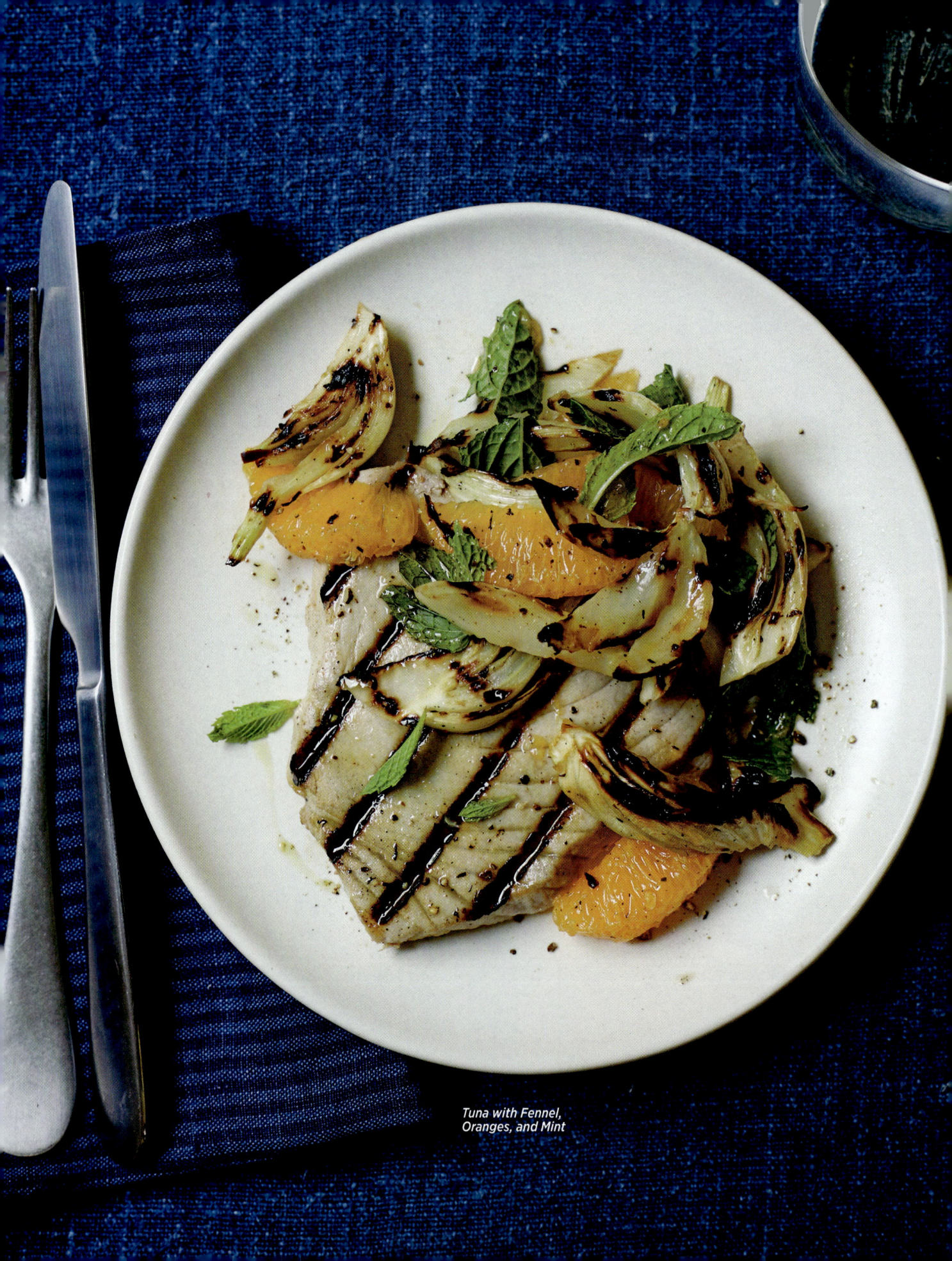

Tuna with Fennel, Oranges, and Mint

TUNA WITH FENNEL, ORANGES, AND MINT

SERVES 4 ● GLUTEN FREE

1 large fennel bulb, trimmed and sliced

4 (5-ounce) tuna steaks

½ teaspoon salt

2 navel oranges, peeled and cut into segments

½ cup fresh mint leaves, torn

2 tablespoons red-wine vinegar

2 teaspoons olive oil

⅛ teaspoon red pepper flakes

1 Spray ridged grill pan with nonstick spray and set over medium heat until hot. Add fennel and grill, turning occasionally, until tender and lightly browned, about 8 minutes. Transfer fennel to cutting board.

2 Sprinkle tuna with ¼ teaspoon salt. Spray same grill pan with nonstick spray. Place tuna on grill pan and grill about 2 minutes on each side for medium.

3 Meanwhile, stir fennel, orange segments, mint, vinegar, oil, red pepper flakes, and remaining ¼ teaspoon salt together in large bowl. Top tuna evenly with fennel mixture.

2 SmartPoints value

Per serving (1 tuna steak with ¾ cup salad): 228 Cal, 4 g Total Fat, 1 g Sat Fat, 375 mg Sod, 13 g Total Carb, 6 g Sugar, 4 g Fib, 35 g Prot.

UP THE PROTEIN

Oranges, fennel, and almonds are a classic Mediterranean combination. You can enjoy it by sprinkling each serving of this savory recipe with 1 tablespoon toasted sliced almonds for an additional 1 SmartPoints value.

THAI TUNA BURGERS

SERVES 4

1 pound skinless tuna steak, cut into chunks

2 tablespoons finely chopped fresh cilantro

1 tablespoon grated peeled fresh ginger

1 tablespoon very finely chopped lemongrass

2 garlic cloves, finely chopped

2 teaspoons Asian fish sauce

1 tablespoon reduced-calorie mayonnaise

¼ teaspoon Sriracha or other hot sauce, or to taste

4 light hamburger rolls or buns, toasted

1 Place tuna in food processor and pulse just until finely chopped, 4 to 5 times. Combine tuna, cilantro, ginger, lemongrass, garlic, and fish sauce in large bowl; divide mixture into 4 equal balls and gently press each ball into patty about 3½ inches in diameter.

2 Combine mayonnaise and Sriracha in small bowl.

3 Coat ridged grill pan with nonstick spray and place over medium-high heat. Cook burgers just until pink in center, about 3 minutes per side. Spread buns with mayonnaise and place 1 burger inside each bun.

4 SmartPoints value

Per serving (1 burger): 225 Cal, 3 g Total Fat, 1 g Sat Fat, 489 mg Sod, 20 g Total Carb, 2 g Sugar, 3 g Fib, 30 g Prot.

COOK'S TIP

Lemongrass stalks are very fibrous, so be sure to only use the inner core of the stalk and mince it. You can also use 1 teaspoon grated lemon zest in its place.

BROILED COD WITH WHITE BEAN AND OLIVE SALAD

SERVES 4 ● GLUTEN FREE ● UNDER 20 MINUTES

1 (15-ounce) can cannellini (white kidney) beans, rinsed and drained

1 cup drained water-packed roasted red bell peppers, chopped

½ small red onion, chopped

½ cup chopped fresh parsley

¼ cup Kalamata olives, pitted and chopped

2 tablespoons finely crumbled feta

1½ teaspoons olive oil

½ teaspoon salt

¼ teaspoon black pepper

4 (5-ounce) skinless cod fillets

Lemon wedges

1 To make salad, stir beans, roasted peppers, onion, parsley, olives, feta, oil, ¼ teaspoon salt, and ⅛ teaspoon black pepper together in large bowl.

2 Spray broiler rack with nonstick spray; preheat broiler. Sprinkle cod fillets with remaining ¼ teaspoon salt and ⅛ teaspoon pepper. Place cod on broiler rack and broil 5 inches from heat just until cod is opaque throughout, about 7 minutes. Serve cod with salad and lemon wedges.

6 SmartPoints value

Per serving (1 fillet and ¾ cup salad): 306 Cal, 5 g Total Fat, 1 g Sat Fat, 1,055 mg Sod, 36 g Total Carb, 5 g Sugar, 7 g Fib, 31 g Prot.

COOK'S TIP

You can make this salad more colorful and filling by adding 1 cup of halved yellow grape tomatoes.

CANTONESE-STYLE WHOLE BRANZINO

SERVES 4 • UNDER 20 MINUTES

¼ **cup dry sherry**

2 **tablespoons reduced-sodium soy sauce**

1 **tablespoon finely chopped pickled ginger**

1 **tablespoon rice vinegar**

2 **garlic cloves, minced**

1 **teaspoon Asian (dark) sesame oil**

Pinch red pepper flakes

2 **(1-pound) whole branzino or striped bass, cleaned and scaled**

1 **bunch scallions, cut diagonally into 2-inch pieces**

1 **teaspoon toasted sesame seeds (optional)**

1 Combine sherry, soy sauce, ginger, vinegar, garlic, oil, and red pepper flakes in small bowl; set aside.

2 Rinse branzino under cold running water and pat dry with paper towels. With sharp knife, make 3 parallel diagonal slashes, down to bone, on each side of fish. Place fish side by side in microwavable baking dish, preferably with lid; tuck tails under or cut tails off if fish does not fit. Pour sherry mixture evenly over fish. Scatter scallions evenly over top. Partially cover dish with lid or cover with wax paper. Microwave on High until fish is just opaque in center, about 6 minutes.

3 Transfer fish to serving platter. Top with scallions, sauce, and sesame seeds (if using). Remove skin before eating.

3 SmartPoints value

Per serving (½ fish and 2 tablespoons scallions, sesame seeds, and sauce): 163 Cal, 4 g Total Fat, 1 g Sat Fat, 372 mg Sod, 5 g Total Carb, 1 g Sugar, 1 g Fib, 22 g Prot.

COOK'S TIP

The microwave is a particularly easy way to cook a whole fish, and if you've never tried it, you should. Microwaving typically leaves the flesh evenly cooked and moist, and you'll have little cleanup and almost no lingering fish odor in your kitchen.

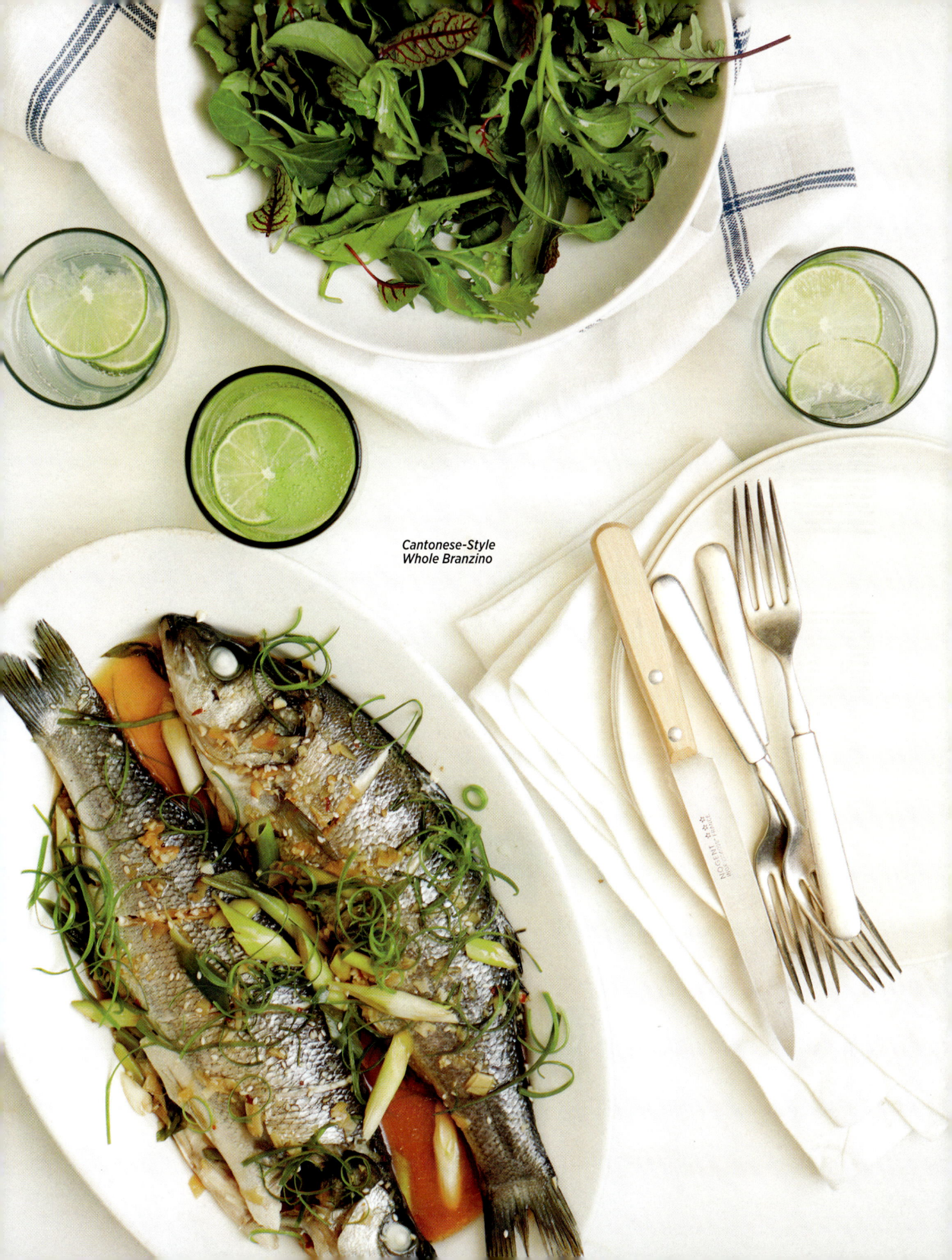

*Cantonese-Style
Whole Branzino*

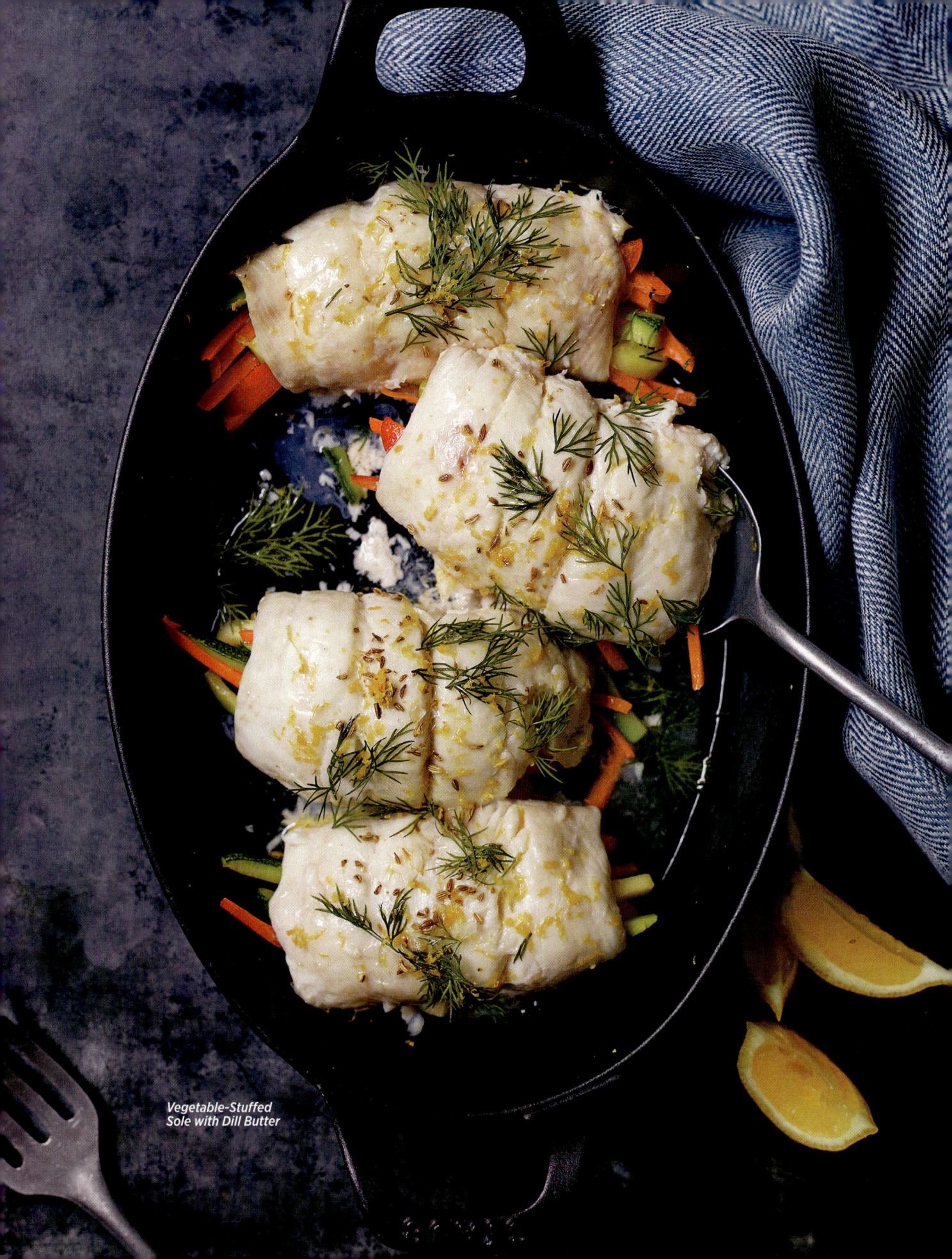

*Vegetable-Stuffed
Sole with Dill Butter*

VEGETABLE-STUFFED SOLE WITH DILL BUTTER

SERVES 4 • GLUTEN FREE

1 large carrot, cut into matchstick strips

½ red bell pepper, cut into matchstick strips

1 zucchini, cut into matchstick strips

2 tablespoons water

¾ teaspoon salt

4 (5-ounce) sole fillets

¼ teaspoon black pepper

4 teaspoons unsalted butter, softened

1 teaspoon grated lemon zest

¼ teaspoon fennel seeds, crushed

2 tablespoons chopped fresh dill

Lemon wedges

1 Preheat oven to 400°F. Spray 7 x 11-inch baking dish with nonstick spray.

2 Combine carrot, bell pepper, zucchini, water, and ¼ teaspoon salt in medium microwavable dish. Cover and microwave on High until crisp-tender, about 3 minutes. Drain and rinse under cold water.

3 Place sole fillets on work surface and sprinkle on all sides with remaining ½ teaspoon salt and black pepper. Place about ½ cup vegetable mixture at wide end of skin side of each fillet. Roll up jelly-roll style and place seam side down in baking dish. Cover dish with foil and bake until sole is just opaque in center, 12–15 minutes.

4 Meanwhile, stir butter, lemon zest, and fennel seeds together in small bowl. Dot evenly over fillets and sprinkle with dill. Serve with lemon wedges.

3 SmartPoints value

Per serving (1 rolled fillet): 185 Cal, 6 g Total Fat, 3 g Sat Fat, 569 mg Sod, 5 g Total Carb, 3 g Sugar, 2 g Fib, 28 g Prot.

COOK'S TIP

You can substitute any thin, mild white fish fillet, such as flounder or fluke, for the sole in this recipe.

STEAMED SOLE AND BROCCOLI WITH BLACK BEAN SAUCE

SERVES 4 • UNDER 20 MINUTES

1 pound fresh broccoli florets (about 5 cups)

1 cup water

4 (5-ounce) sole fillets

1½ teaspoons Asian (dark) sesame oil

3 scallions, chopped

⅓ cup reduced-sodium chicken broth

2 tablespoons rice vinegar

1 tablespoon reduced-sodium soy sauce

2 teaspoons black bean sauce

2 teaspoons minced peeled fresh ginger

1 garlic clove, minced

1 teaspoon cornstarch

1 Combine broccoli and water in 10-inch skillet, spreading broccoli in even layer.

2 Spray bottom of steamer basket with nonstick spray. Brush sole fillets with 1 teaspoon oil, sprinkle one side with scallions, and fold each fillet in half lengthwise. Place in steamer basket and set basket in skillet. Cover and bring to boil. Reduce heat and simmer until broccoli is tender and sole is just opaque throughout, 6–8 minutes.

3 Meanwhile, whisk broth, vinegar, soy sauce, black bean sauce, ginger, garlic, cornstarch, and remaining ½ teaspoon oil together in small saucepan until smooth. Set over medium-high heat and cook, stirring often, until mixture comes to boil and thickens, about 2 minutes.

4 Place 1 fillet on each of 4 plates. Remove steamer basket from skillet and drain broccoli. Divide broccoli evenly among plates; drizzle sauce evenly over sole and vegetables.

2 SmartPoints value

Per serving (1 fillet, ¾ cup broccoli, and scant 2 tablespoons sauce): 199 Cal, 4 g Total Fat, 1 g Sat Fat, 376 mg Sod, 10 g Total Carb, 2 g Sugar, 3 g Fib, 31 g Prot.

COOK'S TIP

To complete the meal, serve the fish and broccoli with brown rice; ½ cup cooked brown rice for each serving will increase the SmartPoints by 4.

CLASSIC PAN-FRIED FLOUNDER

SERVES 4 • UNDER 20 MINUTES

¼ cup yellow cornmeal

2 tablespoons grated Parmesan

1 tablespoon finely chopped fresh thyme or 1 teaspoon dried

½ teaspoon salt, or to taste

½ teaspoon black pepper

1 large egg white

4 (¼-pound) skinless flounder fillets, patted dry

1 tablespoon Dijon mustard

1 tablespoon canola oil or olive oil

4 lemon wedges

1 Combine cornmeal, Parmesan, thyme, salt, and pepper on wax paper. Whisk egg white in wide flat bowl until it forms soft peaks.

2 Place flounder fillets on plate and coat both sides with mustard. Dip fillets into egg white and dredge in cornmeal mixture, coating both sides.

3 Spray large skillet with nonstick spray and set over medium-high heat; add oil and heat until very hot. Add fillets to skillet; cook until undersides are browned, 2–3 minutes. Turn fillets and cook until browned on other side and just opaque throughout, 2–3 minutes longer, lowering heat if fish browns too quickly. Serve fillets with lemon wedges.

4 SmartPoints value

Per serving (1 fillet): 195 Cal, 6 g Total Fat, 1 g Sat Fat, 540 mg Sod, 10 g Total Carb, 1 g Sugar, 1 g Fib, 24 g Prot.

COOK'S TIP

Thin, tender flounder fillets are a classic for pan-searing, but sole, tilapia, or catfish can be substituted. Fish cooks most evenly and flips more easily if your skillet is not overcrowded; if necessary, cook the fish in two batches, using half the amount of oil in each batch.

GRILLED MAHIMAHI WITH LEMON-HERB AÏOLI

SERVES 4 • GLUTEN FREE • UNDER 20 MINUTES

4 (6-ounce) skinless mahimahi fillets

1 teaspoon olive oil

¼ teaspoon salt, or to taste

⅛ teaspoon black pepper, or to taste

2 tablespoons reduced-fat mayonnaise

1 tablespoon chopped fresh chives

1 tablespoon water

1 teaspoon chopped fresh tarragon

½ teaspoon finely grated lemon zest

½ teaspoon lemon juice

¼ teaspoon minced garlic

1 Preheat outdoor grill to medium-high or place ridged grill pan over medium-high heat.

2 Brush fillets with oil and sprinkle with salt and pepper. Stir mayonnaise, chives, water, tarragon, lemon zest, lemon juice, and garlic together in small bowl; set aside.

3 Grill fillets, turning once, just until cooked through, 8–10 minutes. Serve drizzled with sauce.

3 SmartPoints value

Per serving (1 fillet and 1 scant tablespoon sauce): 178 Cal, 5 g Total Fat, 1 g Sat Fat, 347 mg Sod, 1 g Total Carb, 0 g Sugar, 0 g Fib, 31 g Prot.

COOK'S TIP

Fish has a reputation for sticking on the grill, but there are things you can do to prevent that. Most important, make sure your grill grate is impeccably clean: Rub it vigorously with a wire brush to remove any debris or corrosion before heating the grill.

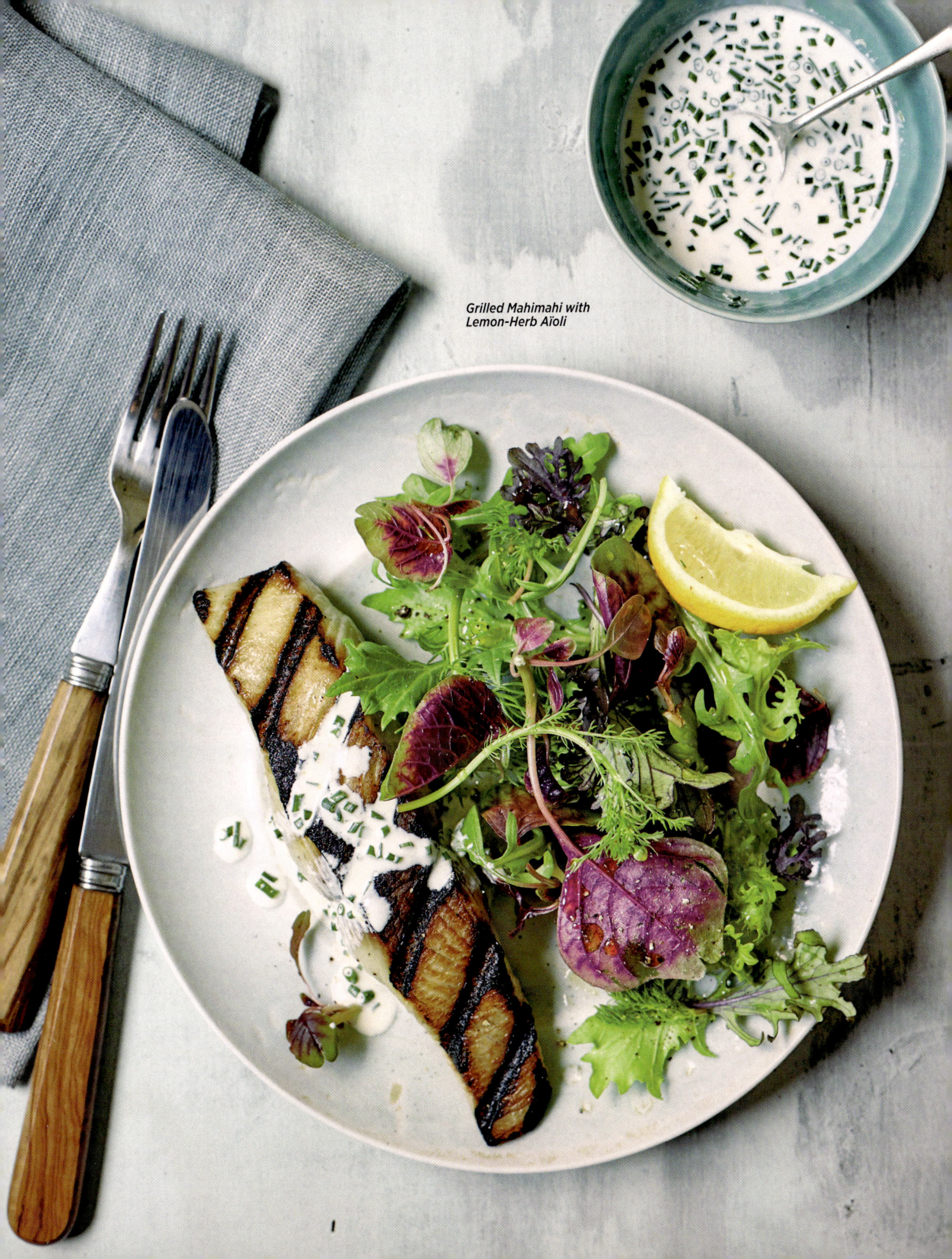

Grilled Mahimahi with Lemon-Herb Aïoli

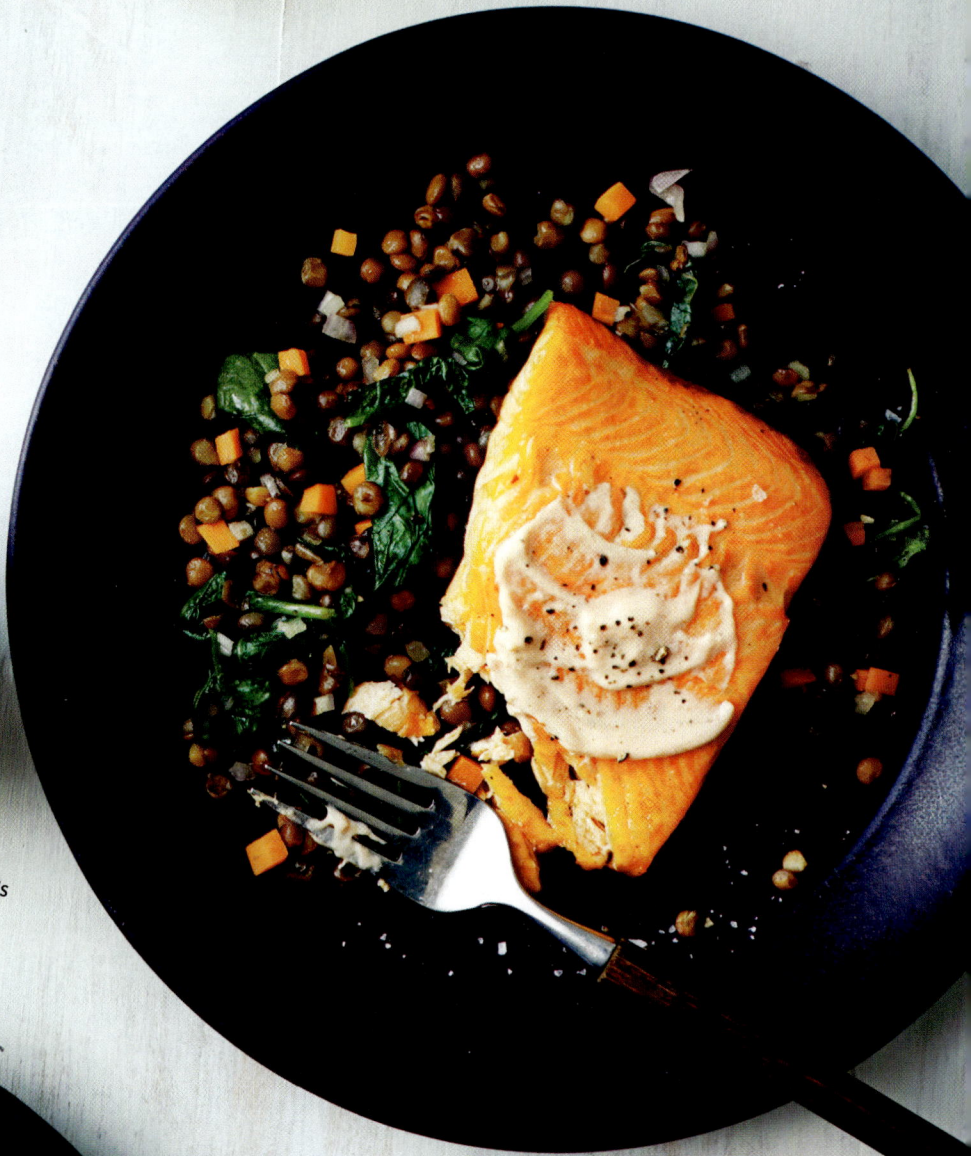

*Arctic Char with Lentils
and Spinach*

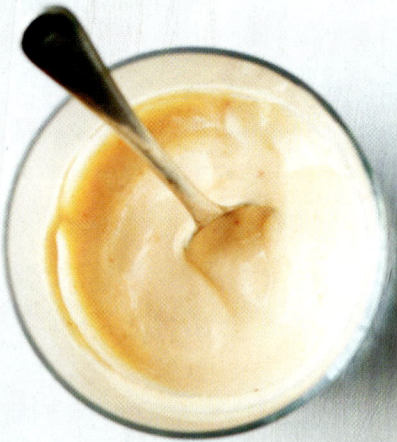

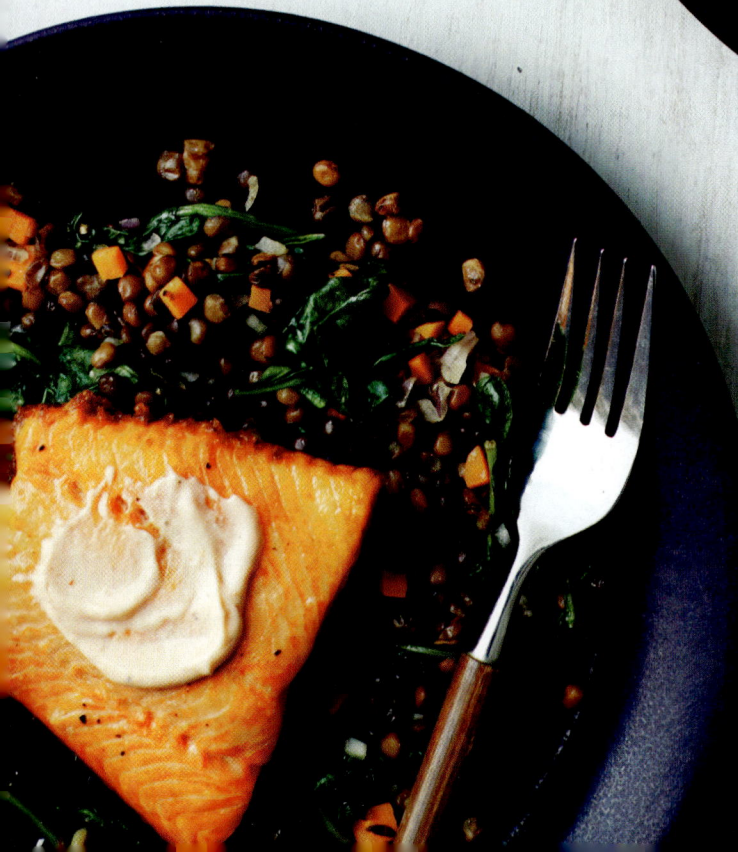

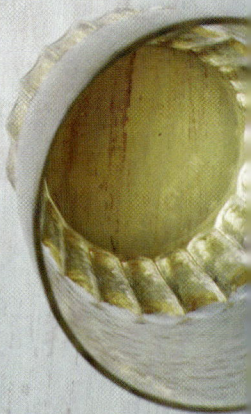

ARCTIC CHAR WITH LENTILS AND SPINACH

SERVES 4 • GLUTEN FREE

2 carrots, finely diced

2 tablespoons water

2 teaspoons olive oil

1 tablespoon finely chopped shallot

2½ cups cooked lentils

1 (6-ounce) bag baby spinach

¼ cup light sour cream

½ teaspoon Sriracha or other hot sauce

Pinch plus ¼ teaspoon salt

4 (¼-pound) skinless arctic char fillets

⅛ teaspoon black pepper

1 Preheat broiler. Line broiler pan with foil and spay with nonstick spray.

2 Mix carrots and water in large microwavable bowl. Cover with plastic wrap, vent one side, and microwave on High until carrots are tender, 5–6 minutes. Drain; stir in oil, shallot, and lentils. Top mixture with spinach. Cover and microwave on High until spinach wilts and lentils are hot, 3–4 minutes. Stir.

3 Meanwhile, mix sour cream, Sriracha, and pinch salt in small bowl. Place fillets on boiler pan; sprinkle with remaining ¼ teaspoon salt and pepper. Broil 5 inches from heat until opaque in center, 4–5 minutes. Serve with lentils and sauce.

7 SmartPoints value

Per serving (1 fillet, ¾ cup lentil mixture, and 1 tablespoon sauce): 322 Cal, 7 g Total Fat, 2 g Sat Fat, 295 mg Sod, 31 g Total Carb, 4 g Sugar, 12 g Fib, 35 g Prot.

COOK'S TIP

Use green, brown, or black lentils in this dish.
Avoid red or orange lentils, however, as they tend to
be too soft for side dishes like this one.

CUBAN-STYLE BRAISED FISH

SERVES 4 • GLUTEN FREE • UNDER 20 MINUTES

1 teaspoon olive oil

1 onion, chopped

2 garlic cloves, chopped

1 (14½-ounce) can diced tomatoes with green chiles

½ cup chicken broth

10 green pimento-stuffed olives, thinly sliced crosswise

4 (6-ounce) skinless halibut fillets

4 tablespoons sliced almonds, toasted

1 Heat oil over medium heat in large skillet. Add onion and cook, stirring, until tender, about 4 minutes. Add garlic and cook 1 minute more.

2 Stir tomatoes, broth, and olives into skillet and bring to simmer. Nestle halibut fillets into skillet. Cover and cook until fillets flake with fork, 8–10 minutes.

3 Transfer fillets to 4 plates. Spoon tomato and olive mixture over fish and sprinkle each with 1 tablespoon almonds.

3 SmartPoints value

Per serving (1 fillet, about ½ cup sauce, and 1 tablespoon almonds): 239 Cal, 7 g Total Fat, 1 g Sat Fat, 636 mg Sod, 8 g Total Carb, 2 g Sugar, 1 g Fib, 35 g Prot.

COOK'S TIP

If you like, serve the fish with steamed broccoli seasoned with a little salt and pepper and a splash of fresh lemon juice.

TILAPIA TACOS WITH CHIPOTLE AÏOLI

SERVES 4 • GLUTEN FREE

AÏOLI:

¼ cup plain low-fat Greek yogurt

¼ cup reduced-fat mayonnaise

1 tablespoon finely chopped canned chipotles en adobo, or to taste

1 tablespoon finely chopped red onion

1 tablespoon chopped fresh cilantro

¼ teaspoon ground cumin

1 teaspoon lime juice

TACOS:

3 tablespoons lime juice

1 tablespoon olive oil

1 teaspoon ground cumin

1 small garlic clove, minced

1 pound tilapia fillets

¾ teaspoon kosher salt

8 small corn tortillas

½ cup packaged coleslaw mix or shredded cabbage

¼ cup finely chopped fresh cilantro

¼ cup finely chopped red onion

1 lime, cut into 8 wedges

1 Combine all aïoli ingredients in small bowl. Cover and refrigerate until ready to serve.

2 Combine lime juice, oil, cumin, and garlic in shallow dish; add tilapia and turn to coat. Cover and refrigerate 30 minutes.

3 Spray ridged grill pan with nonstick spray and place over high heat. Remove tilapia from marinade; discard marinade. Grill fish until it flakes easily with fork, 3–4 minutes per side; sprinkle with salt and slice tilapia into 8 equal pieces.

4 While tilapia cooks, wrap tortillas in paper towel and microwave until warm, about 30 seconds.

5 Top each tortilla with 1 tablespoon slaw, 1 piece tilapia, and 1 heaping tablespoon aïoli; garnish with cilantro and onion. Place 2 tacos on each plate and serve with lime wedges.

7 SmartPoints value

Per serving (2 tacos): 294 Cal, 9 g Total Fat, 2 g Sat Fat, 575 mg Sod, 28 g Total Carb, 3 g Sugar, 4 g Fib, 26 g Prot.

COOK'S TIP

You can make the aïoli up to 4 days ahead if you like.

HADDOCK AND POTATO STEW WITH SAFFRON

SERVES 4 • GLUTEN FREE

½ fennel bulb, finely chopped

2 garlic cloves, chopped

1½ cups canned crushed tomatoes

½ cup dry white wine

¼ teaspoon saffron threads

½ teaspoon salt, or to taste

¼ teaspoon black pepper

2 (8-ounce) russet potatoes, peeled and cut into ½-inch cubes

1 pound haddock fillet or other firm white fish, cut into large chunks

1 tablespoon chopped fresh parsley

4 lemon wedges

1 Spray large saucepan with nonstick spray and place over medium-high heat. Add fennel and garlic and cook, stirring, until fennel is just softened, about 5 minutes. Stir in tomatoes, wine, saffron, salt, and pepper and bring to boil.

2 Stir in potatoes and simmer, covered, until potatoes are just tender, about 12 minutes.

3 Gently stir in haddock and simmer, covered, until fish is firm and opaque, about 6 minutes. Ladle stew into serving bowls and sprinkle with parsley. Serve with lemon wedges

4 SmartPoints value

Per serving (1½ cups): 227 Cal, 1 g Total Fat, 0 g Sat Fat, 685 mg Sod, 28 g Total Carb, 4 g Sugar, 4 g Fib, 22 g Prot.

COOK'S TIP

Saffron is a classic spice for fish stews, adding golden color to the broth and a deep, earthy flavor. You can, however, substitute a few pinches of turmeric, or just leave it out completely.

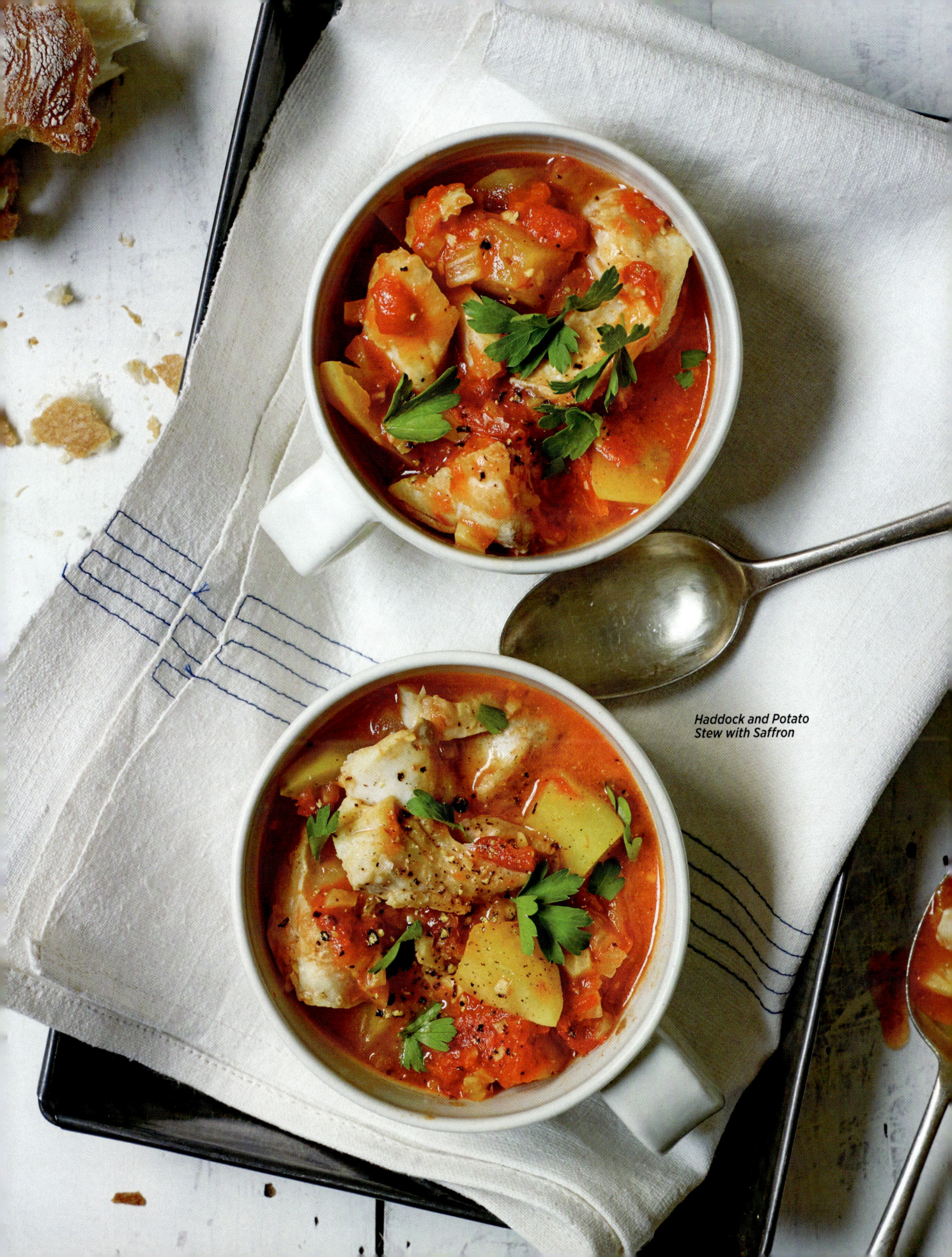

Haddock and Potato Stew with Saffron

SMOKED SALMON SCRAMBLE WITH POTATOES AND DILL SAUCE

SERVES 4 • GLUTEN FREE

1 pound red potatoes, cut into ¾-inch wedges

1 teaspoon salt

¾ cup plain fat-free yogurt

1 tablespoon chopped fresh dill

⅛ teaspoon black pepper

2 large eggs

4 large egg whites

1 tablespoon prepared horseradish, drained

3 teaspoons olive oil

1 cup halved cherry tomatoes

1 medium sweet white onion, chopped

2 ounces sliced smoked salmon, cut into ½-inch pieces

1 Combine potatoes and enough cold water to cover by 1 inch in medium saucepan. Add ½ teaspoon salt and bring to boil. Reduce heat; partially cover and simmer until potatoes are fork-tender, about 8 minutes. Drain and keep warm.

2 Meanwhile, stir yogurt, dill, and pepper together in small bowl. Transfer 2 tablespoons yogurt mixture to medium bowl. Add eggs, egg whites, and ¼ teaspoon salt to yogurt mixture in medium bowl and whisk until smooth. To make sauce, stir horseradish and remaining ¼ teaspoon salt into yogurt mixture in small bowl.

3 Heat 1 teaspoon oil in medium nonstick skillet over medium heat. Add tomatoes and cook, stirring frequently, just until softened, 2–3 minutes. Cover and keep warm.

4 Heat remaining 2 teaspoons oil in large nonstick skillet over medium heat. Add onion and cook, stirring frequently, until softened and lightly browned, about 5 minutes. Add salmon and cook, turning gently with tongs, until it begins to turn white, 2–3 minutes. Add egg mixture and cook, stirring frequently, just until set, 2–3 minutes. Drizzle horseradish sauce evenly over potatoes and top with tomatoes. Serve egg mixture with potatoes.

6 SmartPoints value

Per serving (½ cup egg mixture, ¾ cup potatoes, 2 tablespoons sauce, and 2 tablespoons tomatoes): 221 Cal, 7 g Total Fat, 1 g Sat Fat, 732 mg Sod, 27 g Total Carb, 8 g Sugar, 3 g Fib, 14 g Prot.

COOK'S TIP

Smoked trout is also a terrific fish to try in this recipe. You can substitute 2 ounces of trout, skin removed and flesh flaked, for the salmon for no change in SmartPoints.

KUNG PAO SHRIMP

SERVES 4

3 tablespoons chicken broth

2 tablespoons balsamic vinegar

1 tablespoon soy sauce

1 teaspoon cornstarch

1 teaspoon sugar

1 teaspoon toasted sesame oil

2 tablespoons peanut oil
or canola oil

1 tablespoon minced garlic

1 tablespoon minced peeled
fresh ginger

¼ teaspoon red pepper
flakes, or to taste

1¼ pounds large shrimp, peeled,
deveined, and patted dry

3 cups sugar snap peas, trimmed

½ teaspoon salt, or to taste

1 red bell pepper, diced

2 scallions, thinly sliced

1 Combine broth, vinegar, soy sauce, cornstarch, sugar, and sesame oil in cup; set aside.

2 Heat wok or large skillet over high heat until drop of water sizzles. Swirl in peanut oil. Add garlic, ginger, and red pepper flakes and stir-fry 10 seconds. Add shrimp and cook, undisturbed, 1 minute, letting shrimp begin to sear. Stir-fry 30 seconds, until shrimp are lightly browned but not cooked through.

3 Add snap peas and salt. Stir-fry 30 seconds or just until combined. Add bell pepper and scallions. Stir broth mixture and add to wok. Stir-fry 1–2 minutes or until shrimp are just cooked and vegetables are crisp-tender.

4 SmartPoints value

Per serving (1⅓ cups): 233 Cal, 10 g Total Fat, 2 g Sat Fat, 1,351 mg Sod, 15 g Total Carb, 5 g Sugar, 4 g Fib, 22 g Prot.

COOK'S TIP

This Chinese classic is nicely spicy. If, however, you prefer a milder dish, you can reduce the amount of red pepper flakes to ⅛ teaspoon, or even omit them entirely.

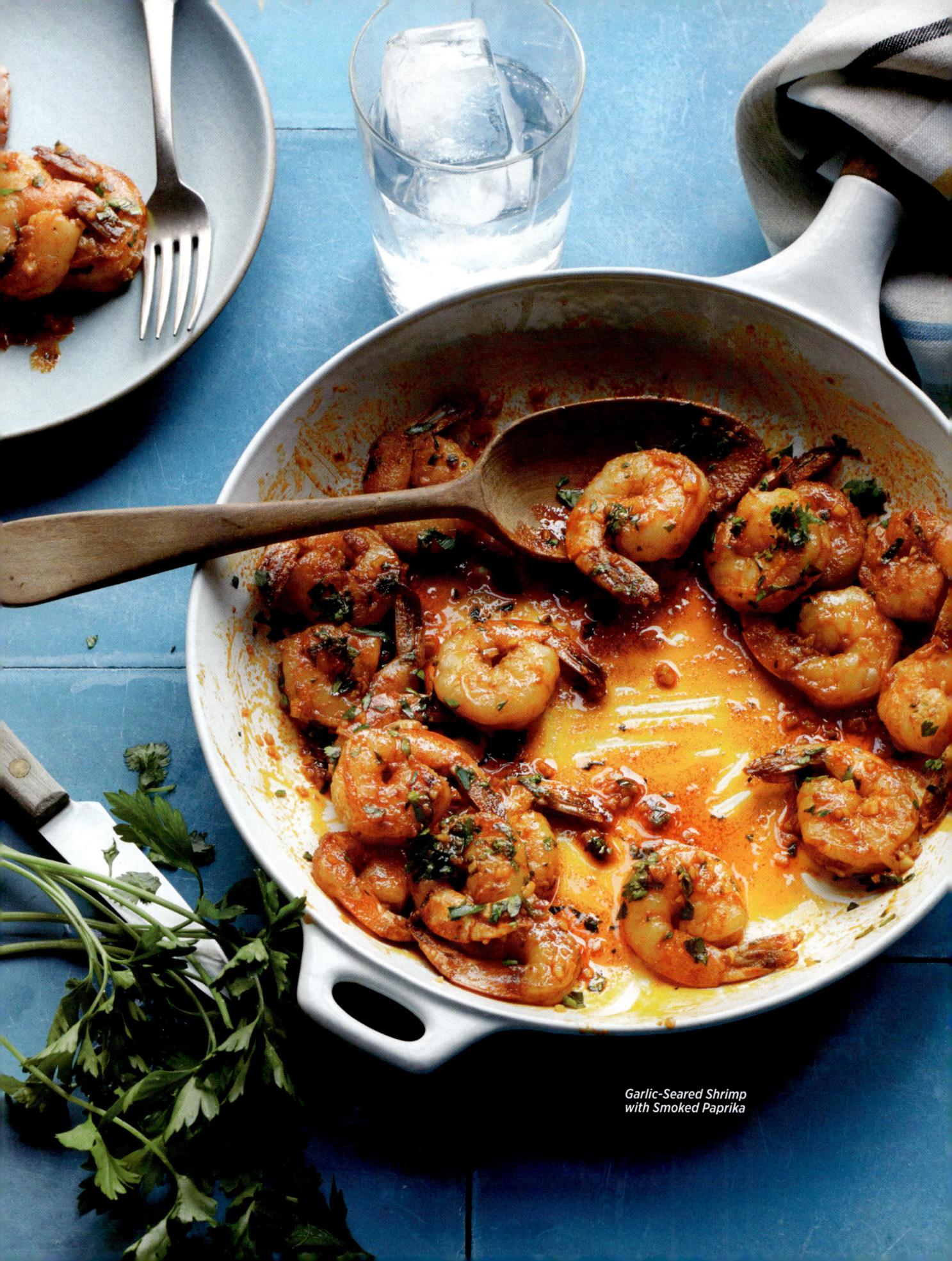

Garlic-Seared Shrimp with Smoked Paprika

GARLIC-SEARED SHRIMP WITH SMOKED PAPRIKA

SERVES 4 • GLUTEN FREE • UNDER 20 MINUTES

1¼ pounds large shrimp, peeled, deveined, and patted dry

¼ teaspoon salt, or to taste

4 teaspoons olive oil

6 garlic cloves, finely chopped

1½ teaspoons sweet smoked paprika

1 tablespoon chopped fresh parsley

1 tablespoon chopped fresh cilantro, plus extra for garnish

½ teaspoon lemon juice

1 Toss shrimp with salt. Heat large heavy skillet over high heat until very hot. Lightly coat bottom of pan with 1 teaspoon oil; heat until lightly smoking. Add half of shrimp in single layer. Cook just until golden and orange, about 10 seconds; turn shrimp quickly. Cook 10 seconds more; immediately transfer to plate. Repeat with remaining shrimp and 1 teaspoon oil.

2 Reduce heat to medium-high; add remaining 2 teaspoons oil. Add garlic and cook, stirring, until light golden but not browned, about 2 minutes. Stir in paprika; return shrimp to pan.

3 Reduce heat slightly and cook until shrimp are just opaque in center, about 1 minute; stir in parsley, cilantro, and lemon juice. Serve shrimp with pan sauce spooned over top and garnish with additional cilantro.

3 SmartPoints value

Per serving (about 7 shrimp): 149 Cal, 6 g Total Fat, 1 g Sat Fat, 951 mg Sod, 3 g Total Carb, 0 g Sugar, 0 g Fib, 20 g Prot.

COOK'S TIP

If you like, serve the shrimp over a bed of steamed spinach drizzled with lemon juice.

KALE CAESAR SALAD WITH GRILLED SHRIMP

SERVES 4 • GLUTEN FREE

1½ pounds large shrimp, peeled and deveined

1 teaspoon grated lemon zest

1 garlic clove, crushed through garlic press

¼ teaspoon salt, or to taste

2 tablespoons fat-free Greek yogurt

2 tablespoons low-fat mayonnaise

2 tablespoons lemon juice

2 teaspoons olive oil

2 anchovies, rinsed and well mashed, or 1 teaspoon anchovy paste

½ teaspoon Dijon mustard

⅛ teaspoon black pepper

¼ cup freshly grated Parmesan

1 (¾-pound) bunch curly kale, stems and tough ribs removed and discarded, leaves thinly sliced (about 12 cups)

½ ounce Parmesan shaved with vegetable peeler

1 Toss shrimp, lemon zest, ¼ teaspoon garlic, and ⅛ teaspoon salt in medium bowl; set aside.

2 To make dressing, whisk yogurt, mayonnaise, lemon juice, oil, anchovies, mustard, pepper, remaining garlic, and remaining ⅛ teaspoon salt together in large bowl. Whisk in grated Parmesan. Add kale and toss with hands thoroughly so kale softens slightly. Cover and refrigerate 20 minutes.

3 Spray grill pan with nonstick spray and place over medium-high heat. Place shrimp on pan and grill just until opaque in center, 2–3 minutes per side.

4 Divide salad and shrimp among 4 plates. Sprinkle with shaved Parmesan.

5 SmartPoints value

Per serving (1¼ cups salad, about 9 shrimp, and about 3 Parmesan shavings): 257 Cal, 10 g Total Fat, 3 g Sat Fat, 1,447 mg Sod, 12 g Total Carb, 3 g Sugar, 3 g Fib, 31 g Prot.

COOK'S TIP

To make turning the shrimp easier, you can thread them on metal skewers if you like.

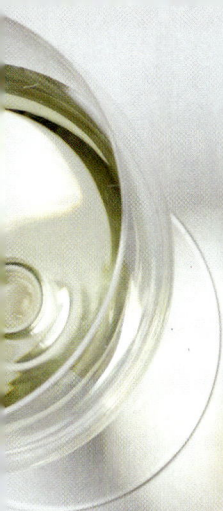

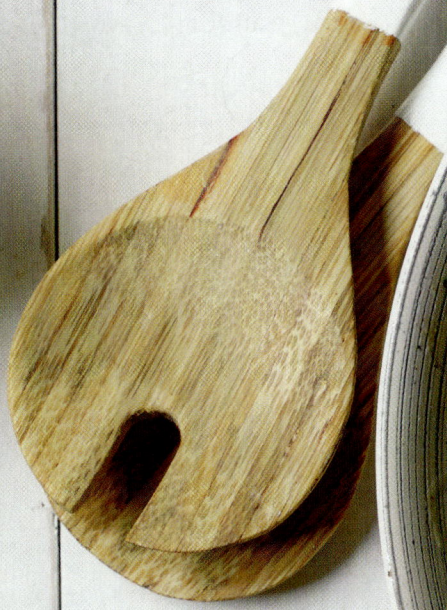

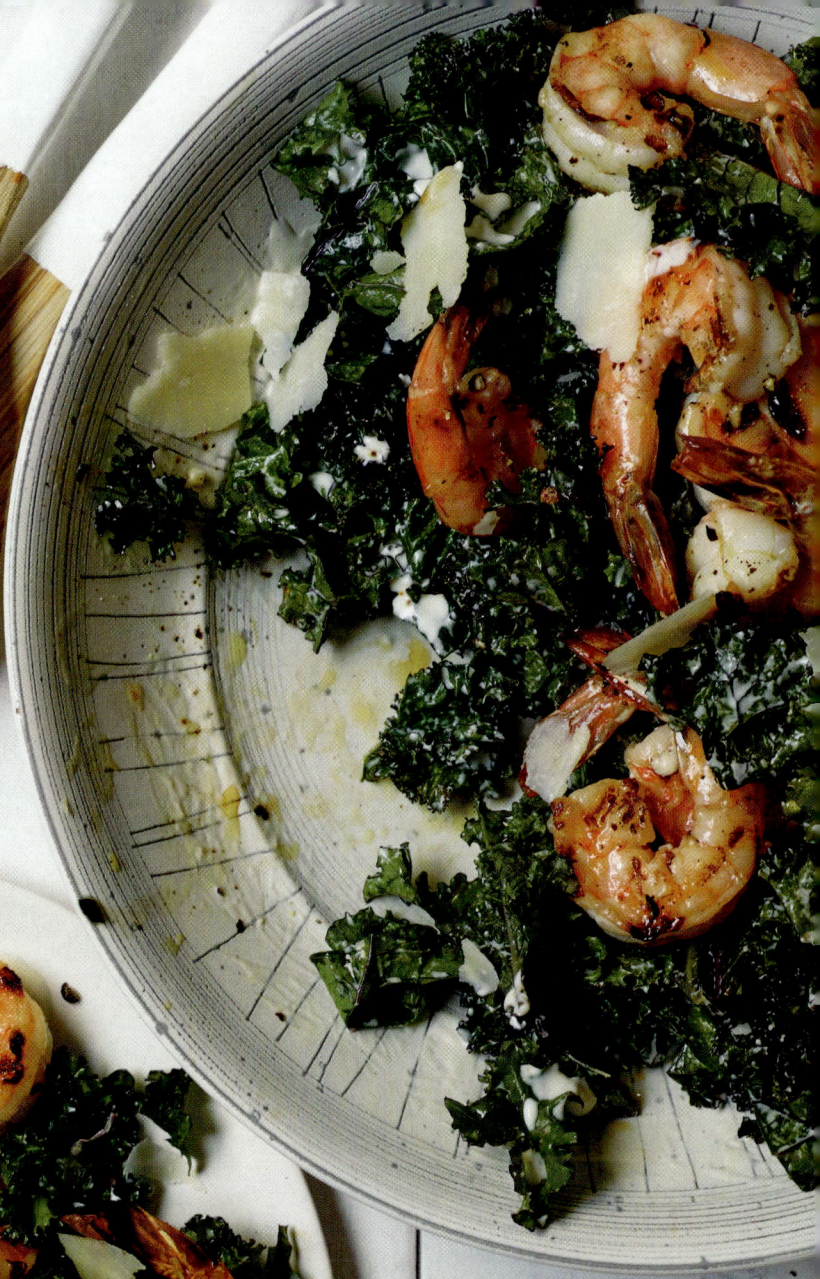

*Kale Caesar Salad
with Grilled Shrimp*

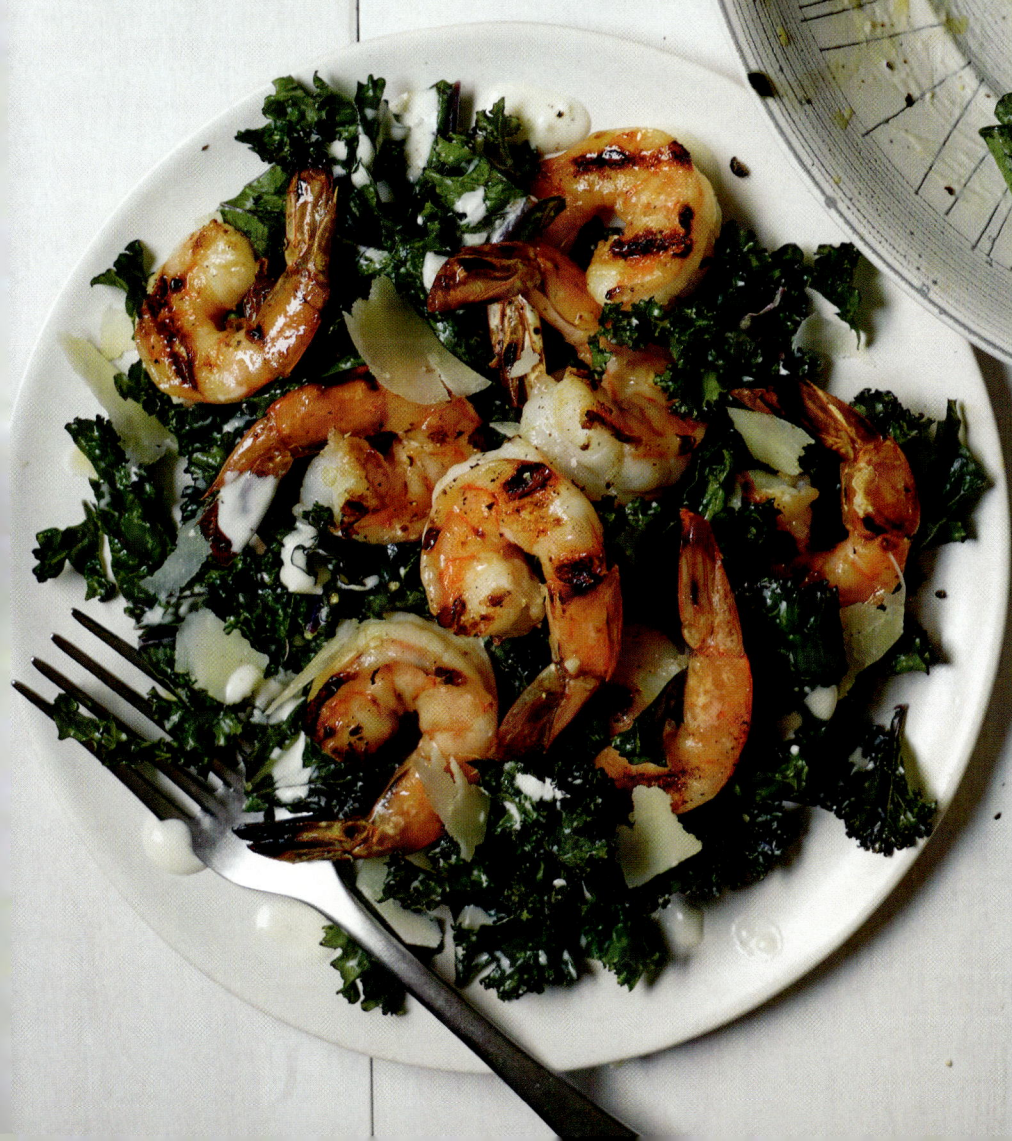

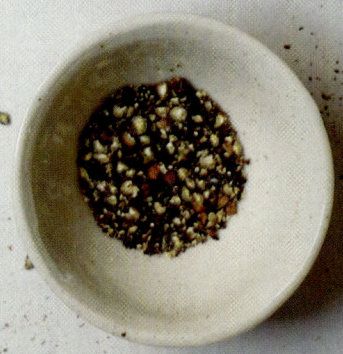

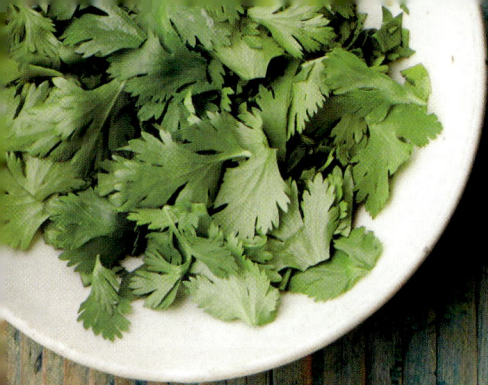

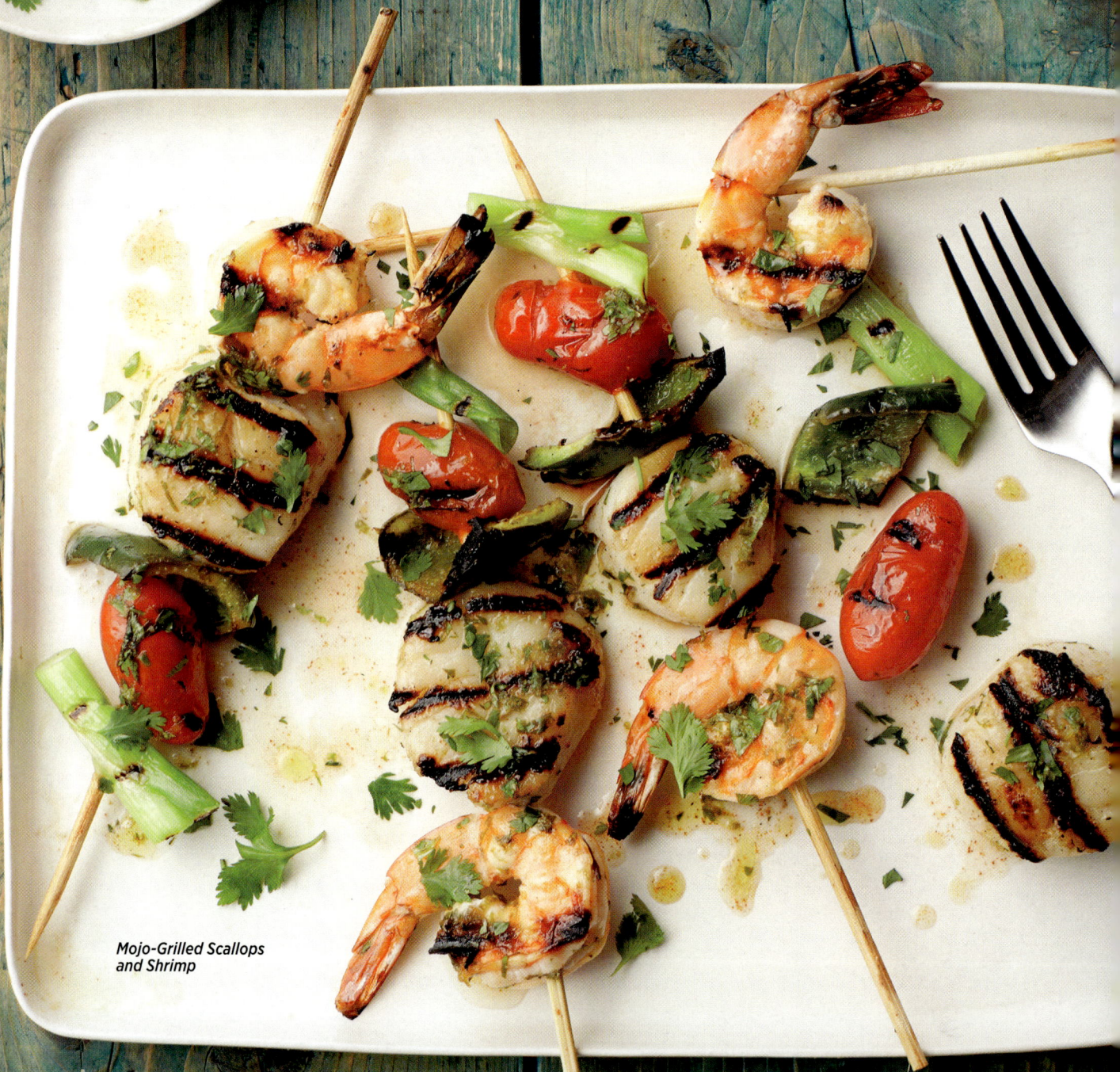

Mojo-Grilled Scallops and Shrimp

MOJO-GRILLED SCALLOPS AND SHRIMP

SERVES 4 • GLUTEN FREE

½ cup lime juice

¼ cup chopped fresh cilantro

1 tablespoon olive oil

2 teaspoons granulated garlic

2 teaspoons grated lime zest, or to taste

¼ teaspoon salt

⅛ teaspoon cayenne, or to taste

16 large sea scallops (about 1 pound)

16 extra large shrimp (about ⅔ pound), peeled, tails left on, and deveined

1 poblano pepper, cut into 16 pieces

16 grape tomatoes or cherry tomatoes

4 scallions, each cut into four 1½-inch pieces

1 Stir lime juice, 2 tablespoons cilantro, oil, garlic, lime zest, salt, and cayenne together in large bowl; remove and reserve 3 tablespoons oil mixture for serving.

2 Add scallops, shrimp, poblano, tomatoes, and scallions to bowl with remaining oil mixture; toss to coat. Let stand, tossing occasionally, about 20 minutes.

3 Preheat outdoor grill to medium-high or place ridged grill pan over medium-high heat.

4 Thread 1 piece each shrimp, scallop, poblano, tomato, and scallion onto 16 short metal skewers. (If using wooden skewers, soak them in water 20 minutes prior to use to prevent charring.) Brush skewers with any remaining oil mixture in bottom of bowl. Grill skewers, turning as needed, just until scallops and shrimp are cooked through, 5–6 minutes.

5 Transfer skewers to serving platter; drizzle with reserved oil mixture and sprinkle with remaining 2 tablespoons cilantro.

3 SmartPoints value

Per serving (4 skewers): 196 Cal, 5 g Total Fat, 1 g Sat Fat, 1,022 mg Sod, 14 g Total Carb, 4 g Sugar, 2 g Fib, 25 g Prot.

COOK'S TIP

We threaded the ingredients onto 16 short skewers for easy flipping on the grill, but you can use 8 long skewers if you prefer.

CHILI-CRUSTED GRILLED SEA SCALLOPS WITH ZUCCHINI

SERVES 4 • GLUTEN FREE • UNDER 20 MINUTES

1 tablespoon light brown sugar

2 teaspoons chili powder

½ teaspoon finely grated lemon zest

½ teaspoon ground cumin

1 teaspoon salt

¼ teaspoon cayenne, or to taste

1¼ pounds (about 20) sea scallops

2 medium (7-ounce) zucchini, cut lengthwise into ¼-inch-thick planks

1 teaspoon olive oil

Lemon wedges for serving

1 Preheat outdoor grill to medium or place ridged grill pan over medium-high heat.

2 Stir brown sugar, chili powder, lemon zest, cumin, ½ teaspoon salt, and cayenne together in small bowl; pat scallops dry and dredge in spice mixture. Toss zucchini with oil and remaining ½ teaspoon salt in large bowl.

3 Grill scallops and zucchini, turning once, until scallops are just opaque in center and zucchini is tender, 3–4 minutes for scallops and 6–8 minutes for zucchini. Serve with lemon wedges.

2 SmartPoints value.

Per serving (5 scallops and about 3 pieces zucchini): 141 Cal, 2 g Total Fat, 0 g Sat Fat, 1,177 mg Sod, 12 g Total Carb, 5 g Sugar, 2 g Fib, 18 g Prot.

UP THE PROTEIN

*Serve the scallops with a side of nutty quinoa.
A ½ cup of cooked quinoa per serving will increase
the SmartPoints value by 3.*

BROWN RICE CALIFORNIA ROLLS

SERVES 4

½ cup short-grain brown rice

1 teaspoon rice vinegar

4 sheets nori seaweed

6 ounces cooked Alaskan king crab leg or 4 (1½-ounce) crabsticks

¼ avocado, thinly sliced

½ cup matchstick strips peeled and seeded cucumber

8 teaspoons reduced-sodium soy sauce

1 Preheat oven to 300°F.

2 Combine 1½ cups water, rice, and vinegar in medium saucepan; set over high heat and bring to boil. Reduce heat to low, and simmer, covered, until liquid is absorbed and rice sticks together, about 30 minutes; remove from heat and let cool.

3 Meanwhile, place seaweed on baking sheet and place in oven. Toast until warm and soft, 1–2 minutes.

4 Arrange seaweed on flat surface or bamboo sushi mat. With damp hands, press about ¼ cup rice over seaweed in even layer, leaving ½-inch border around edges. Arrange one-quarter of crab, avocado, and cucumber down center of each sheet. Starting from one end and pressing down gently, roll up seaweed into tight roll.

5 With damp knife, slice each roll crosswise into 4 or 5 pieces (slice off and discard ends if they have no rice or filling). Serve rolls with soy sauce on the side.

4 SmartPoints value

Per serving (1 roll and 2 teaspoons soy sauce): 155 Cal, 3 g Total Fat, 0 g Sat Fat, 809 mg Sod, 20 g Total Carb, 1 g Sugar, 2 g Fib, 11 g Prot.

COOK'S TIP

Dab these whole-grain rolls with wasabi paste for spicy, classically Japanese flavor.

MEXICAN-SPICED CRAB BURGERS

SERVES 6

1 pound lump crabmeat, picked over for pieces of shell and cartilage

⅔ cup panko (Japanese bread crumbs)

¾ cup finely chopped red onion

¼ cup finely chopped fresh cilantro

2 tablespoons reduced-fat mayonnaise

2 large eggs, lightly beaten

1 teaspoon ground cumin

½ teaspoon kosher salt

⅛ teaspoon cayenne, or to taste

6 light English muffins, split and toasted

6 tablespoons store-bought guacamole

6 romaine lettuce leaves

6 slices fresh tomato

1 Preheat oven to 400°F. Line baking pan with parchment paper.

2 Combine crabmeat, panko, onion, cilantro, mayonnaise, eggs, cumin, salt, and cayenne in medium bowl. Scoop up heaping ½ cup crab mixture and form into ¾-inch-thick patty; repeat with remaining mixture to make 6 patties. Spray patties on both sides with nonstick spray and place on prepared pan. Bake until undersides are browned, about 10 minutes; carefully turn and cook until browned on other side, about 10 minutes.

3 Place a burger on each muffin bottom; top each with 1 tablespoon guacamole, 1 lettuce leaf, and 1 tomato slice and cover with muffin top.

7 SmartPoints value

Per serving (1 burger): 285 Cal, 8 g Total Fat, 1 g Sat Fat, 825 mg Sod, 35 g Total Carb, 3 g Sugar, 7 g Fib, 23 g Prot.

COOK'S TIP

Panko bread crumbs give seafood burgers a particularly light texture. You'll find them in most supermarkets.

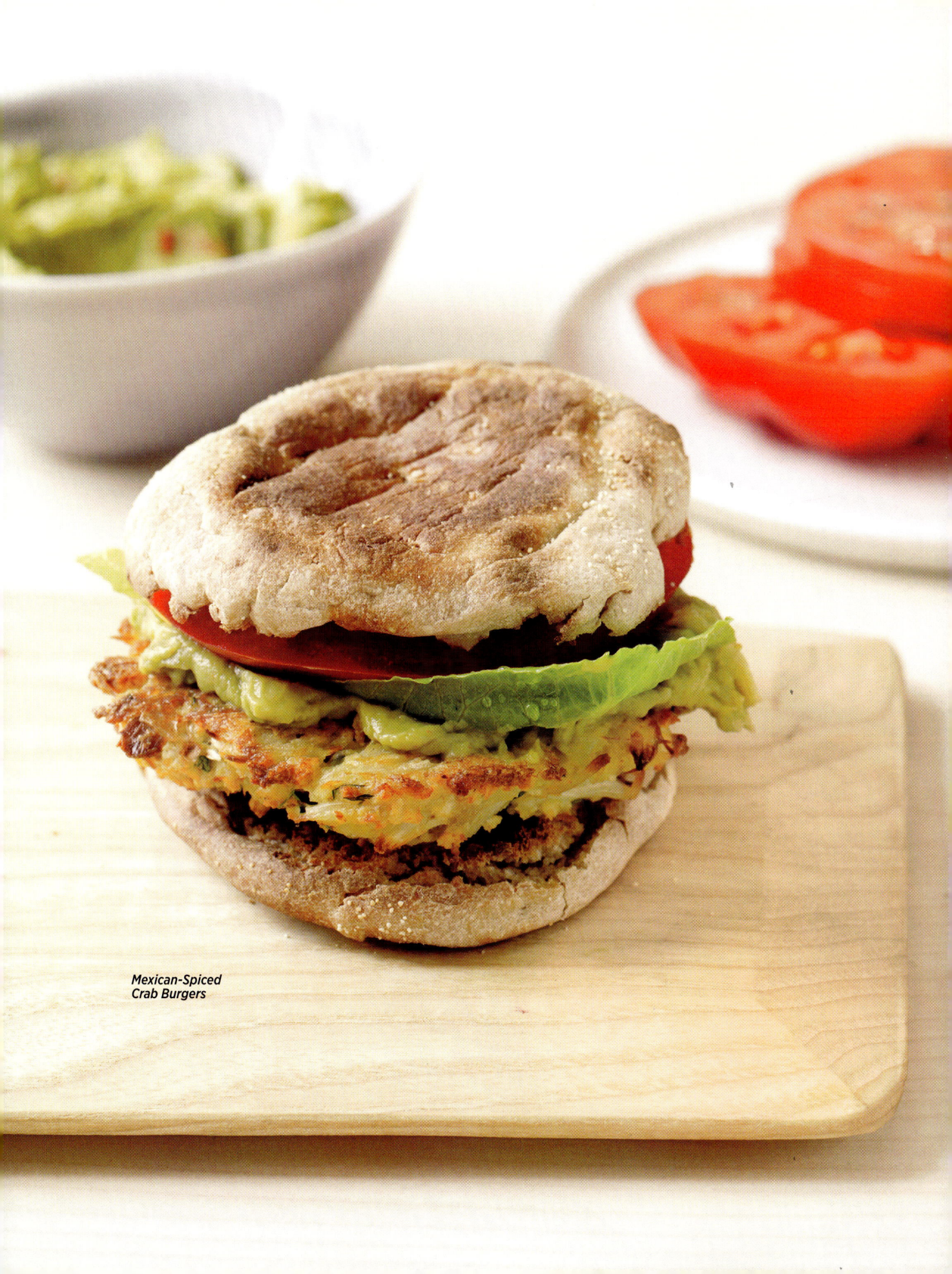

*Mexican-Spiced
Crab Burgers*

CAJUN SHRIMP SAUTÉ

SERVES 4 ● GLUTEN FREE

½ teaspoon paprika

½ teaspoon dried oregano

½ teaspoon kosher salt, or to taste

¼ teaspoon cayenne

¼ teaspoon black pepper

1½ pounds large shrimp, peeled, deveined, and patted dry

1 tablespoon plus 1 teaspoon olive oil

1 large onion, coarsely chopped

1 tablespoon chopped garlic

2 large yellow bell peppers, coarsely chopped

1 large Cubanelle pepper, cut into ½-inch dice

½ cup roughly chopped fresh parsley

½ lemon, cut into 4 wedges

1 Stir paprika, oregano, salt, cayenne, and black pepper together in small bowl. Place shrimp in large bowl; toss with half of spice mixture and set aside.

2 Heat large nonstick skillet over medium-high heat; add 1 tablespoon of oil and swirl to coat pan. When oil is hot, add onion; cook, stirring frequently, just until softened, about 3 minutes. Add garlic and cook, stirring, until fragrant, about 1 minute. Add bell peppers and Cubanelle pepper; sprinkle with remaining spice mixture and cook until crisp-tender and lightly golden, 4–5 minutes. Transfer mixture to bowl; cover and set aside.

3 Set same skillet over medium-high heat; add remaining 1 teaspoon oil and swirl to coat pan. Add shrimp in single layer; cook 2 minutes, then turn shrimp. Cook, stirring, until shrimp are just opaque in center, 2 minutes more; add pepper mixture and toss to heat through. Sprinkle with parsley and serve with lemon wedges.

3
SmartPoints
value

Per serving (1½ cups): 218 Cal, 7 g Total Fat, 1 g Sat Fat, 1,093 mg Sod, 15 g Total Carb, 3 g Sugar, 3 g Fib, 25 g Prot.

COOK'S TIP

Cubanelle peppers, also known as Cuban peppers or frying peppers, are mild and richly flavored. If you can't find them, you can substitute a small green bell pepper or, for a little heat, a fresh poblano pepper.

FRESH MANHATTAN CLAM CHOWDER

SERVES 6 • GLUTEN FREE

5 slices turkey bacon

2 teaspoons olive oil

1 large onion, diced

2 large carrots, diced

4 celery stalks, diced

½ pound Yukon Gold potatoes, cut into ½-inch pieces

4 cups bottled clam juice

32 ounces canned crushed tomatoes in tomato puree

1½ tablespoons fresh thyme leaves

1 bay leaf

½ teaspoon salt

½ teaspoon black pepper

3 pounds littleneck clams, scrubbed

¼ cup fresh parsley

1 Place large skillet over medium-high heat. Add bacon and cook, turning once or twice, until crispy, 5–6 minutes. Cool bacon on paper towel–lined plate and crumble; set aside.

2 In same skillet, heat oil over medium heat about 1 minute. Add onion, carrots, celery, and potato; stir vegetables, scraping bacon drippings from bottom of skillet with wooden spoon. Cook, stirring occasionally, until vegetables soften, 10–15 minutes; add clam juice, tomatoes, thyme, bay leaf, salt, and pepper. Bring to boil, then reduce heat to medium-low. Simmer, uncovered, until potatoes are tender, about 30 minutes.

3 Add clams, cover, and increase heat to high. Boil just until clams open, 6–8 minutes. Discard any clams that do not open. Remove clams from shells, discard shells, and place clams back in soup. Sprinkle with parsley and bacon.

3 SmartPoints value

Per serving (about 1½ cups): 154 Cal, 5 g Total Fat, 1 g Sat Fat, 1,099 mg Sod, 19 g Total Carb, 7 g Sugar, 5 g Fib, 11 g Prot.

UP THE PROTEIN

White beans are a delicious addition to seafood soups and add a good amount of fiber and protein. You can add 1 cup of rinsed and drained beans to the soup with the clams for an additional 1 SmartPoints per serving.

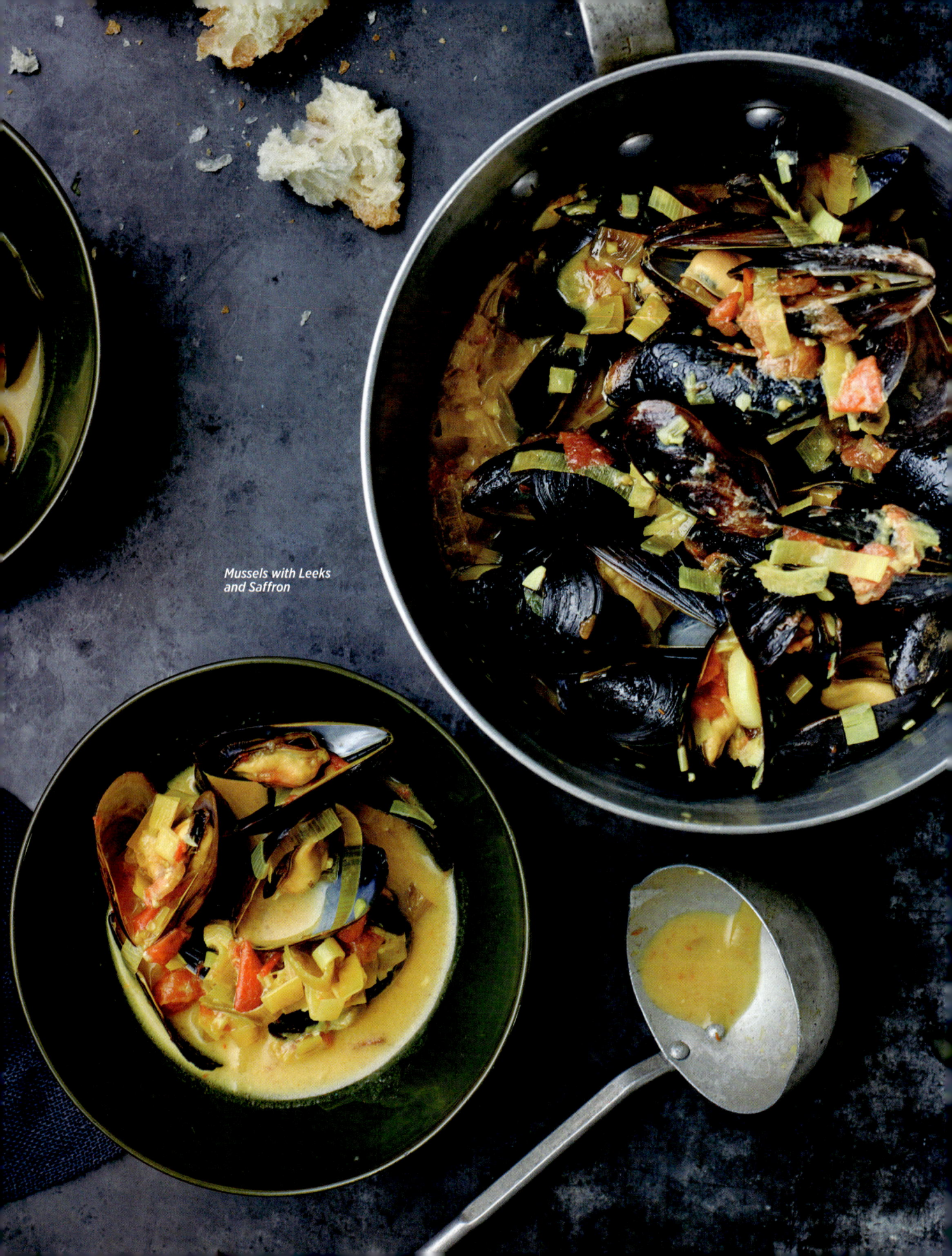

*Mussels with Leeks
and Saffron*

MUSSELS WITH LEEKS AND SAFFRON

SERVES 4 • GLUTEN FREE

2 teaspoons olive oil

2 large leeks, white and light-green parts only, halved lengthwise, thinly sliced and rinsed well

3 garlic cloves, minced

1 cup dry white wine

½ cup chicken broth

2 tomatoes, chopped

½ teaspoon saffron threads, crumbled

⅛ teaspoon cayenne, or to taste

3 pounds mussels, scrubbed and debearded

½ cup silken tofu

⅛ teaspoon salt, or to taste

1 tablespoon chopped fresh parsley

1 Heat oil in large Dutch oven over medium-low heat. Add leeks and cook, stirring occasionally, until softened, about 6 minutes. Stir in garlic and cook until fragrant, about 1 minute.

2 Stir in wine, broth, tomato, saffron, and cayenne; bring to boil. Add mussels, cover, and cook until mussels open, about 4 minutes. Discard any mussels that do not open. Transfer mussels with slotted spoon to large bowl; cover with foil to keep hot.

3 Return Dutch oven to medium heat and simmer until mixture is slightly thickened, about 6 minutes. Pour ½ cup pan juices into blender. Add tofu and salt and puree. Return mixture to Dutch oven and bring to boil.

4 Divide mussels among 4 bowls. Pour pan juices over mussels, dividing evenly. Sprinkle with parsley.

8 SmartPoints value

Per serving (about 24 mussels with pan juices): 427 Cal, 11 g Total Fat, 2 g Sat Fat, 1,150 mg Sod, 25 g Total Carb, 5 g Sugar, 2 g Fib, 44 g Prot.

COOK'S TIP

Silken tofu imparts creaminess and richness to the mussel broth, and also adds protein.

LINGUINE WITH RED CLAM SAUCE

SERVES 4

24 littleneck clams, scrubbed

½ cup dry white wine

1 tablespoon fresh thyme
or 1 teaspoon dried

1 tablespoon chopped fresh
oregano or 1 teaspoon dried

4 garlic cloves, finely chopped

6 ounces linguine

1 tablespoon olive oil

8 plum tomatoes, chopped

2 tablespoons chopped
fresh basil

3 tablespoons chopped
fresh parsley

¼ teaspoon red pepper flakes

½ teaspoon salt

1 (6.5-ounce) can chopped
clams and juice

1 Scrub clams well under cold running water. Place in large pot of cold water; let soak a few minutes to release any residual grit, then drain. Repeat for several changes of water until no sand falls to bottom of pot.

2 Combine clams, wine, thyme, oregano, and garlic in large saucepan. Cover and cook over medium heat until clams open, about 5 minutes. Discard any clams that do not open. When cool enough to handle, remove clam meat from 12 shells and coarsely chop. Reserve remaining clams with meat still inside for garnish; reserve cooking liquid (including the garlic and herbs) separately.

3 Cook linguine according to package directions. Drain and place in warmed serving bowl; keep warm.

4 Meanwhile, heat oil in medium nonstick skillet over medium heat. Add tomatoes, 1 tablespoon basil, 2 tablespoons parsley, red pepper flakes, and salt. Cook, stirring, over medium heat, until tomatoes begin to break down, 5–10 minutes. Add reserved clam cooking liquid and canned clams and juice; reduce heat and simmer until thickened. Stir in chopped clam meat and heat through, about 1 minute. Pour over linguine, toss to coat, and garnish with reserved clam shells. Sprinkle with remaining 1 tablespoon parsley and 1 tablespoon basil and serve at once.

8 SmartPoints value

Per serving (about 1⅔ cups): 376 Cal, 6 g Total Fat, 1 g Sat Fat, 684 mg Sod, 48 g Total Carb, 8 g Sugar, 4 g Fib, 27 g Prot.

COOK'S TIP

*Using both fresh and canned clams in this sauce
makes it particularly rich and delicious.*

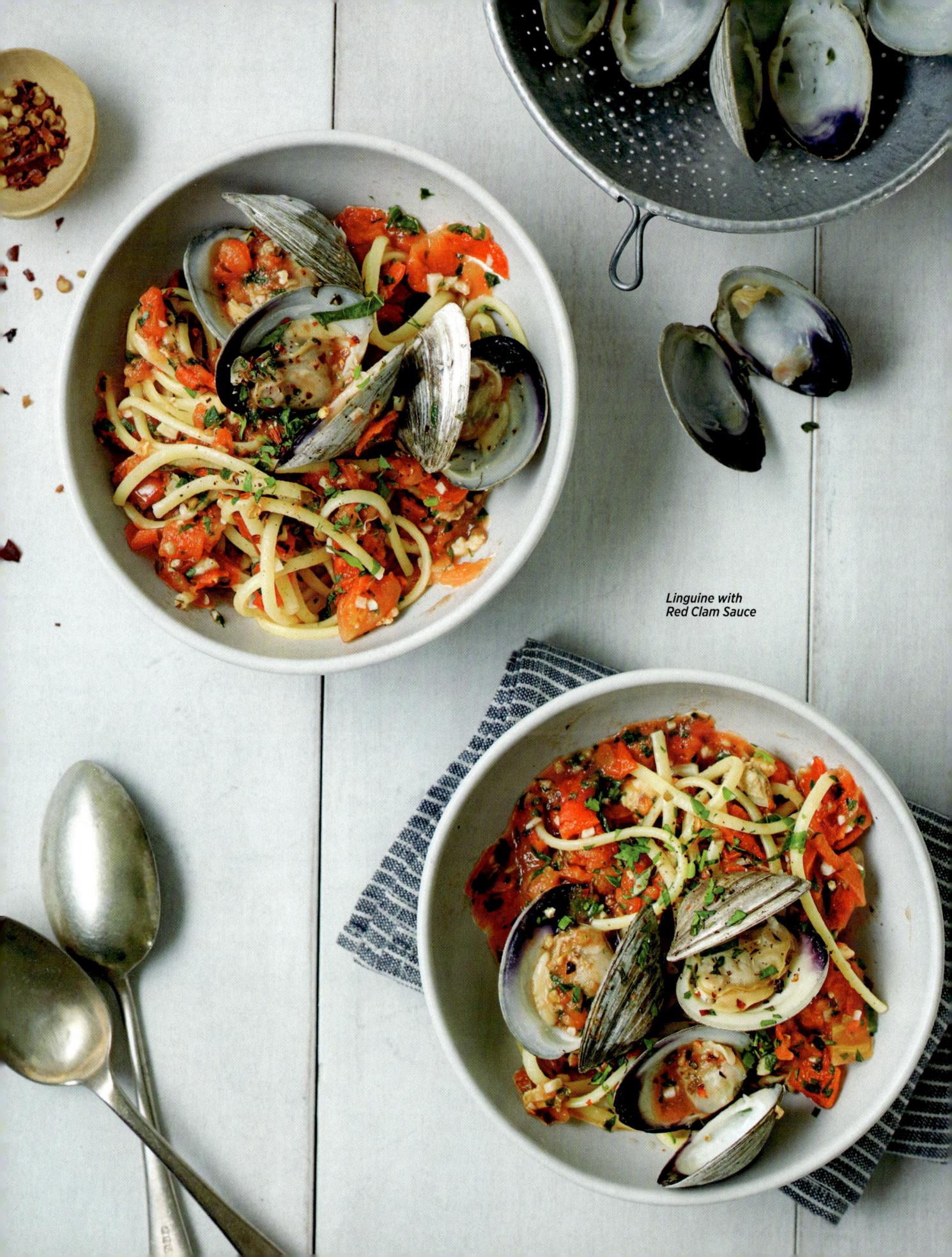

*Linguine with
Red Clam Sauce*

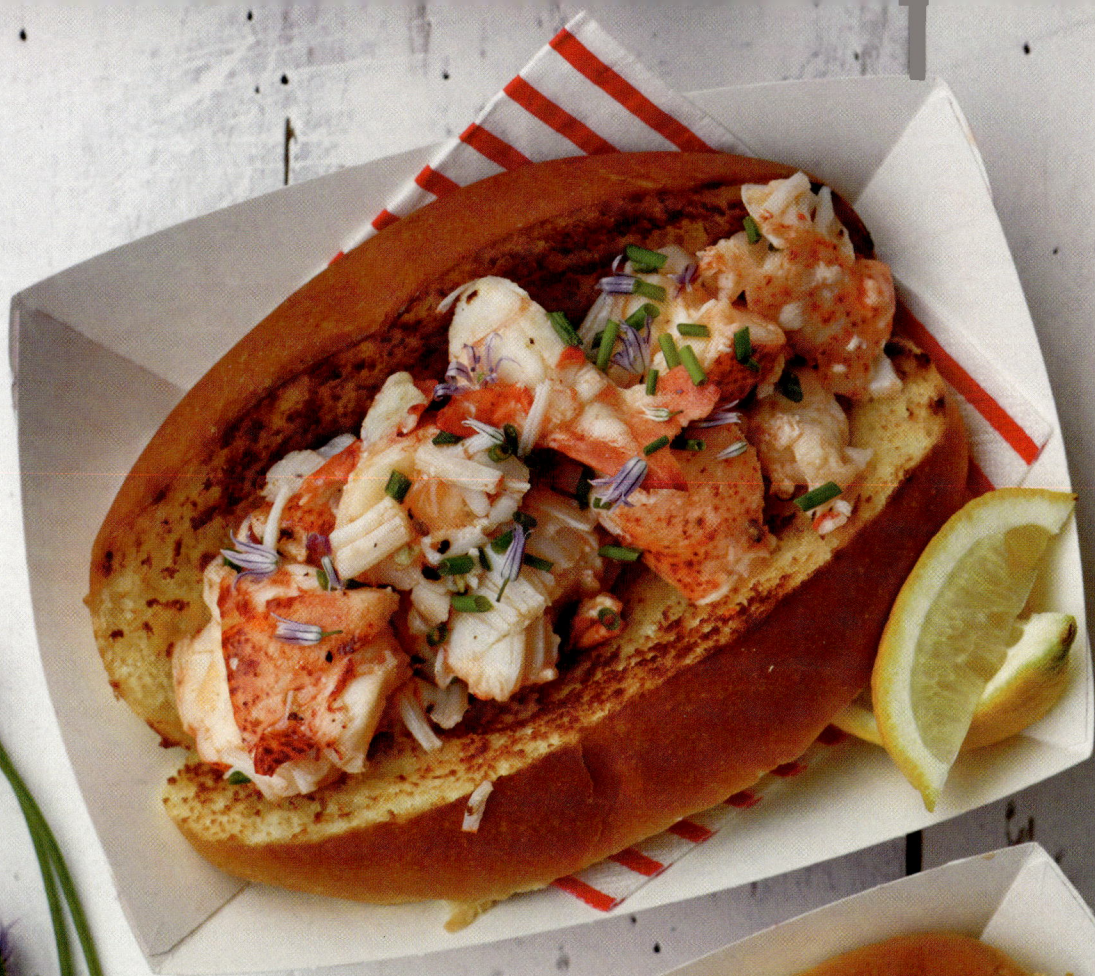

Lobster Rolls

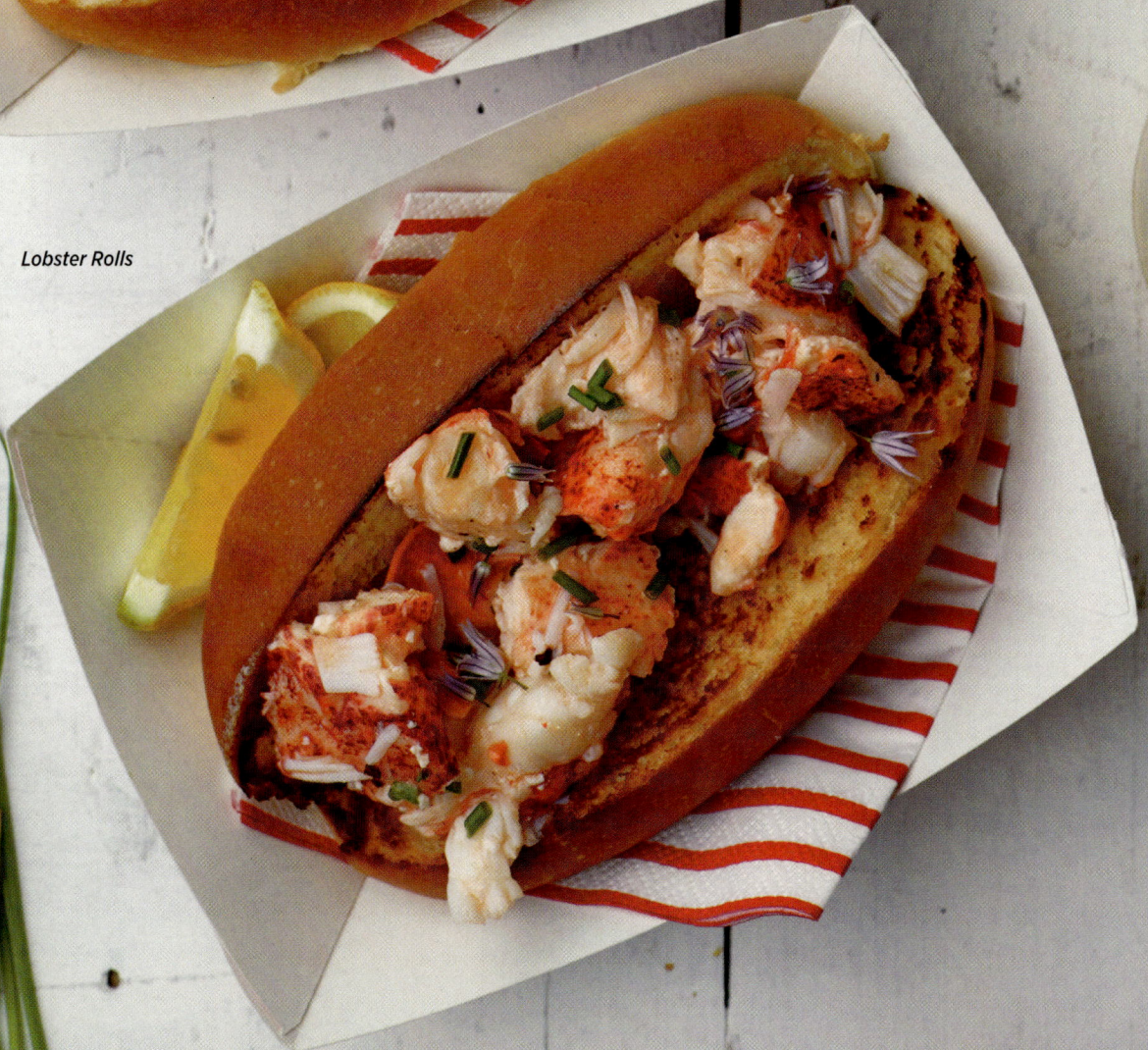

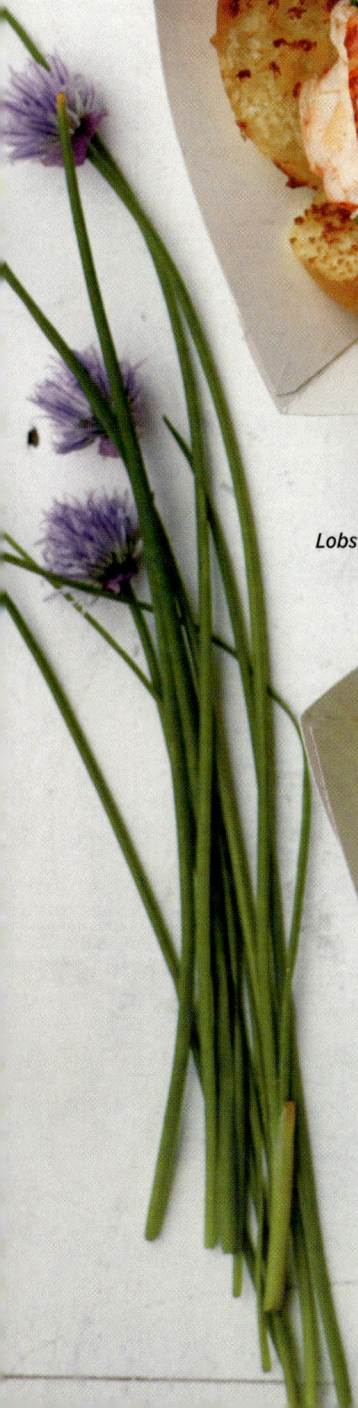

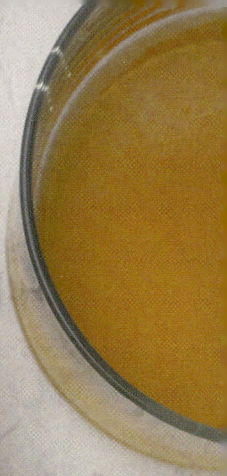

LOBSTER ROLLS

SERVES 4 • UNDER 20 MINUTES

3½ tablespoons unsalted butter

4 reduced-calorie hot dog buns, split

1 pound fresh or frozen thawed lobster meat (2–3 tails)

¼ teaspoon salt

¼ teaspoon black pepper

2 teaspoons lemon juice

Chopped chives for garnish

4 lemon wedges

1 Melt 1½ tablespoons butter; brush on insides of split hot dog buns and set aside.

2 Slice lobster into bite-size pieces. Heat large skillet over medium-low heat; add remaining 2 tablespoons butter, salt, and pepper. Melt butter; add lobster and cook until pink, about 4 minutes. Add lemon juice, then transfer lobster and any liquid in pan to bowl.

3 Wipe skillet clean; set over medium heat. Toast hot dog buns, buttered-side down, until golden. Lay each toasted bun open on plate and fill with lobster and any sauce. Sprinkle with chives and serve rolls with lemon wedges.

8 SmartPoints value

Per serving (1 lobster roll): 264 Cal, 12 g Total Fat, 7 g Sat Fat, 796 mg Sod, 19 g Total Carb, 2 g Sugar, 3 g Fib, 22 g Prot.

COOK'S TIP

To remove the meat from a raw lobster tail, turn tail upside down and make a slit with a sharp knife in the underside of the shell from top to bottom. Hold shell with both hands and crack shell backward so you can pull lobster meat out of the shell in one piece.

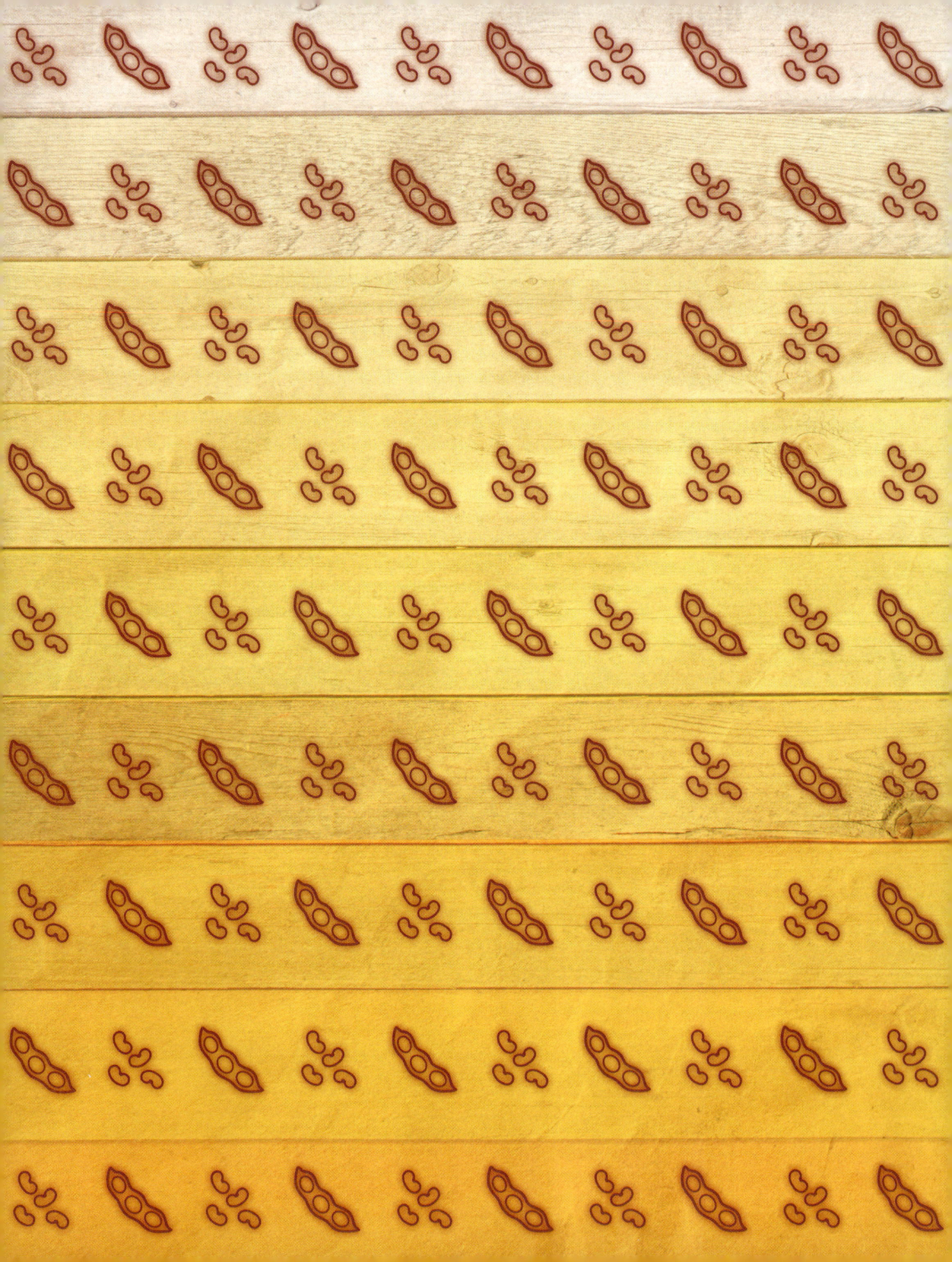

TOFU BEANS LENTILS & OTHER VEGGIE PROTEINS

SOBA NOODLES WITH TOFU AND SPINACH

SERVES 4 • VEGETARIAN • UNDER 20 MINUTES

6 ounces soba noodles

2 tablespoons rice wine vinegar

2 tablespoons soy sauce

2 teaspoons honey

1 scallion, thinly sliced

1 teaspoon Asian (dark) sesame oil

1 garlic clove, finely chopped

1 (4-ounce) container fresh spinach leaves, rinsed but not dried

1 (8-ounce) package baked teriyaki tofu

1 Cook noodles according to package directions (do not overcook or noodles will be gummy). Drain and place in large bowl. While noodles are still warm, add vinegar, soy sauce, honey, and scallion; toss to coat.

2 Meanwhile, spray large skillet or wok with nonstick spray; add oil and place skillet over medium-high heat. When oil is hot, add garlic; cook, stirring, until fragrant, about 30 seconds. Add spinach; cook, covered, until spinach wilts, 3–5 minutes. Add spinach mixture to noodle mixture and toss; keep warm.

3 Add tofu to skillet and cook, tossing, until heated through, about 1 minute. Sprinkle tofu over noodles and spinach.

6 SmartPoints value

Per serving (about 1⅓ cups): 212 Cal, 3 g Total Fat, 0 g Sat Fat, 904 mg Sod, 40 g Total Carb, 4 g Sugar, 2 g Fib, 11 g Prot.

UP THE PROTEIN

Add 1⅓ cups shelled cooked edamame to the skillet along with the spinach in Step 2 for an additional 2 SmartPoints per serving.

EDAMAME AND CHICKPEA SALAD WITH MISO DRESSING

SERVES 4 • VEGETARIAN • UNDER 20 MINUTES

1 (10-ounce) package frozen shelled edamame

2 tablespoons white miso

1 teaspoon grated lemon zest

2 tablespoons lemon juice

1 tablespoon olive oil

½ teaspoon grated peeled fresh ginger

¼ teaspoon salt

1 (15-ounce) can chickpeas, rinsed and drained

½ English (seedless) cucumber, halved lengthwise and sliced

1 carrot, shredded

3 tablespoons chopped red onion

1 Bring medium saucepan of water to boil. Add edamame and cook 5 minutes; drain and rinse under cold running water.

2 Whisk miso, lemon zest, lemon juice, oil, and ginger together in large bowl until smooth. Add edamame, chickpeas, cucumber, carrot, and onion and stir to combine. Let stand at room temperature 10 minutes before serving, or cover and refrigerate up to 2 hours and serve chilled.

6 SmartPoints value

Per serving (1 cup): 235 Cal, 9 g Total Fat, 1 g Sat Fat, 815 mg Sod, 27 g Total Carb, 5 g Sugar, 9 g Fib, 15 g Prot.

UP THE PROTEIN

If you like, sprinkle a finely diced peeled hard-cooked egg over each serving of the salad for an additional 2 SmartPoints per serving.

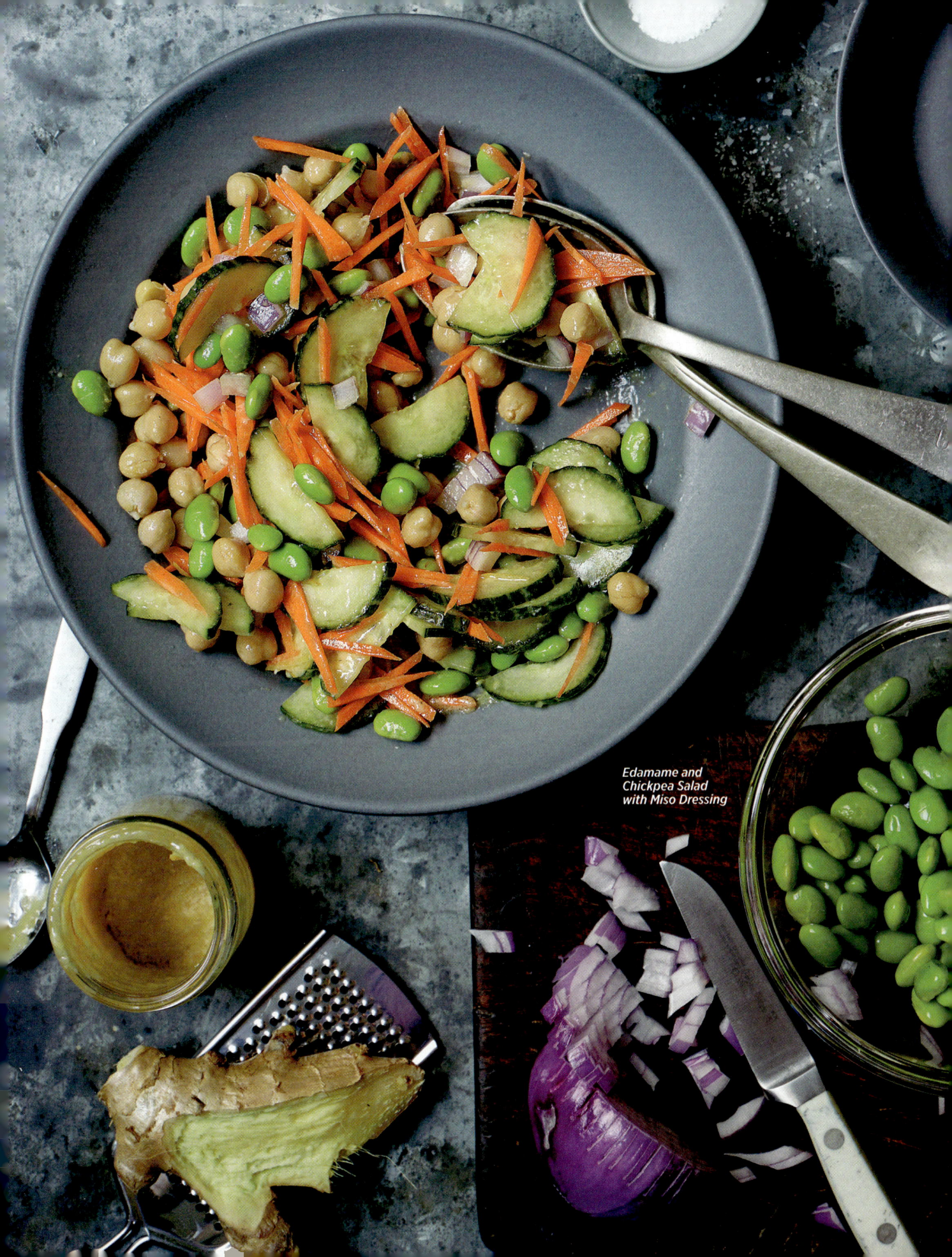

*Edamame and
Chickpea Salad
with Miso Dressing*

SOY AND HONEY-GLAZED TOFU-VEGETABLE SKEWERS

SERVES 4 • VEGETARIAN

½ cup quinoa, rinsed well

3 tablespoons soy sauce

1 tablespoon honey

1 tablespoon lime juice

1 (16-ounce) container extra-firm tofu, drained and cut into 1-inch cubes

1 yellow bell pepper, cut into 1-inch pieces

1 green bell pepper, cut into 1-inch pieces

1 small red onion, quartered and separated into pieces

8 grape tomatoes

1 Cook quinoa according to package directions.

2 Meanwhile, stir soy sauce, honey, and lime juice together in cup; set aside.

3 Spray ridged grill pan with nonstick spray and set over medium-high heat. Thread tofu, yellow and green bell peppers, onion, and tomatoes onto 8 (12-inch) metal skewers (if using wooden skewers, soak them in water 20 minutes prior to use to prevent charring); brush with soy sauce mixture. Place skewers in pan and cook, turning, until tofu is browned and vegetables are softened, about 10 minutes. Serve over quinoa.

6 SmartPoints value

Per serving (2 skewers and about ⅓ cup quinoa): 237 Cal, 8 g Total Fat, 1 g Sat Fat, 662 mg Sod, 29 g Total Carb, 8 g Sugar, 5 g Fib, 17 g Prot.

COOK'S TIP

For variety, try red or black quinoa or a blend of red, black, and white quinoa.

ROASTED CAULIFLOWER AND TOFU CURRY

SERVES 4 • GLUTEN FREE • VEGETARIAN

1 pound extra-firm tofu, cut into 1-inch cubes

2 teaspoons olive oil

2 tablespoons Madras curry powder

1 teaspoon ground cumin

1 teaspoon ground ginger

1 teaspoon salt

1 large onion, halved and sliced ¼ inch thick

1 head cauliflower, cut into 1½-inch pieces

2 cups cooked warm brown rice

1 Preheat oven to 450°F. Gently press tofu between several layers of paper towels to remove excess water; set aside.

2 Heat oil in large nonstick skillet over medium-high heat. Add curry powder, cumin, ginger, and salt; swirl skillet to combine. Add onion and cook, stirring often, until onion is browned, 8–9 minutes.

3 Combine cauliflower and tofu in large bowl. Pour onion mixture into bowl and spray with nonstick spray; stir to combine. Spread mixture onto baking sheet in even layer. Roast, stirring every 10 minutes, until cauliflower and tofu are golden brown, 25–35 minutes. Serve over rice.

7 SmartPoints value

Per serving (1¾ cups curry and ½ cup rice): 318 Cal, 10 g Total Fat, 1 g Sat Fat, 636 mg Sod, 43 g Total Carb, 6 g Sugar, 9 g Fib, 19 g Prot.

COOK'S TIP

Madras curry powder is a medium-hot variety, a little fierier than most curry powders sold in the United States. You can taste the vegetables before serving them and add a little more curry powder or a little cayenne if you'd like a spicier dish.

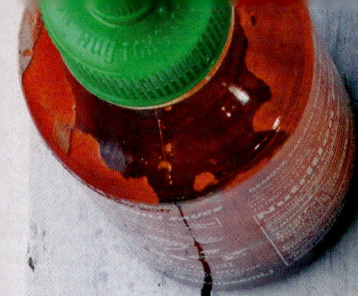

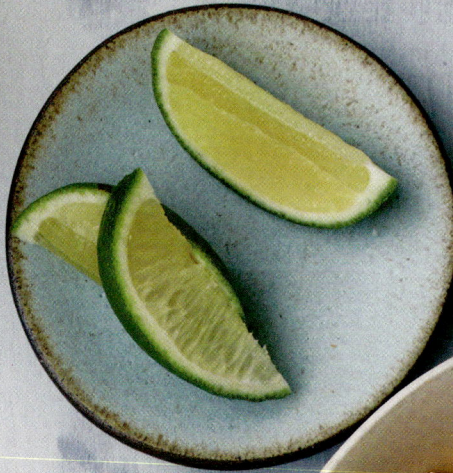

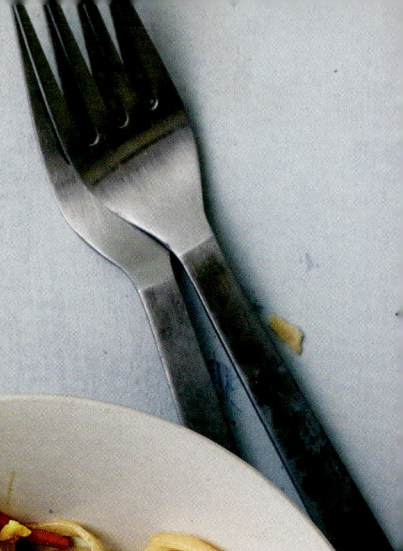

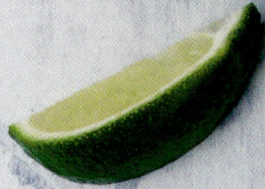

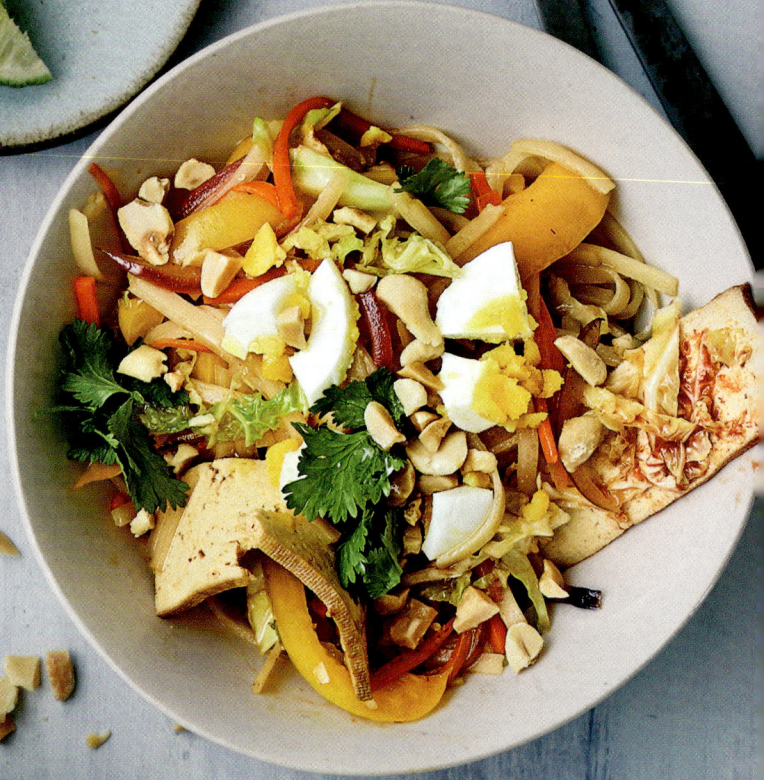

*Vegetable
Pad Thai*

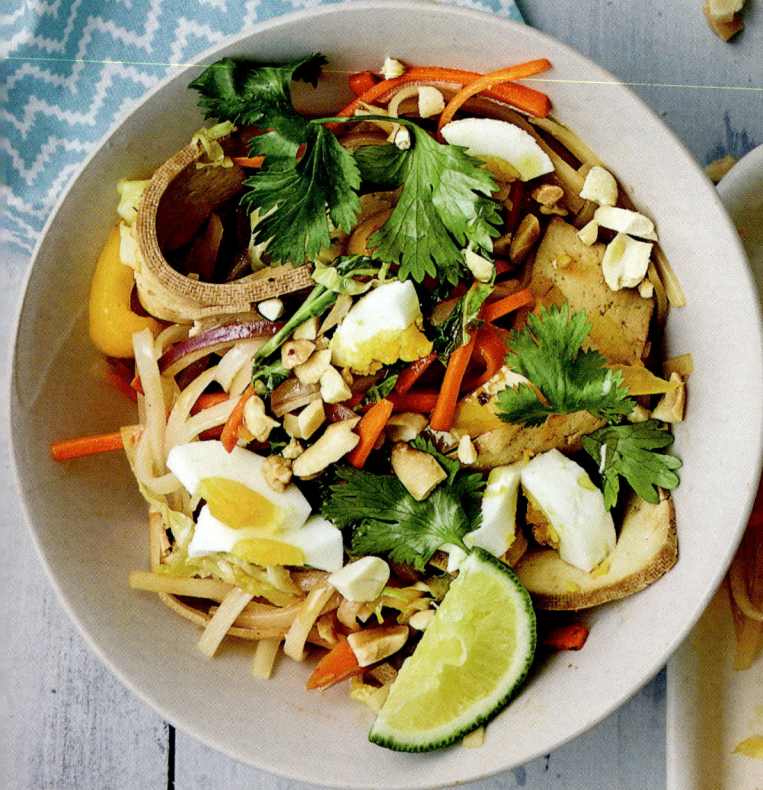

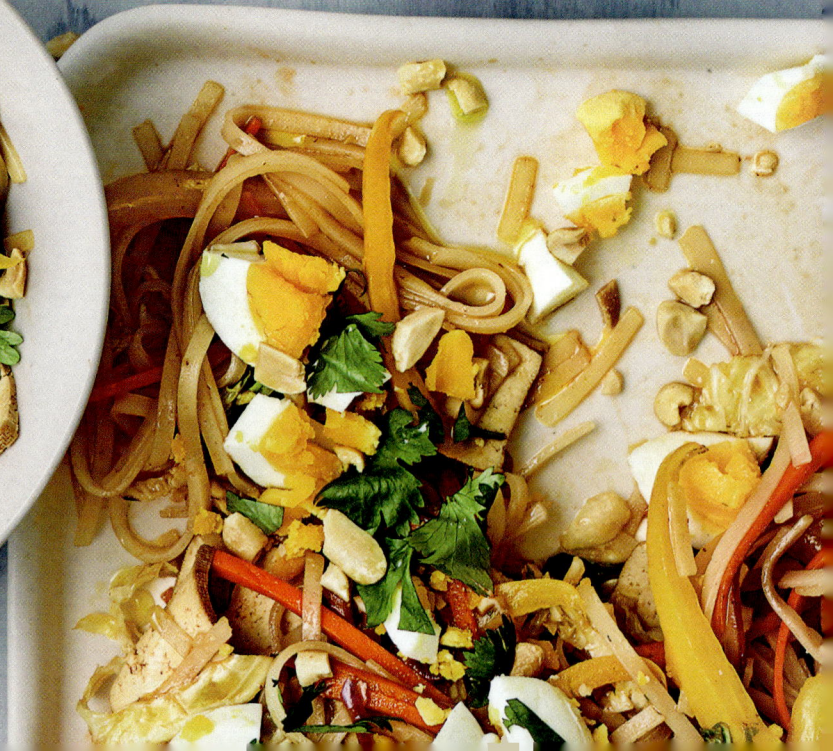

VEGETABLE PAD THAI

SERVES 6 • VEGETARIAN

4 ounces flat rice stick noodles

2 teaspoons canola oil

1 red or yellow bell pepper, cut into thin strips

1 small red onion, thinly sliced

2 carrots, cut into thin strips

1½ cups thinly sliced cabbage

2 garlic cloves, finely chopped

2 tablespoons Asian fish sauce

1 tablespoon sugar

2 tablespoons reduced-sodium soy sauce

8 ounces baked or smoked tofu, cut into thin strips

1½ teaspoons Sriracha

2 large hard-cooked eggs, chopped

½ cup chopped fresh cilantro

2 tablespoons dry-roasted peanuts, chopped

Lime wedges

1 Place noodles in large bowl. Add enough boiling water to cover; let stand until noodles are softened but still firm at the center, 3–7 minutes. Drain in colander and rinse under cold running water. Drain again.

2 Meanwhile, heat oil in large skillet over medium-high heat. Add bell pepper, onion, and carrots; cook, stirring frequently, until vegetables are crisp-tender, 2–3 minutes. Add cabbage and garlic; cook, stirring frequently, until fragrant, about 1 minute. Add fish sauce, sugar, and soy sauce; cook, stirring, until sugar dissolves, about 30 seconds. Add noodles and tofu; cook, tossing gently to mix, until heated through, 2–3 minutes.

3 Remove pan from heat. Add Sriracha and toss gently. Transfer noodles to platter; sprinkle with eggs, cilantro, and peanuts. Serve with lime wedges.

6 SmartPoints value

Per serving (about 1 cup noodles and 1 teaspoon peanuts): 228 Cal, 8 g Total Fat, 2 g Sat Fat, 916 mg Sod, 29 g Total Carb, 7 g Sugar, 3 g Fib, 7 g Prot.

COOK'S TIP

Rice noodles can vary in thickness, so for best results, start checking for doneness after 3 minutes. The texture should be cooked through but firm, not mushy. If the noodles need more soaking time, check again every minute and add a little more water if needed.

TEMPEH AND SNOW PEAS IN ORANGE SAUCE

SERVES 4 • VEGETARIAN • UNDER 20 MINUTES

Zest and juice of ½ orange

1½ teaspoons cornstarch

1 tablespoon Asian (dark) sesame oil

3 scallions, minced

½ shallot, minced

1 tablespoon minced peeled fresh ginger

¼ teaspoon red pepper flakes

¾ pound fresh snow peas, trimmed

1 red bell pepper, diced

1 (8-ounce) package tempeh, diced

½ cup vegetable broth

2 tablespoons soy sauce

1 tablespoon hoisin sauce

1 Whisk orange juice and cornstarch together in small bowl until smooth.

2 Heat wok over medium-high heat until drop of water sizzles in pan. Add oil and swirl to coat pan. Add scallions, shallot, ginger, and red pepper flakes; stir-fry until scallions begin to soften, about 30 seconds. Add snow peas and bell pepper; stir-fry until snow peas turn bright green, about 1 minute. Add tempeh and stir-fry until heated through, about 2 minutes.

3 Stir in broth, soy sauce, hoisin sauce, and orange zest; bring to boil. Whisk orange juice mixture again and add to wok. Stir-fry until mixture is bubbling and thickened, about 1 minute.

4 SmartPoints value®

Per serving (1¼ cups): 212 Cal, 10 g Total Fat, 2 g Sat Fat, 595 mg Sod, 20 g Total Carb, 7 g Sugar, 7 g Fib, 14 g Prot.

COOK'S TIP

If you don't have a wok, use a large heavy skillet for cooking this dish. The deeper the skillet the easier it will be to stir-fry your ingredients.

DELICATA SQUASH, CHARD, AND CHICKPEA CURRY

SERVES 4 • VEGETARIAN

1 pound delicata squash (unpeeled)

1 cup light (low-fat) coconut milk

1 tablespoon tomato paste

2 teaspoons reduced-sodium soy sauce

1 tablespoon olive oil

½ cup diced onion

2 garlic cloves, smashed

1 tablespoon Madras curry powder

2 cups torn young Swiss chard leaves

1 (15-ounce) can chickpeas, rinsed and drained

½ teaspoon salt

1 Cut squash in half lengthwise; remove and discard seeds and stringy flesh. Place each squash half, cut side down, on cutting board; slice each half into quarters and then cut each quarter into ¼-inch-thick slices.

2 Combine coconut milk, tomato paste, and soy sauce in small bowl; set aside.

3 Heat oil over medium heat in large saucepan. Add onion and garlic; cook, stirring frequently, until onion softens, about 1 minute. Add curry powder and stir until fragrant, about 10 seconds. Add squash, Swiss chard, and coconut milk mixture; increase heat to medium-high and bring to boil. Reduce heat to medium-low and cover; simmer, stirring occasionally, until squash is tender when pierced with knife, 5–7 minutes. Add chickpeas and salt; increase heat to medium and stir until chickpeas are heated through, 2–3 minutes.

6 SmartPoints value

Per serving (1¼ cups): 233 Cal, 9 g Total Fat, 3 g Sat Fat, 757 mg Sod, 34 g Total Carb, 4 g Sugar, 8 g Fib, 8 g Prot.

UP THE PROTEIN

Top each serving of curry with 2 tablespoons chopped cashews for an additional 3 SmartPoints.

BELL PEPPERS WITH CHICKPEA MASH, EGGS, AND HARISSA

SERVES 6 • GLUTEN FREE • VEGETARIAN

6 bell peppers, assorted colors

1 onion, diced

¾ teaspoon salt, or to taste

½ teaspoon black pepper, or to taste

½ teaspoon ground turmeric

½ teaspoon garlic powder

¼ teaspoon ground cumin

¼ teaspoon cinnamon

3 cups baby spinach, chopped

¾ cup canned chickpeas, rinsed and drained, mashed slightly with fork

6 large eggs

6 teaspoons finely chopped fresh chives or cilantro

6 tablespoons harissa paste, mild or hot

1 Preheat oven to 425°F. Line baking sheet with foil and spray foil with nonstick spray.

2 Slice lengthwise piece off each bell pepper, leaving stem and bottom intact, creating a boat shape from each; reserve cut pieces of bell pepper. Carefully scoop out membrane and seeds from peppers with melon baller or teaspoon. Set bell peppers on prepared pan, cut side up. Loosely cover with foil; bake 15 minutes.

3 Meanwhile, dice reserved bell pepper pieces. Spray large skillet with nonstick spray and place over medium-low heat. Add diced bell peppers, onion, ½ teaspoon salt, and ¼ teaspoon black pepper; cook, stirring frequently, until tender, about 7 minutes. Add turmeric, garlic powder, cumin, and cinnamon and toss to combine. Add spinach and chickpeas; toss to combine and remove from heat.

4 Remove bell peppers from oven and reduce heat to 375°F. Place peppers in baking dish. Divide chickpea mixture evenly among peppers; crack 1 egg onto each pepper and sprinkle with remaining ¼ teaspoon salt and remaining ¼ teaspoon black pepper. Bake, uncovered, until egg whites are set, about 20 minutes. Sprinkle with chives and spoon harissa paste over top.

3 SmartPoints value

Per serving (1 stuffed pepper): 143 Cal, 6 g Total Fat, 2 g Sat Fat, 494 mg Sod, 14 g Total Carb, 4 g Sugar, 4 g Fib, 10 g Prot.

COOK'S TIP

Harissa is a spicy condiment commonly found in North African cuisine that can range from mild to fiery hot. Look for one that meets your spice threshold.

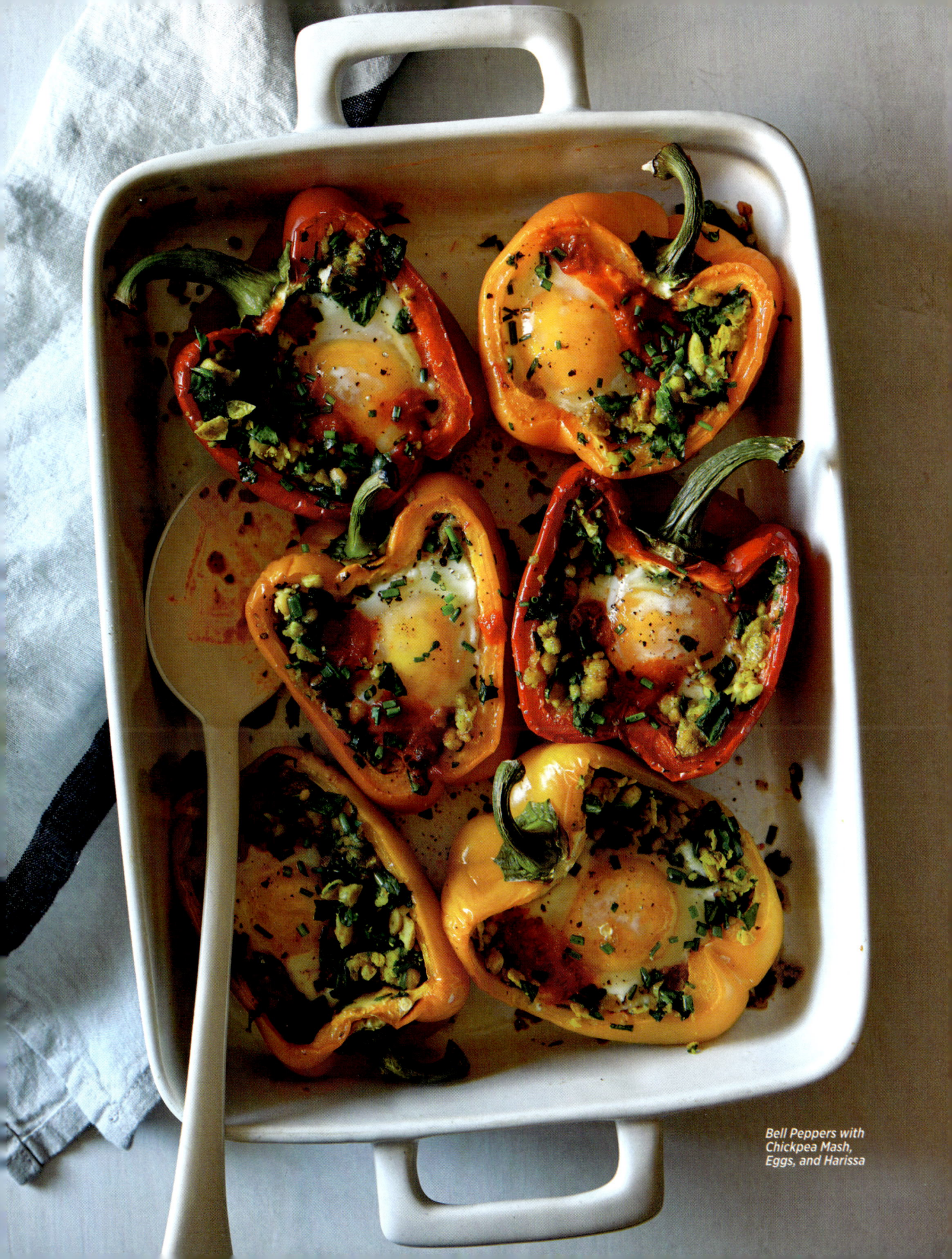

Bell Peppers with
Chickpea Mash,
Eggs, and Harissa

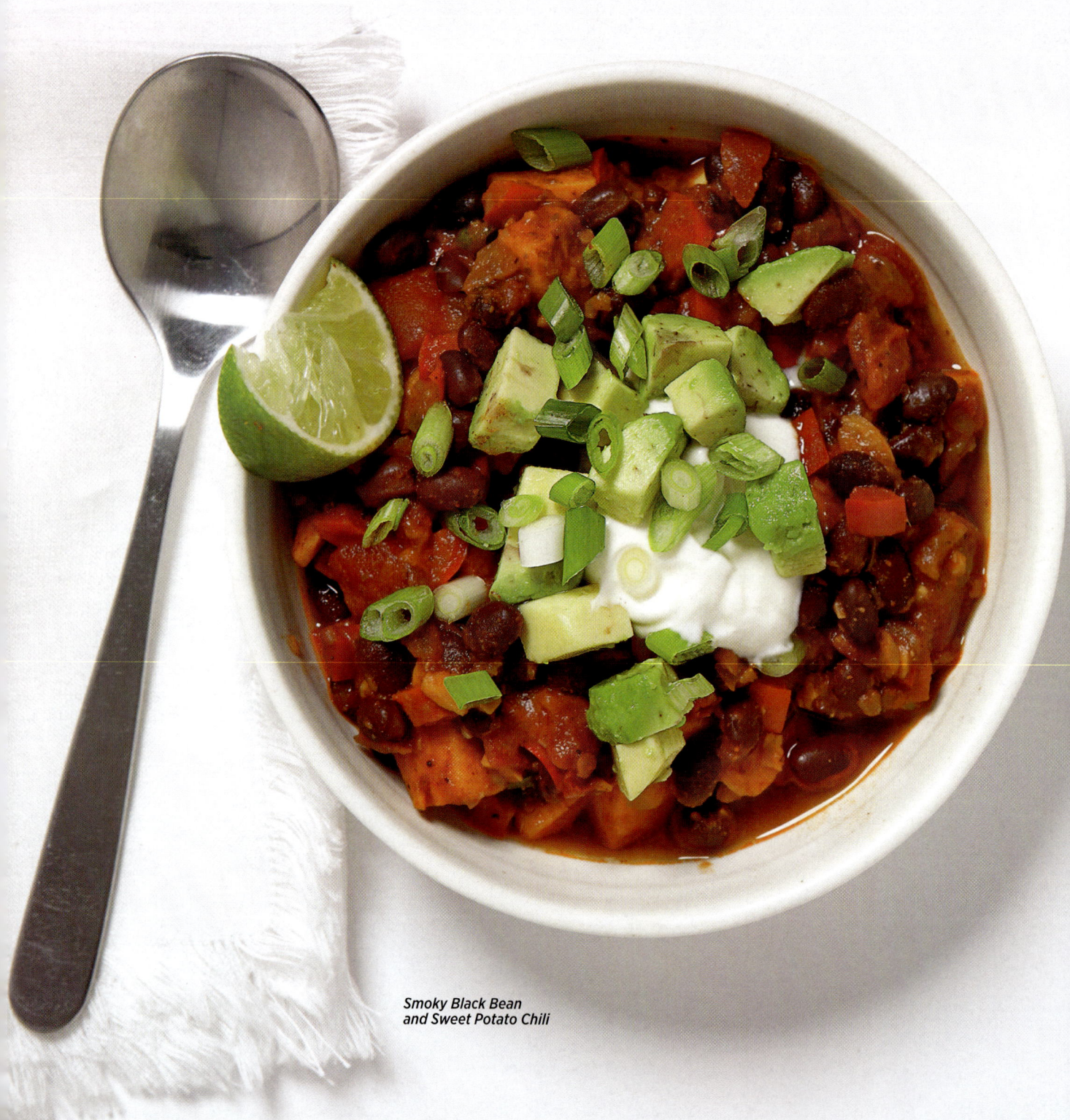

*Smoky Black Bean
and Sweet Potato Chili*

SMOKY BLACK BEAN AND SWEET POTATO CHILI

SERVES 4 • GLUTEN FREE • VEGETARIAN

1 tablespoon olive oil

1 onion, diced

1 large red bell pepper, diced

1 medium (8-ounce) sweet potato, peeled and cut into ¼-inch cubes

3 garlic cloves, finely chopped

2 tablespoons chili powder, or to taste

1 teaspoon ground cumin

1 teaspoon ground coriander

1 teaspoon dried oregano

½ teaspoon salt, or to taste

1 (14½-ounce) can diced tomatoes, with juice

1 cup vegetable broth

1 teaspoon finely chopped canned chipotles en adobo

1 (15-ounce) can black beans, rinsed and drained

½ avocado, diced

4 tablespoons light sour cream

1 scallion, thinly sliced

4 lime wedges

1 Heat oil in large heavy pot or Dutch oven over medium heat. Add onion and bell pepper; cook, stirring occasionally, until softened, 3–5 minutes.

2 Stir in sweet potato, garlic, chili powder, cumin, coriander, oregano, and salt; cook 1 minute. Add tomatoes and their juice, broth, and chipotles; bring to boil. Reduce heat, and simmer, covered, for 20 minutes. Stir in beans; simmer until sweet potato is tender and beans are heated through, about 3 minutes.

3 Serve topped with avocado, sour cream, scallions, and lime wedges.

7 SmartPoints value

Per serving (about 1½ cups chili, 2 tablespoons avocado, and 1 tablespoon sour cream): 296 Cal, 10 g Total Fat, 2 g Sat Fat, 1,173 mg Sod, 45 g Total Carb, 9 g Sugar, 15 g Fib, 11 g Prot.

COOK'S TIP

This vegetarian chili packs some heat. To make yours milder, scrape the seeds out of the chipotle and discard before chopping the pepper.

GREEK PORTOBELLO-CHICKPEA BURGERS

SERVES 6 ● VEGETARIAN

1 (15-ounce) can chickpeas, rinsed and drained

1 cup cooked whole wheat couscous

½ cup shredded carrot

½ cup crumbled feta

3 tablespoons chopped fresh dill

8 Kalamata olives, pitted and chopped

1 large egg white

¼ teaspoon salt, or to taste

6 (3½-inch) Portobello mushroom caps

6 tablespoons plain fat-free Greek yogurt

6 (¼-inch-thick) slices red onion

6 Boston lettuce leaves

6 thin slices tomato

1 Place chickpeas in food processor and pulse until finely chopped. Transfer chickpeas to medium bowl; stir in couscous, carrot, feta, 2 tablespoons dill, olives, egg white, and salt, stirring until mixture clumps together. Shape mixture into 6 (3-inch) patties. Spray patties with nonstick spray.

2 Spray large ridged grill pan with nonstick spray and place over medium-high heat. Place patties in pan and grill until golden brown and heated through, 3–4 minutes per side.

3 Meanwhile, scrape away gills from under mushroom caps with spoon. Mix yogurt and remaining 1 tablespoon dill in small bowl.

4 Place 1 chickpea patty in each upturned mushroom cap, gently pressing each to fill caps. Return burgers to one side of grill pan, mushroom side down. Spray onion slices with nonstick spray and add to other side of pan. Grill burgers until mushrooms are tender and onions are lightly charred, about 8 minutes, turning onions halfway through grilling time.

5 Serve each burger topped with 1 lettuce leaf, 1 tomato slice, 1 grilled onion slice, and 1 tablespoon yogurt-dill sauce.

4 SmartPoints value

Per serving (1 burger): 190 Cal, 5 g Total Fat, 2 g Sat Fat, 506 mg Sod, 27 g Total Carb, 6 g Sugar, 7 g Fib, 11 g Prot.

COOK'S TIP

You can also use cannellini beans in place of chickpeas for this recipe.

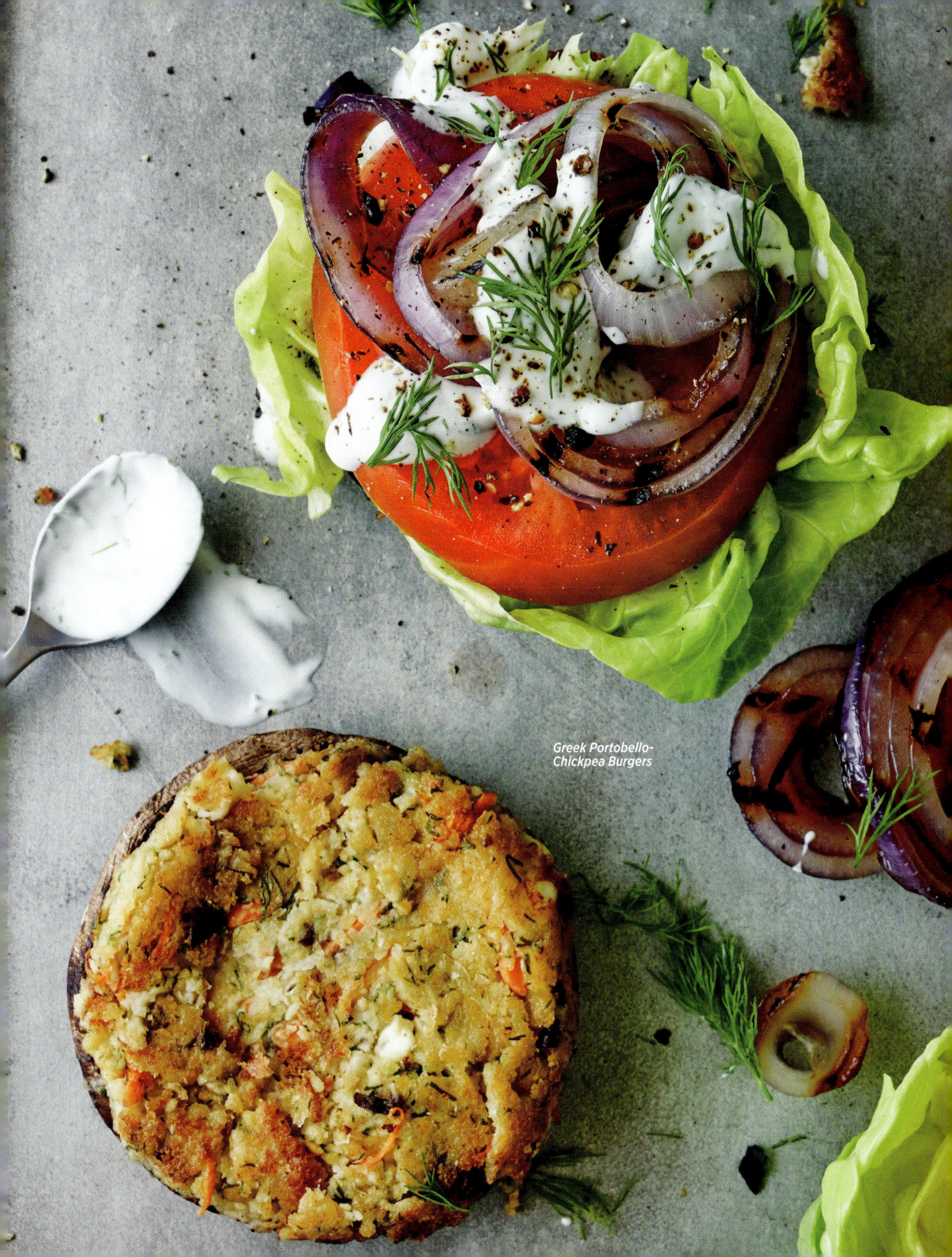

Greek Portobello-Chickpea Burgers

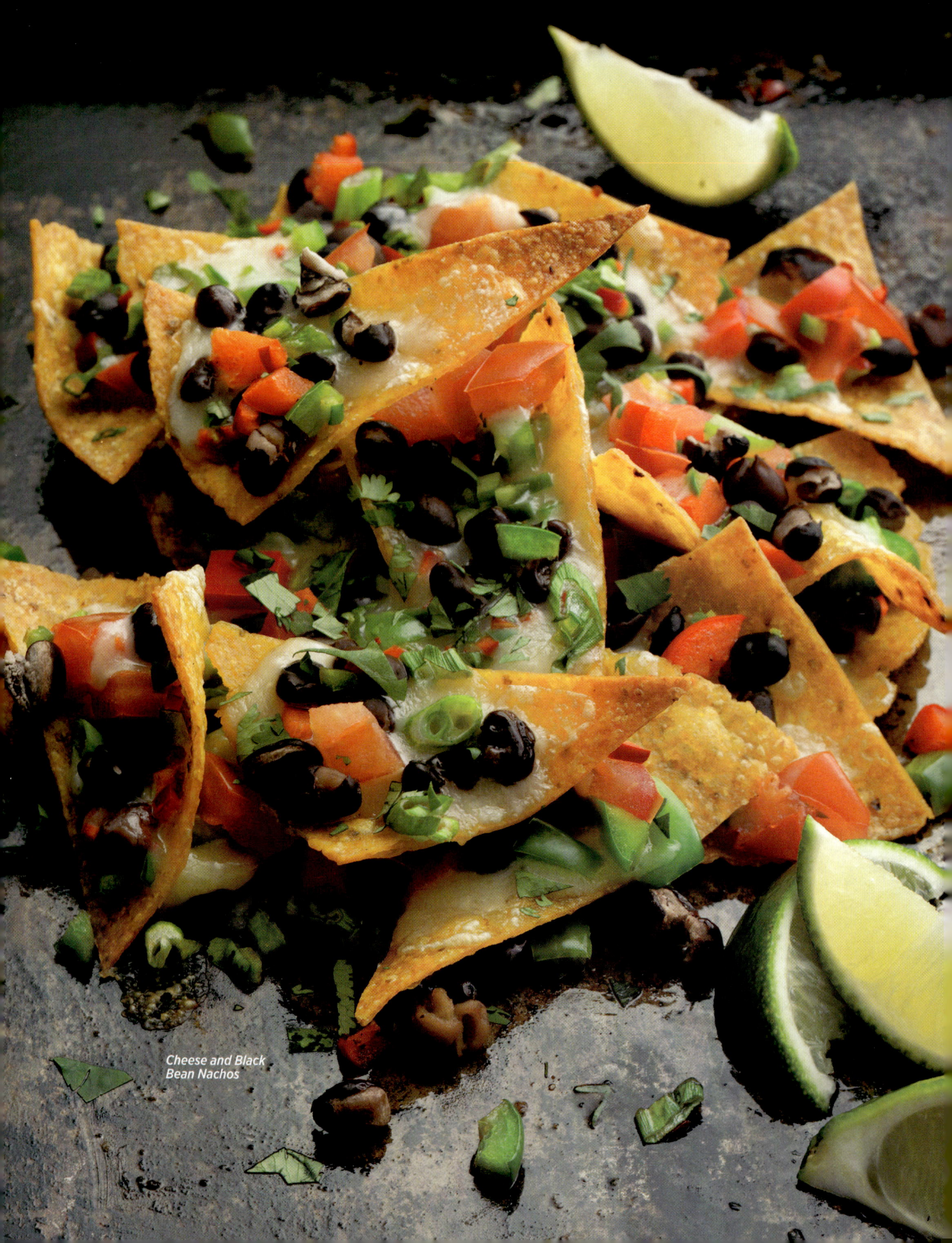

*Cheese and Black
Bean Nachos*

CHEESE AND BLACK BEAN NACHOS

SERVES 6 • GLUTEN FREE • VEGETARIAN

36 baked low-fat tortilla chips

1 (15-ounce) can black beans, rinsed and drained

2 scallions, thinly sliced

1 jalapeño pepper, seeded and minced

⅓ cup light sour cream

1 cup shredded fat-free Monterey Jack

2 plum tomatoes, seeded and chopped

3 tablespoons chopped fresh cilantro

Lime wedges

1 Preheat oven to 400°F. Spray 13 x 9-inch baking dish lightly with nonstick spray.

2 Arrange 24 tortilla chips in single layer in baking dish. Top with beans, scallions, and jalapeño, and dollop with sour cream.

3 Crush remaining 12 tortilla chips and sprinkle over sour cream. Top evenly with Monterey Jack. Bake until heated through and cheese is melted and bubbling, about 20 minutes. Sprinkle with tomatoes and cilantro. Serve with lime wedges.

6 SmartPoints value

Per serving (⅙ of dish): 217 Cal, 7 g Total Fat, 4 g Sat Fat, 508 mg Sod, 27 g Total Carb, 2 g Sugar, 7 g Fib, 12 g Prot.

UP THE PROTEIN

Sprinkle the nachos with 4 ounces crumbled or diced soy chorizo before baking for an additional 2 SmartPoints per serving.

CURRIED LENTILS WITH BUTTERNUT, KALE, AND COCONUT

SERVES 4 • VEGETARIAN

2 teaspoons olive oil

1 large onion, chopped

1 leek, halved lengthwise, rinsed, thinly sliced, and rinsed again

1 (32-ounce) container vegetable broth

1 pound peeled, halved, seeded, and diced butternut squash (about 2½ cups)

1 tablespoon curry powder

½ teaspoon ground cumin

½ teaspoon salt

Pinch cayenne

1 cup red lentils, picked over, rinsed and drained

3 cups lightly packed coarsely chopped kale leaves

½ cup light (low-fat) coconut milk

1 Heat oil in Dutch oven over medium-high heat. Add onion and leek and cook, stirring, until softened, about 3 minutes. Stir in broth, squash, curry powder, cumin, salt, and cayenne. Bring to boil. Adjust heat and simmer until squash begins to soften, about 10 minutes.

2 Stir in lentils and kale and cook until lentils begin to fall apart and vegetables are tender, 10–12 minutes. Stir in coconut milk and heat through.

3 SmartPoints value

Per serving (1½ cups): 165 Cal, 5 g Total Fat, 1 g Sat Fat, 992 mg Sod, 29 g Total Carb, 7 g Sugar, 5 g Fib, 5 g Prot.

UP THE PROTEIN

This delicious stew combines a host of terrific flavors. If you like, you can stir in 1⅓ cups rinsed and drained canned chickpeas for an additional 2 SmartPoints per serving.

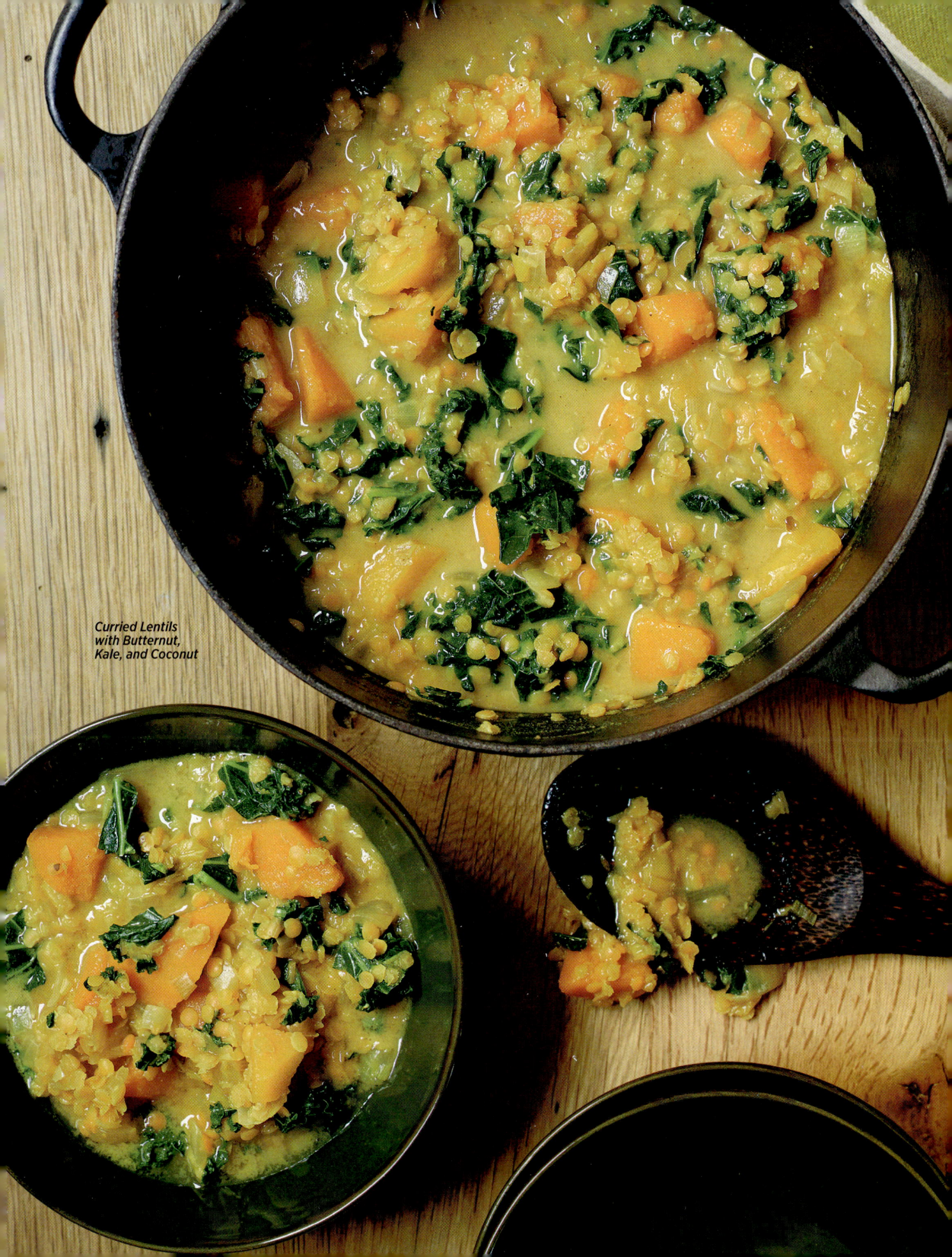

Curried Lentils with Butternut, Kale, and Coconut

LENTIL SALAD WITH FRESH
MINT AND GOAT CHEESE

SERVES 6 • GLUTEN FREE • VEGETARIAN

1½ cups dry green (French) lentils, picked over and rinsed

2 bay leaves

½ small red onion, coarsely chopped

¼ cup fresh mint leaves, coarsely chopped

½ teaspoon salt, or to taste

¼ teaspoon black pepper

½ cup semisoft goat cheese, crumbled

1 Place lentils in medium saucepan and add enough water to cover lentils by 2–3 inches. Add bay leaves and bring to boil over high heat. Reduce heat to medium and partially cover pan; simmer until lentils are tender, 15–20 minutes. Drain; discard bay leaves and transfer lentils to large bowl.

2 While lentils are still warm, stir in onion, mint, salt, and pepper. Sprinkle goat cheese over salad just before serving; serve warm or chilled.

7 SmartPoints value

Per serving (about ¾ cup lentil salad and scant 1½ tablespoons cheese): 235 Cal, 6 g Total Fat, 4 g Sat Fat, 276 mg Sod, 28 g Total Carb, 1 g Sugar, 15 g Fib, 17 g Prot.

COOK'S TIP

Green French lentils, sometimes called Le Puy lentils, hold their shape better than most other varieties, making them ideal for salads like this one. Black lentils are also a good option.

STUFFED PEPPERS WITH SAVORY QUINOA

SERVES 4 • GLUTEN FREE • VEGETARIAN

1 teaspoon olive oil

1 small onion, diced

1½ teaspoons kosher salt, or to taste

1 teaspoon minced garlic

1 (14½-ounce) can Italian-style diced tomatoes

1 cup quinoa, rinsed well

1 cup water

4 red bell peppers

10 Kalamata olives, pitted and chopped

1 cup canned chickpeas, rinsed and drained

1½ tablespoons prepared pesto

⅓ cup crumbled feta

1 Preheat oven to 375°F. Line baking sheet with foil and spray with nonstick spray.

2 Heat oil in medium saucepan over medium heat. Add onion and ½ teaspoon salt; cook, stirring occasionally, until onion softens, 5–7 minutes. Add garlic and cook, stirring, 30 seconds more. Add tomatoes and their liquid, quinoa, water, and remaining 1 teaspoon salt; stir to combine. Increase heat to high and bring to boil; reduce heat to low and simmer, covered, until quinoa is tender, about 15 minutes.

3 Meanwhile, slice top off each bell pepper and remove core, ribs, and seeds; reserve tops for another use. Cut thin slice from bottom of each pepper so they sit flat; place on prepared baking sheet.

4 Combine quinoa mixture, olives, chickpeas, and pesto. Spoon about 1 cup mixture into each bell pepper; bake, uncovered, 25 minutes. Remove from oven and sprinkle each pepper with a heaping tablespoon of feta; return peppers to oven and continue baking until cheese is slightly melted, about 5 minutes more.

6 SmartPoints value

Per serving (1 stuffed pepper): 224 Cal, 7 g Total Fat, 2 g Sat Fat, 683 mg Sod, 32 g Total Carb, 4 g Sugar, 6 g Fib, 9 g Prot.

COOK'S TIP

Quinoa grows with a bitter, protective coating called saponin on its grains, so giving it a good rinse in a fine-mesh sieve is essential before cooking.

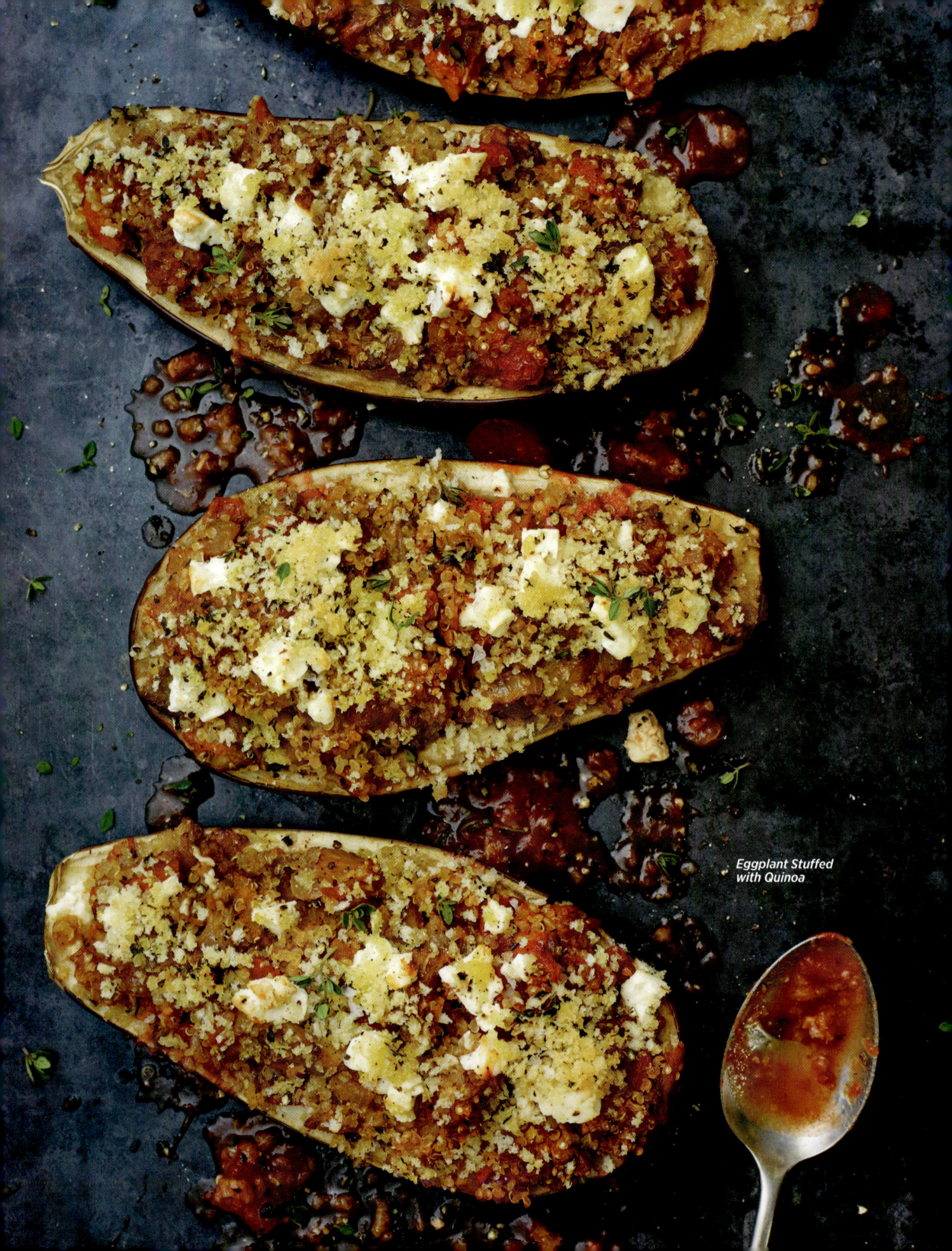

Eggplant Stuffed with Quinoa

EGGPLANT STUFFED WITH QUINOA

SERVES 4 ● VEGETARIAN

2 small (12-ounce) eggplants, halved lengthwise, stem end trimmed

3 teaspoons olive oil

1 onion, chopped

3 garlic cloves, finely chopped

¾ teaspoon salt

1 (14½-ounce) can diced tomatoes, drained and juice reserved

1 cup refrigerated meatless veggie sausage

¾ cup cooked quinoa

¼ teaspoon black pepper

⅓ cup crumbled reduced-fat feta

¼ cup whole wheat panko (Japanese bread crumbs)

1 teaspoon chopped fresh thyme

1 Preheat oven to 400°F. Spray 9 x 13-inch baking dish lightly with nonstick spray.

2 Run paring knife around inside of each eggplant ½ inch from edge. Scoop out flesh with spoon leaving ½-inch-thick shells. Coarsely chop flesh.

3 Heat 2 teaspoons oil in large nonstick skillet over medium heat. Add onion and cook, covered, until softened, about 4 minutes. Stir in garlic and cook until fragrant, about 1 minute. Stir in chopped eggplant and ¼ teaspoon salt; cover and cook, stirring occasionally, until eggplant is tender, about 7 minutes. Remove skillet from heat and stir in tomatoes, veggie sausage, quinoa, pepper, and ¼ teaspoon salt.

4 Sprinkle eggplant shells with remaining ¼ teaspoon salt. Spoon filling into shells and place in prepared baking dish; sprinkle evenly with feta. Add enough water to reserved tomato juice to equal ¾ cup. Pour around eggplant into bottom of baking dish. Mix panko, thyme, and remaining 1 teaspoon oil in small bowl. Sprinkle over filling. Cover baking dish with foil. Bake 25 minutes. Uncover and bake until eggplant shells are tender and crumbs are browned, about another 15 minutes.

5 SmartPoints value

Per serving (1 stuffed eggplant half): 268 Cal, 9 g Total Fat, 2 g Sat Fat, 966 mg Sod, 34 g Total Carb, 8 g Sugar, 9 g Fib, 17 g Prot.

COOK'S TIP

Browned, crunchy panko crumbs are a delicious topping for this dish. If you'd like yours even crisper, you can place the baked eggplants under the broiler for 1 to 2 minutes.

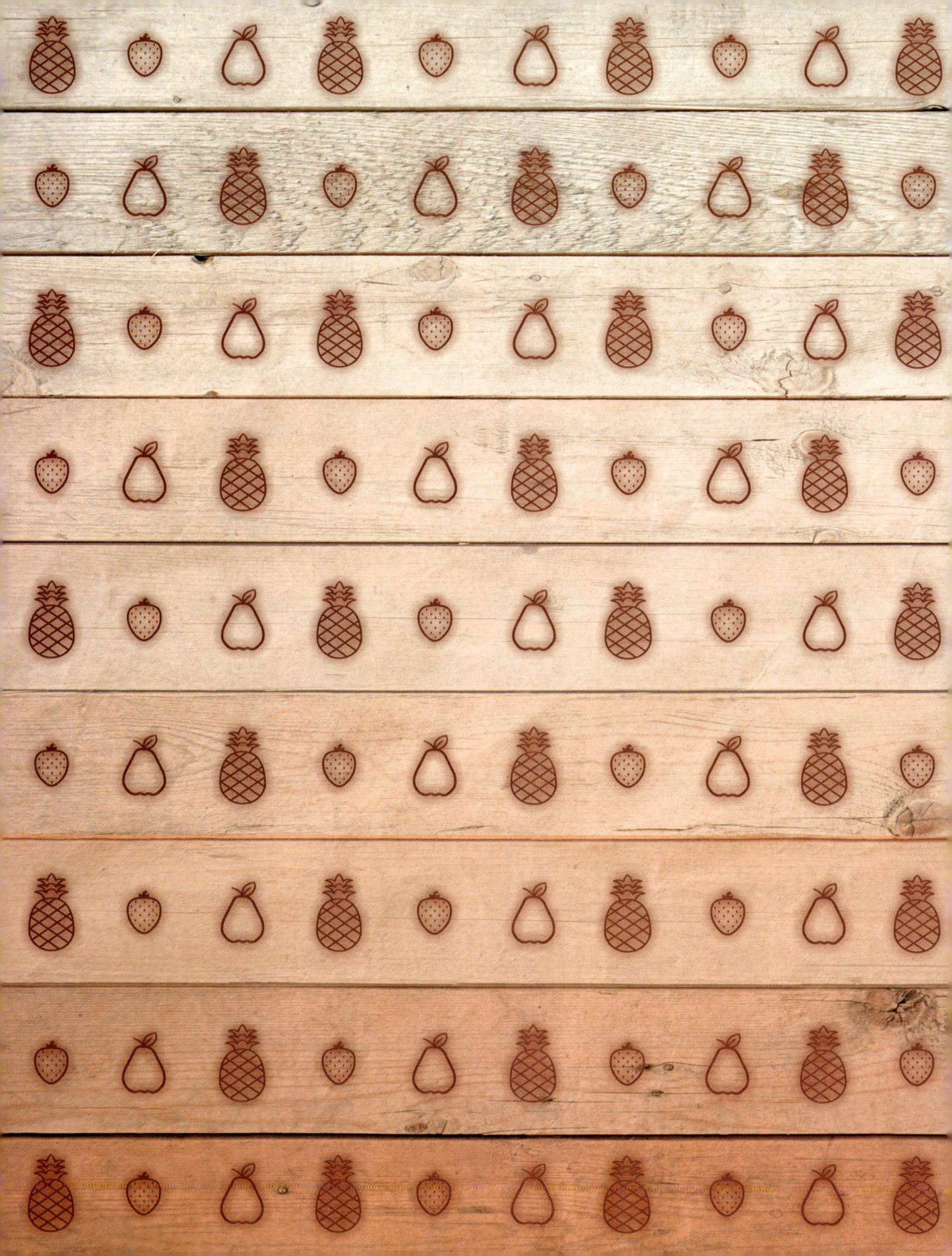

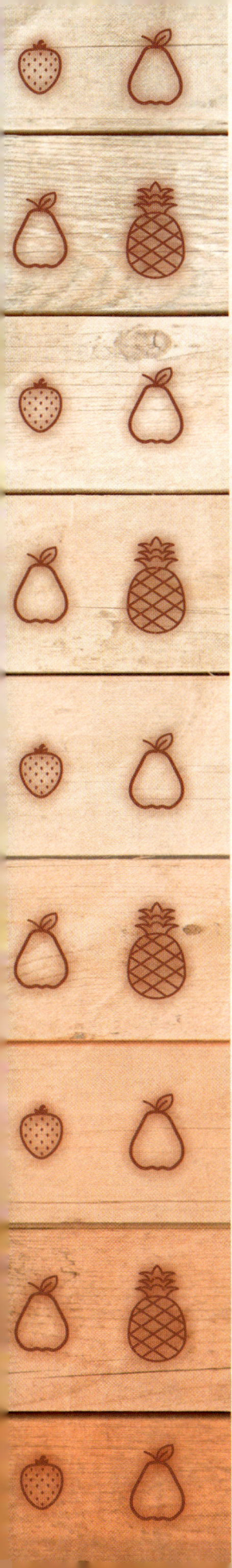

CHAPTER 6

FRUIT DESSERTS: CAKES TARTS & MORE

IN THIS CHAPTER

APRICOT-CHERRY CLAFOUTI

SERVES 8 • VEGETARIAN

5 ripe apricots, halved and pitted

1 cup fresh or frozen unsweetened cherries

⅓ cup granulated sugar

3 tablespoons all-purpose flour

⅛ teaspoon salt

2 large eggs

½ cup low-fat (1%) milk

¼ cup light sour cream

1 teaspoon vanilla extract

2 teaspoons confectioners' sugar

1 Preheat oven to 350°F. Spray 10-inch pie plate with nonstick spray.

2 Arrange apricots, cut side up, in pie plate. Place cherries around apricots.

3 Whisk granulated sugar, flour, and salt together in large bowl. Whisk eggs, milk, sour cream, and vanilla together in small bowl. Add egg mixture to sugar mixture and whisk until blended. Pour batter over fruit. Bake until puffed and golden brown, 40–45 minutes.

4 Sprinkle top of clafouti with confectioners' sugar. Cut into 8 wedges and serve warm.

4 SmartPoints value

Per serving: (1 wedge): 105 Cal, 3 g Total Fat, 1 g Sat Fat, 65 mg Sod, 17 g Total Carb, 14 g Sugar, 1 g Fib, 3 g Prot.

COOK'S TIP

You can substitute plums or quartered peaches or nectarines for the apricots in this recipe.

ANGEL FOOD CAKE WITH PEACH-BOURBON SAUCE

SERVES 16 • VEGETARIAN

1¼ cups sugar

1 cup cake flour

¼ teaspoon salt

12 large egg whites

1½ teaspoons cream of tartar

1½ teaspoons vanilla extract

¼ teaspoon almond extract

6 cups thinly sliced peaches

2 tablespoons packed brown sugar

1 tablespoon bourbon

1 Position oven rack in lower third of oven; preheat oven to 350°F.

2 Put sugar in food processor and pulse for 1 minute. Remove and reserve ¾ cup. Add flour and salt to remaining sugar in processor and pulse about 30 seconds.

3 With electric mixer on medium-low speed, beat egg whites in large bowl until foamy, about 1 minute. Beat in cream of tartar. Increase speed to mediumand beat in reserved ¾ cup sugar, 1 tablespoon at a time, beating well after each addition. Once all sugar has been added, increase speed to medium- high and beat until stiff peaks form when beaters are lifted. Beat in vanilla and almond extracts.

4 Sift flour mixture, one-third at a time, over beaten egg whites, gently folding with rubber spatula just until blended. (Be careful not to overmix.) Scrape batter into ungreased 10-inch tube pan with removable bottom. Spread evenly. Bake until cake springs back when lightly pressed, 35–40 minutes.

5 Meanwhile, combine peaches, brown sugar, and bourbon in medium bowl. Let stand at least 10 minutes, or refrigerate up to 2 days.

6 When cake is done, immediately invert pan onto its legs or over neck of bottle and let cool completely. Run thin knife around sides and center tube of pan. Remove cake from pan and transfer to serving plate. Cut into 16 slices and serve with peach mixture.

5 SmartPoints value

Per serving (1 slice cake and ¼ cup peaches): 119 Cal, 0 g Total Fat, 0 g Sat Fat, 78 mg Sod, 25 g Total Carb, 18 g Sugar, 0 g Fib, 3 g Prot.

COOK'S TIP

Processing sugar in a food processor makes it superfine, giving this cake a finer texture. Processing the sugar again with the flour helps aerate it, keeping the cake light.

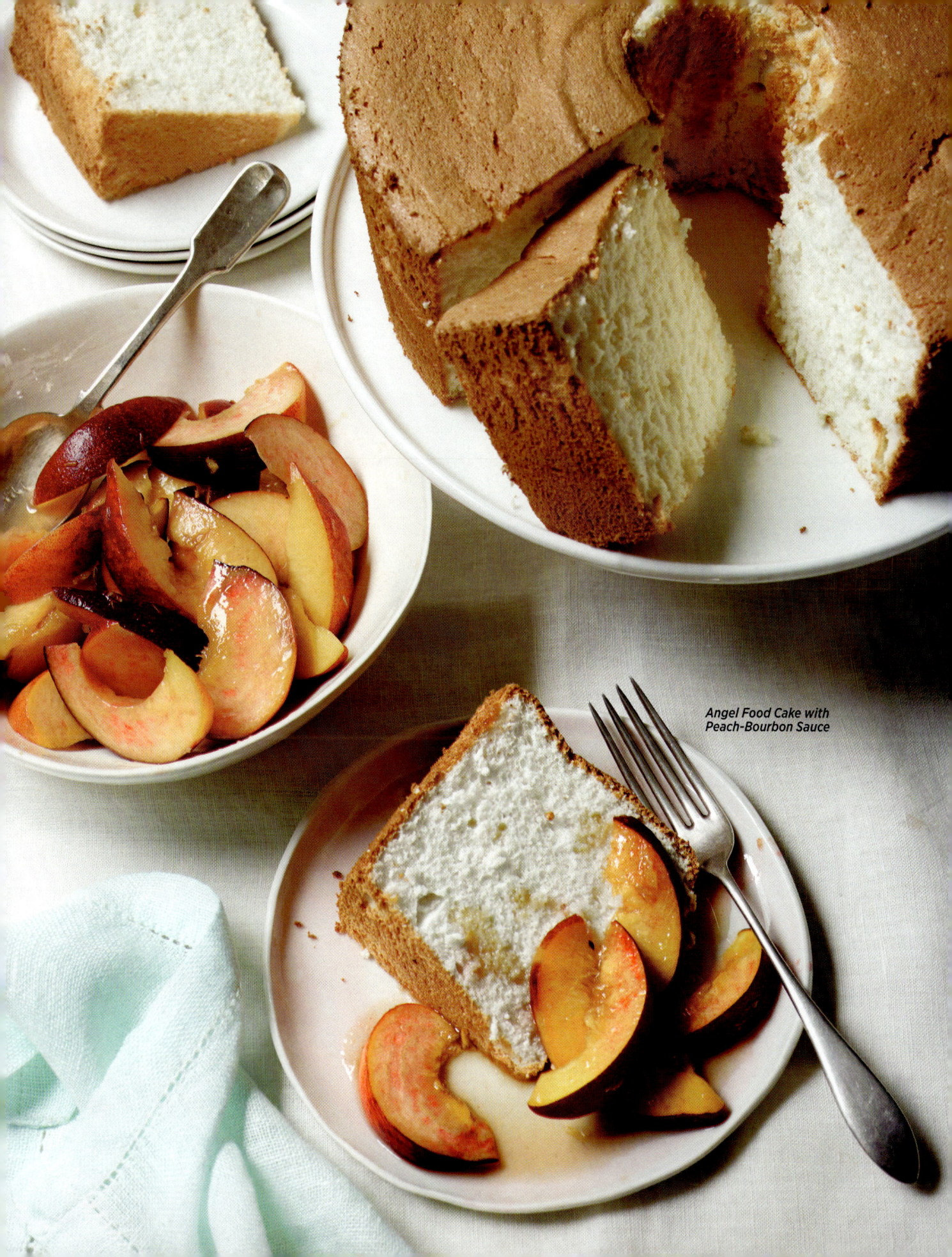

Angel Food Cake with
Peach-Bourbon Sauce

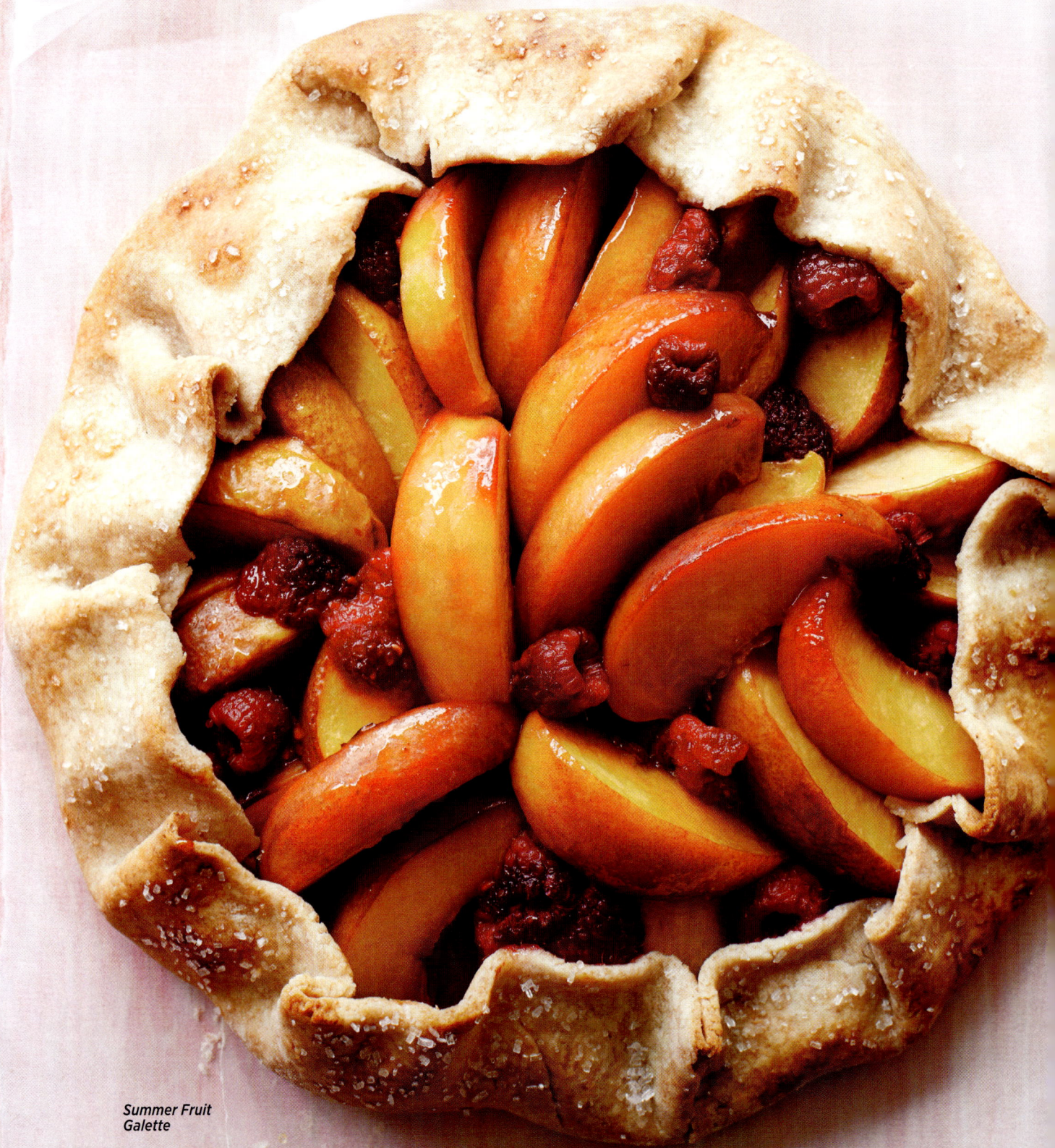

*Summer Fruit
Galette*

SUMMER FRUIT GALETTE

SERVES 10 • VEGETARIAN

CRUST:

1¼ cups white whole wheat flour

1 tablespoon sugar

½ teaspoon salt

3 tablespoons canola oil

1 tablespoon cold butter, cut into pieces

3–4 tablespoons ice water

FILLING:

1¼ pounds nectarines, halved, pitted, and cut into ½-inch wedges

6 ounces raspberries

⅓ cup plus 1 teaspoon sugar

1 teaspoon lemon juice

Pinch salt

2 teaspoons fat-free milk

1 To make crust, pulse flour, sugar, and salt in food processor until blended. Add oil and butter; pulse until mixture resembles coarse crumbs. Add 3 tablespoons ice water through feed tube and pulse until dough forms; if dough doesn't come together, add remaining 1 tablespoon water and pulse. Shape dough into disk, wrap in plastic, and refrigerate until firm, at least 30 minutes or up to 1 day.

2 To make filling, combine nectarines, raspberries, ⅓ cup sugar, lemon juice, and salt in medium bowl.

3 Preheat oven to 375°F. Cover large baking sheet with parchment paper.

4 On lightly floured surface with lightly floured rolling pin, roll out dough to 13-inch round; transfer to baking sheet. Mound filling over dough leaving 3-inch border. Fold edge of dough up and over filling, pleating as you go. Brush edges of dough with milk; sprinkle with remaining 1 teaspoon sugar.

5 Bake until filling is tender and crust is browned, 35–40 minutes. Slide galette and parchment onto rack. Slip out parchment and discard. Cool galette and cut into 10 wedges.

5 SmartPoints value

Per serving (1 wedge): 167 Cal, 6 g Total Fat, 1 g Sat Fat, 155 mg Sod, 27 g Total Carb, 15 g Sugar, 2 g Fib, 3 g Prot.

COOK'S TIP

You can also use peaches and blueberries in this delicious free-form tart.

TROPICAL CHEESECAKE TARTS

SERVES 30 • VEGETARIAN

30 mini phyllo shells

1 large mango, ½ cut in 30 small chunks, ½ sliced

8 ounces light cream cheese (Neufchâtel), at room temperature

2 tablespoons confectioners' sugar

1 teaspoon lime juice, or more to taste

½ teaspoon grated lime zest, plus extra for garnish

1 Preheat oven to 350°F. Place phyllo shells on baking sheet and bake until lightly toasted, about 5 minutes; let cool.

2 Puree sliced mango in food processor or mini chopper; place in medium bowl. Add cream cheese, confectioners' sugar, lime juice, and lime zest and stir until smooth.

3 Fill baked phyllo shells evenly with cream cheese mixture. (To fill shells quickly, spoon mixture into plastic zip-close bag, snip off one corner, and pipe mixture into shells.) Garnish each shell with mango chunk. Refrigerate until filling firms slightly, about 30 minutes. Garnish with lime zest before serving.

1 SmartPoints value

Per serving (1 tart): 42 Cal, 2 g Total Fat, 1 g Sat Fat, 37 mg Sod, 5 g Total Carb, 3 g Sugar, 0 g Fib, 1 g Prot.

COOK'S TIP

Try other tropical fruits such as pineapple or papaya in these easy tropical treats.

PEAR CRISP WITH STAR ANISE

SERVES 8 • VEGETARIAN

5 medium Bartlett or Anjou pears, cored, cut in ¼-inch-thick slices

¼ cup packed dark brown sugar

1½ teaspoons lemon juice

½ tablespoon pear brandy or regular brandy

¼ cup old-fashioned oats

2 tablespoons all-purpose flour

½ teaspoon finely ground star anise

½ teaspoon cinnamon

¼ teaspoon salt

1 tablespoon unsalted butter, melted

1 Preheat oven to 375°F.

2 Place pears in 8-inch-square baking dish; sprinkle with 2 teaspoons brown sugar. Drizzle lemon juice and brandy over top; gently toss to coat and arrange pear slices in even layer.

3 Combine oats, remaining brown sugar, flour, star anise, cinnamon, and salt in food processor; pulse a few times to blend. Add butter; pulse until mixture is crumbly, then scatter mixture evenly over pears.

4 Bake until pears are tender and top is golden and bubbling, about 45 minutes. Cut into 8 pieces; serve warm or at room temperature.

3 SmartPoints value

Per serving (1 piece): 128 Cal, 2 g Total Fat, 1 g Sat Fat, 76 mg Sod, 27 g Total Carb, 17 g Sugar, 4 g Fib, 1 g Prot.

COOK'S TIP

Star anise is a star-shaped, dark brown pod. It lends wonderful flavor to baked goods thanks to its strong flavor. If you can't find it ground, you can also substitute Chinese five-spice powder in this recipe.

STRAWBERRY NAPOLEON

SERVES 12 • VEGETARIAN

6 sheets phyllo, thawed if frozen

6 teaspoons plus 3 tablespoons granulated sugar

3 ounces light cream cheese (Neufchâtel), softened

½ cup light sour cream

2 teaspoons finely grated lemon zest

¾ cup light whipped topping

4 cups strawberries, hulled and thinly sliced

1 teaspoon confectioners' sugar

1 Preheat oven to 350°F. Place 1 sheet phyllo on baking sheet, spray with nonstick spray and sprinkle with 1 teaspoon granulated sugar; repeat with remaining phyllo sheets and another 5 teaspoons granulated sugar, spraying each with nonstick spray and stacking them. Cut the stacked phyllo lengthwise into 3 strips and prick all over with fork. Bake 12–15 minutes or until golden; transfer to wire rack to cool completely.

2 With electric mixer on medium speed, beat cream cheese in bowl until fluffy. Add remaining 3 tablespoons granulated sugar, sour cream, and lemon zest. Continue to beat until light and airy; fold in whipped topping with rubber spatula.

3 Carefully place 1 phyllo strip on serving platter and spread with half the cream cheese mixture; top with half the strawberries. Repeat with second phyllo strip and remaining cheese mixture and berries. Top with third phyllo strip and sprinkle with confectioner's sugar. Cut into 12 pieces with serrated knife.

4 SmartPoints value

Per serving (1 piece): 109 Cal, 4 g Total Fat, 2 g Sat Fat, 83 mg Sod, 16 g Total Carb, 9 g Sugar, 1 g Fib, 2 g Prot.

COOK'S TIP

To give desserts an even, professional-looking finish, put confectioners' sugar in a small metal strainer; hold the strainer about 8 inches above the dessert and very gently tap the edge of the strainer as you move it slowly over the top.

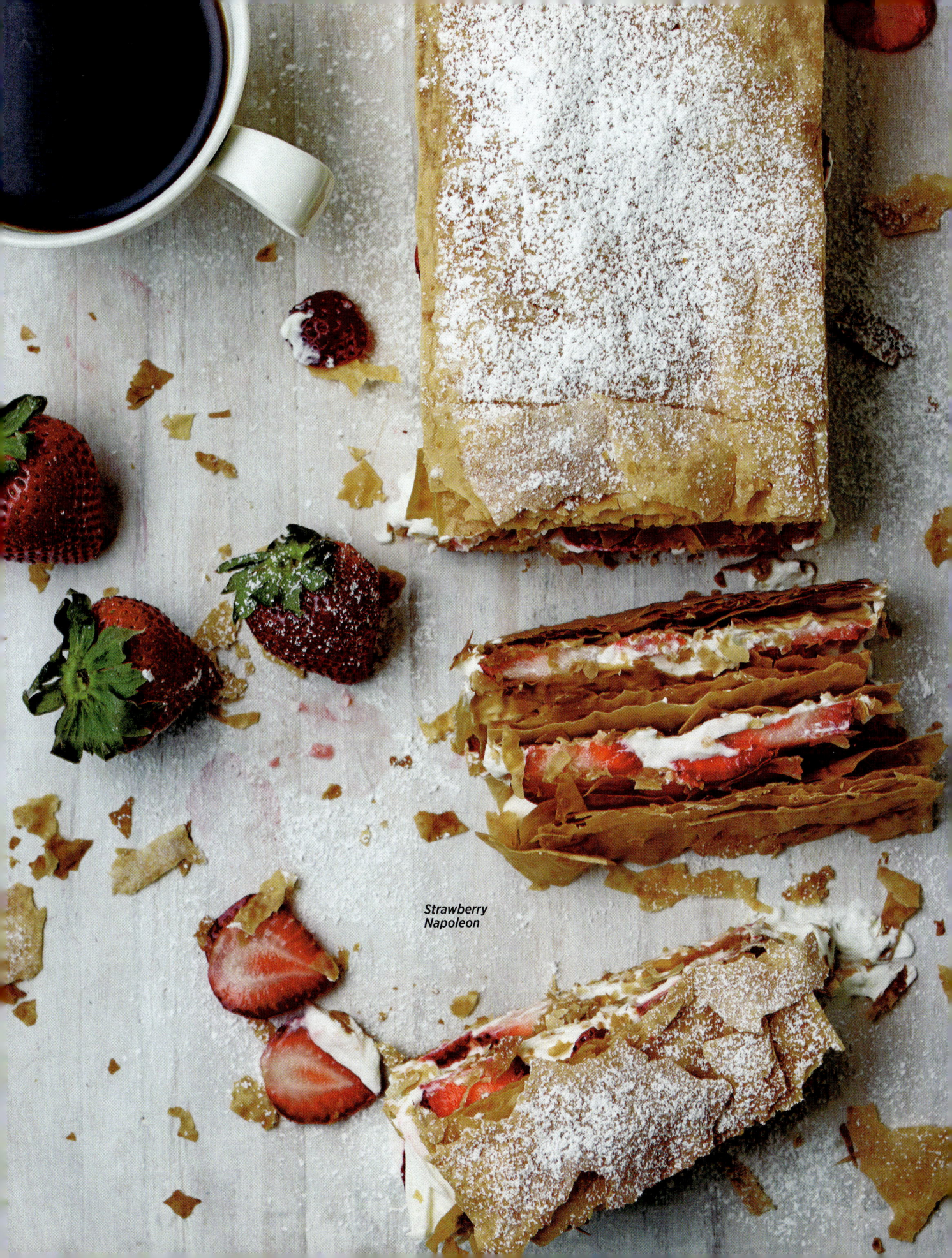

*Strawberry
Napoleon*

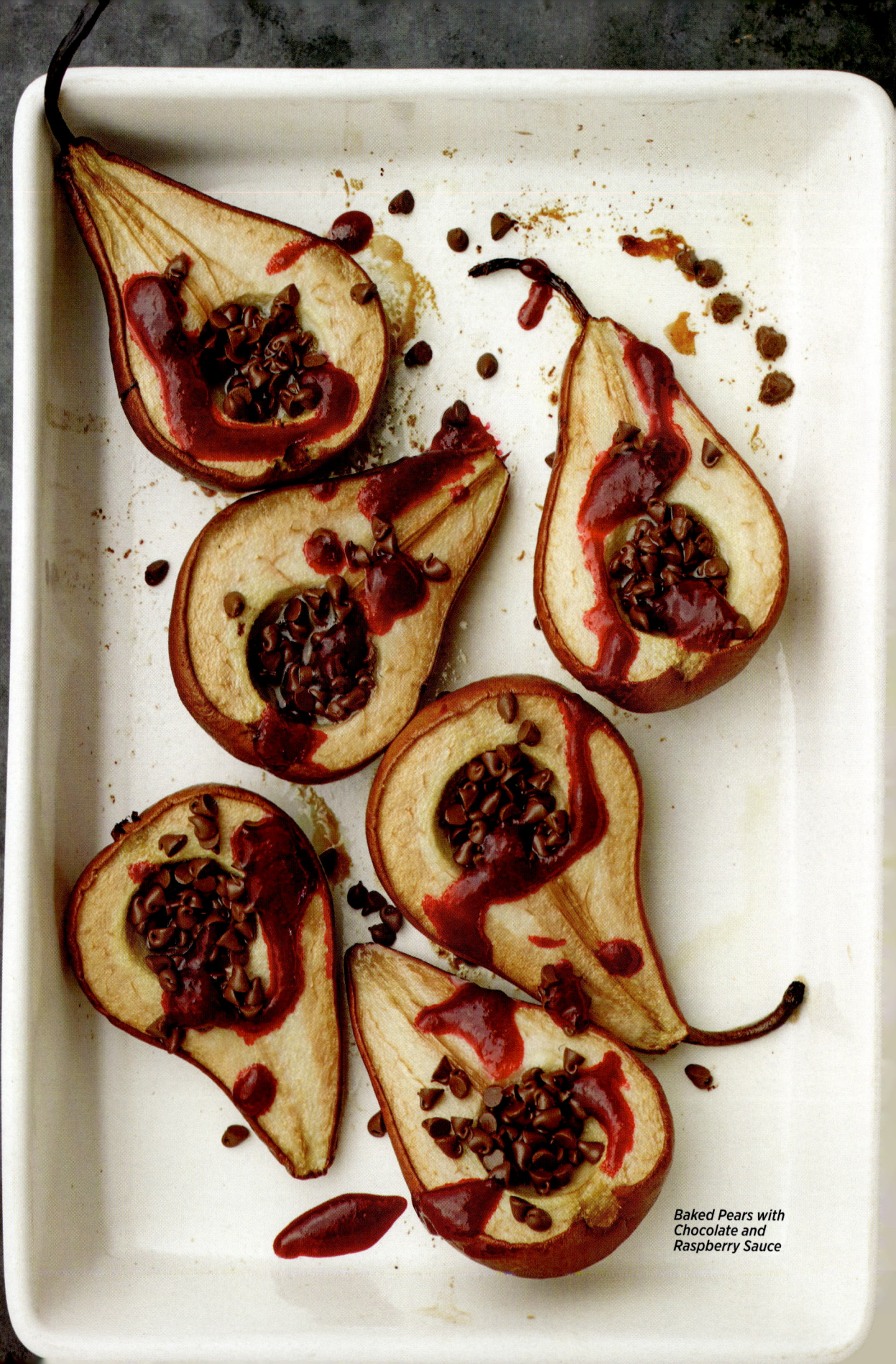

Baked Pears with Chocolate and Raspberry Sauce

BAKED PEARS WITH CHOCOLATE AND RASPBERRY SAUCE

SERVES 6 • GLUTEN FREE • VEGETARIAN

3 medium ripe but firm pears, halved and cored

½ teaspoon salted butter, melted

1 cup unsweetened frozen raspberries

1 tablespoon sugar

2 tablespoons semisweet chocolate chips, chopped, or mini chocolate chips

1 Preheat oven to 350°F.

2 Arrange pears, cut sides up, in shallow baking dish; brush with melted butter. Bake until tender, 30–35 minutes.

3 Meanwhile, put raspberries and sugar in small saucepan; bring to simmer over medium-high heat, mashing berries with wooden spoon against bottom and sides of pan. Reduce heat to low; simmer until raspberries are very soft, about 2 minutes. Remove pan from heat and strain sauce through sieve, pressing on mixture to extract as much liquid as possible; set aside.

4 When pears are finished baking, turn off oven. Remove baking dish from oven and fill each pear cavity with ½ teaspoon chocolate chips; return to oven until chocolate melts, about 5 minutes.

5 Remove pears from oven; let stand 1 minute. Drizzle with raspberry sauce or spoon sauce on plates and place pear half on top.

2 SmartPoints value **Per serving** (1 pear half and 2 teaspoons raspberry sauce): 88 Cal, 2 g Total Fat, 1 g Sat Fat, 4 mg Sod, 20 g Total Carb, 13 g Sugar, 4 g Fib, 1 g Prot.

COOK'S TIP

Roasting pears intensifies their sweetness. Filling their core with chocolate and drizzling them with raspberry sauce is a wonderful finishing touch.

FRESH STRAWBERRY CRÊPES

SERVES 8 • VEGETARIAN

5 large egg whites

1 cup fat-free milk

1½ tablespoons unsalted butter, melted

1 teaspoon vanilla extract

⅛ teaspoon salt

1 cup all-purpose flour

1 pound strawberries, hulled and sliced very thin (about 3 cups)

¼ cup confectioners' sugar

1 Whisk egg whites, milk, melted butter, vanilla, and salt together in medium bowl. Whisk in flour just until combined.

2 Spray 8- or 9-inch skillet or crêpe pan with nonstick spray; set over medium heat. When pan is hot, add ¼ cup batter and swirl to coat bottom of pan with thin layer of batter. Cook 2 minutes; flip crêpe. Top with about ⅓ cup strawberries; cook 2 minutes more. Fold crêpe over and slide onto serving plate; cover to keep warm. Repeat with remaining ingredients. Sprinkle crêpes with confectioners' sugar.

4 SmartPoints value

Per serving (1 crêpe): 131 Cal, 3 g Total Fat, 1 g Sat Fat, 85 mg Sod, 22 g Total Carb, 8 g Sugar, 2 g Fib, 5 g Prot.

UP THE PROTEIN

These crêpes make a terrific not-too-sweet dessert. You can make them more substantial by filling each one with an added 2 tablespoons part-skim ricotta for an additional 1 SmartPoints or with 2 tablespoons (1 ounce) goat cheese for 3 SmartPoints more.

MAPLE-PECAN GRILLED BANANAS

SERVES 4 • GLUTEN FREE • VEGETARIAN

2 large medium-ripe bananas
2 tablespoons chopped pecans
¼ teaspoon cinnamon
2 teaspoons maple syrup

1 Trim stem ends of bananas; halve lengthwise through peels (leave peels on) and set aside.

2 Put pecans in small nonstick skillet; cook over medium heat, shaking pan frequently, until pecans smell toasted, about 4 minutes. Remove from heat; set aside.

3 Off heat, spray an outdoor grill rack or ridged stovetop grill pan with nonstick spray; heat to medium.

4 Sprinkle cut sides of bananas with cinnamon; lightly brush with 1 teaspoon maple syrup. Cook bananas, cut sides down, until grill marks appear, 2–3 minutes. Turn and cook until bananas start to pull away from peel and soften, 3–5 minutes.

5 Transfer bananas to serving platter. Brush cut sides of bananas with remaining 1 teaspoon maple syrup; sprinkle with pecans (dust with additional cinnamon if desired).

1 SmartPoints value · **Per serving** (1 banana half with ½ tablespoon pecans): 93 Cal, 3 g Total Fat, 0 g Sat Fat, 1 mg Sod, 18 g Total Carb, 10 g Sugar, 2 g Fib, 1 g Prot.

COOK'S TIP

Bananas grill right in their skins and become deliciously caramelized with a coating of maple syrup. They're a terrific light dessert by themselves, or you can chop them and serve over Greek yogurt, low-fat ice cream, or whole-grain waffles.

BROILED PINEAPPLE WITH CANDIED GINGER YOGURT CREAM

SERVES 4 • GLUTEN FREE • VEGETARIAN • UNDER 20 MINUTES

¼ cup plain low-fat Greek yogurt

1 tablespoon minced crystallized ginger

1 medium pineapple, peeled, cored, and cut into 12 rounds

1½ tablespoons light brown sugar

½ teaspoon ground allspice

Fresh mint leaves (optional)

1 Set oven rack about 5 inches from broiler; preheat broiler.

2 Place yogurt in small bowl and stir in ginger; set aside.

3 Place 3 slices pineapple in each of 4 small (10-inch) oval gratin dishes, overlapping them slightly; sprinkle with brown sugar and allspice. Broil pineapple until bubbling and lightly caramelized, about 8 minutes (check once or twice to make sure pineapple isn't getting too dark).

4 Remove pineapple from oven; top each dish with 1 rounded tablespoon yogurt. Garnish with mint (if using) and serve warm.

1 SmartPoints value

Per serving (3 slices pineapple with 1 tablespoon topping): 85 Cal, 0 g Total Fat, 0 g Sat Fat, 8 mg Sod, 20 g Total Carb, 16 g Sugar, 1 g Fib, 2 g Prot.

COOK'S TIP

Crystallized ginger imparts a ton of fabulous flavor to yogurt. It's a wonderful topping for almost any type of broiled or baked fruit. Look for it in the bulk-foods section of natural foods stores so you don't have to buy more then you need.

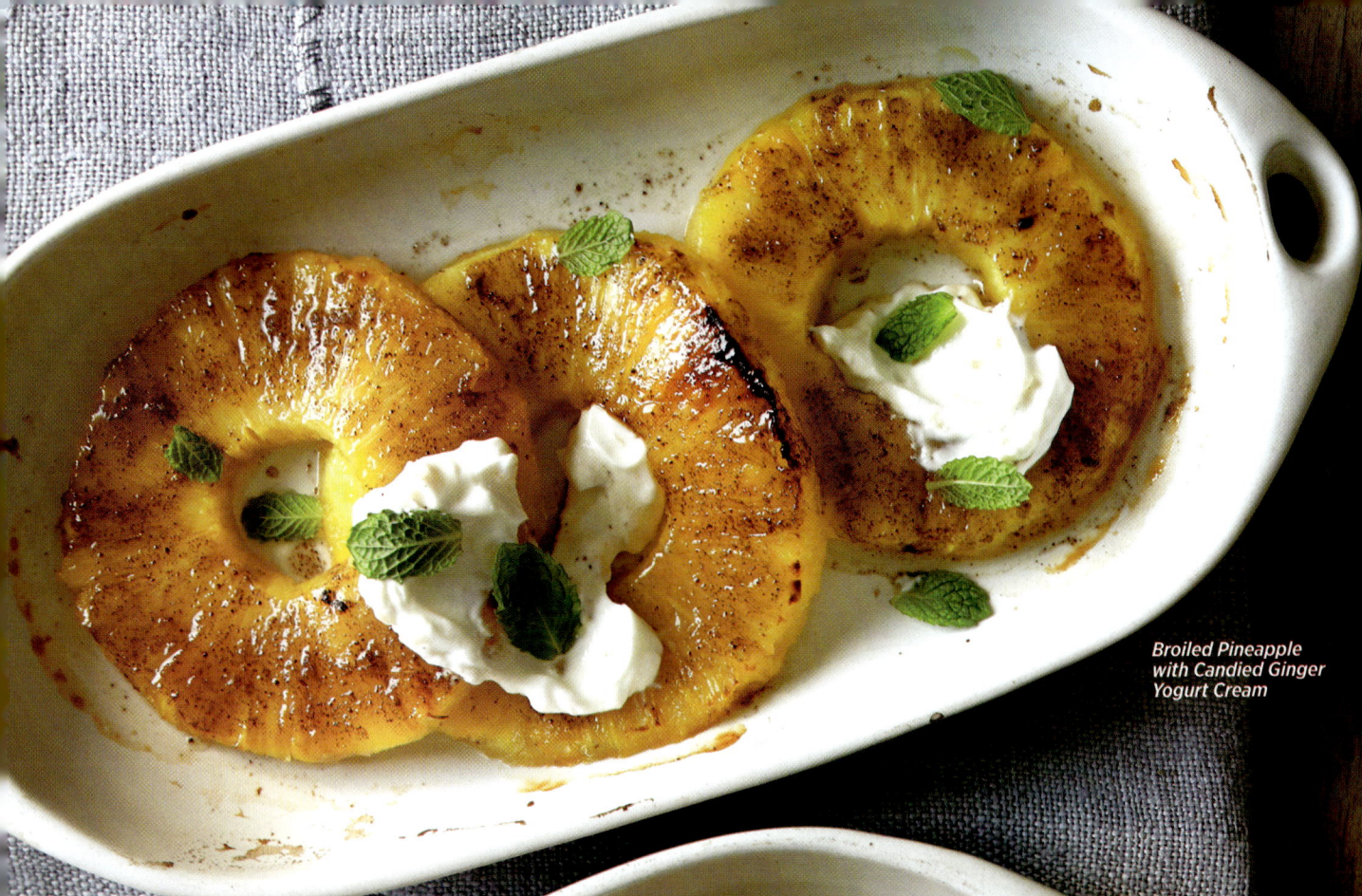

Broiled Pineapple
with Candied Ginger
Yogurt Cream

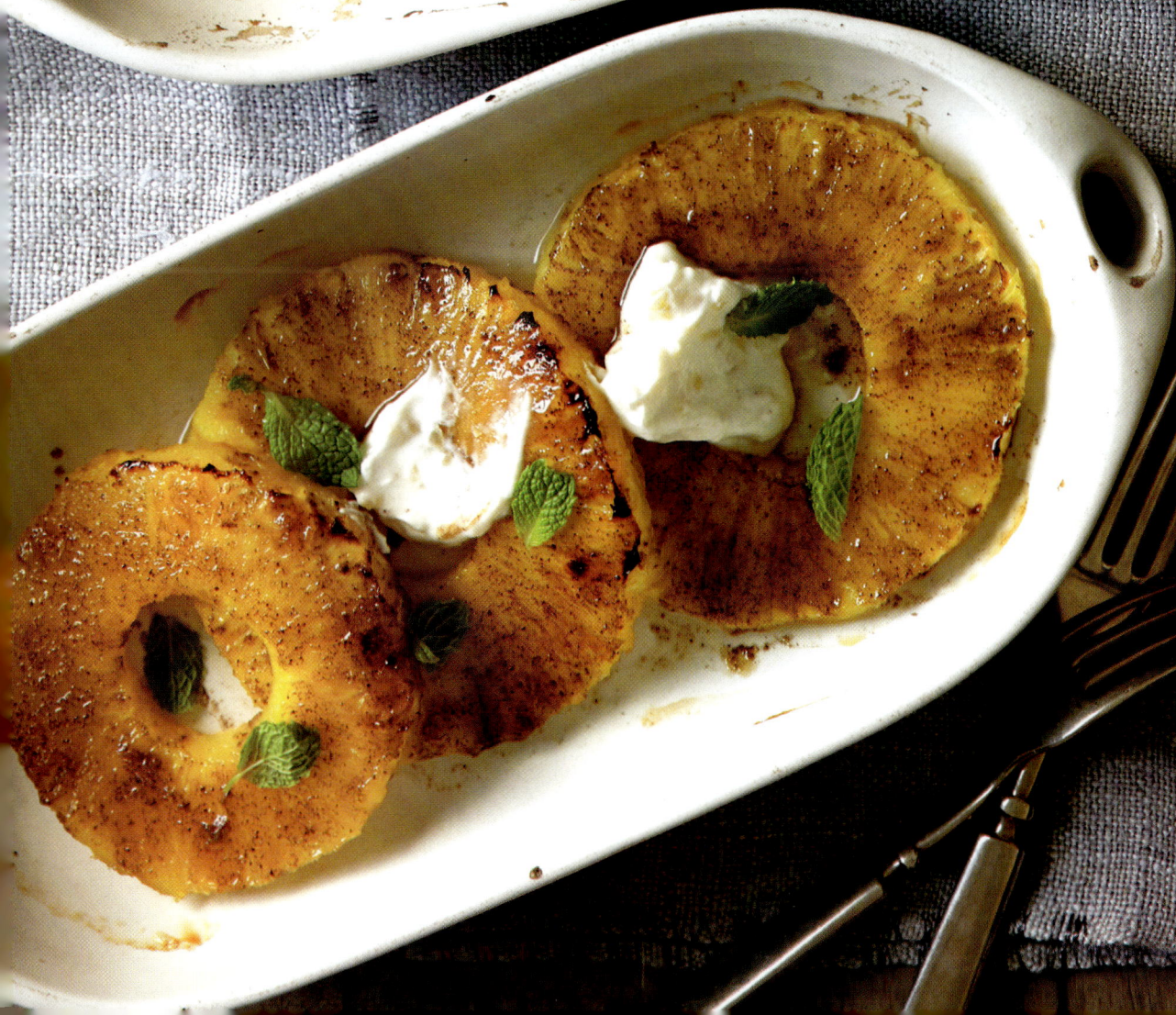

BLUEBERRY-CHEESECAKE YOGURT BARK

SERVES 8 • VEGETARIAN • NO COOK

1 cup plain low-fat Greek yogurt

1 tablespoon agave nectar

½ teaspoon grated lemon zest

½ teaspoon lemon juice

1 cup blueberries

3 squares graham crackers, crushed

1 Line 9 x 5-inch loaf pan with foil so foil hangs over edges of pan.

2 Combine yogurt, agave nectar, lemon zest, and lemon juice in small bowl; fold in blueberries and 3 tablespoons crushed graham crackers. Using back of spoon, spread evenly in prepared loaf pan; sprinkle with remaining graham cracker crumbs. Cover pan with foil; freeze at least 1 hour.

3 Remove from freezer, uncover pan, and lift bark from pan holding edges of foil. Cut into 8 even squares and then slice each square into triangle (if bark is too hard to cut, let sit for a few minutes to soften slightly). Keep triangles stored in freezer in sealed container until ready to serve.

Per serving (2 triangles): 49 Cal, 1 g Total Fat, 0 g Sat Fat, 23 mg Sod, 8 g Total Carb, 5 g Sugar, 1 g Fib, 3 g Prot.

COOK'S TIP

All the flavors of cheesecake come together in this delicious and simple chilled treat. Make up a batch to have at the ready for snacking anytime.

FIGS STUFFED WITH HONEY AND GOAT CHEESE

SERVES 8 • GLUTEN FREE • VEGETARIAN • UNDER 20 MINUTES • NO COOK

16 medium fresh figs, washed and patted dry, each sliced in half lengthwise

6 tablespoons part-skim ricotta

2 tablespoons crumbled goat cheese

2 tablespoons chopped fresh thyme

2 tablespoons honey

½ teaspoon black pepper, or to taste

Place figs on large serving platter, cut side up. Combine ricotta, goat cheese, and thyme in small bowl. Spoon about ¾ teaspoon cheese mixture over each fig half; drizzle with honey and sprinkle with pepper.

2 SmartPoints value

Per serving (4 fig halves): 120 Cal, 3 g Total Fat, 1 g Sat Fat, 29 mg Sod, 24 g Total Carb, 21 g Sugar, 3 g Fib, 4 g Prot.

COOK'S TIP

This is a super-easy way to prepare fresh figs when they're in season. They make a great dessert treat, or serve them as an appetizer with white wine spritzers.

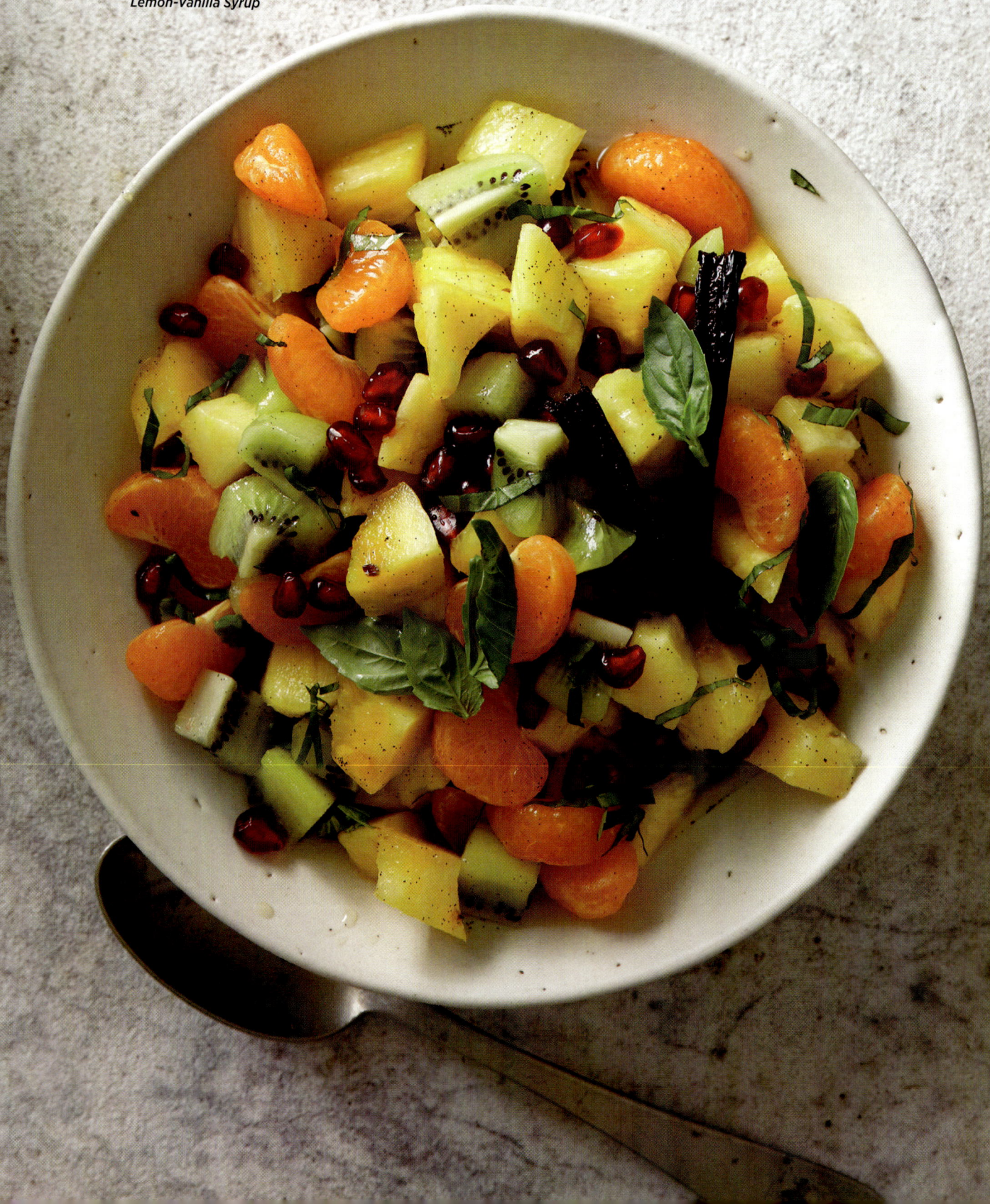

*Brilliant Fruit Salad with
Lemon-Vanilla Syrup*

BRILLIANT FRUIT SALAD
WITH LEMON-VANILLA SYRUP

SERVES 10 • GLUTEN FREE • VEGETARIAN

⅓ cup sugar

¾ cup water

½ vanilla bean, split lengthwise

1 lemon

4 large clementines, peeled and separated into segments

3 cups diced pineapple

3 kiwifruit, peeled and diced

1 cup pomegranate seeds

6 basil leaves or mint leaves, cut into thin strips (optional)

1 Combine sugar and water in medium saucepan. Scrape seeds from vanilla bean with tip of paring knife and add to pan; add vanilla pod to pan.

2 Using vegetable peeler, remove zest from lemon in long strips, avoiding as much white pith as possible; add zest to pan with 1 tablespoon lemon juice. Bring mixture to boil over high heat; reduce heat to medium and simmer, uncovered, until mixture thickens slightly, about 5 minutes. Remove syrup from heat; refrigerate until cool.

3 Place clementines, pineapple, kiwifruit, and pomegranate seeds in large serving bowl. Remove lemon zest from syrup; pour syrup over fruit (leave vanilla bean in to continue to impart flavor) and toss to coat. Cover; refrigerate at least 30 minutes or up to 1 day.

2 SmartPoints value

Per serving (½ cup): 108 Cal, 0 g Total Fat, 0 g Sat Fat, 3 mg Sod, 28 g Total Carb, 21 g Sugar, 3 g Fib, 1 g Prot.

COOK'S TIP

If you like, you can make the lemon-vanilla syrup up to 1 week ahead and store it in an airtight container in the refrigerator.

SUMMER FRUITS WITH LIMONCELLO

SERVES 6 • GLUTEN FREE • VEGETARIAN • UNDER 20 MINUTES • NO COOK

2 tablespoons honey

3 tablespoons lemon-flavored Italian liqueur (such as limoncello)

1 teaspoon grated lemon zest

1 tablespoon lemon juice

3 cups cubed honeydew

2 peaches, peeled, pitted, and sliced

2 cups strawberries, hulled and quartered

1 cup fresh blueberries

3 tablespoons thinly sliced fresh basil leaves

Stir honey, liqueur, lemon zest, and lemon juice together in large bowl. Add honeydew, peaches, strawberries, and blueberries; toss to combine. Serve at once, or cover and refrigerate up to 4 hours and serve chilled. Stir in basil just before serving.

3 SmartPoints value ®

Per serving (generous 1 cup): 126 Cal, 1 g Total Fat, 0 g Sat Fat, 17 mg Sod, 29 g Total Carb, 25 g Sugar, 3 g Fib, 2 g Prot.

COOK'S TIP

To add more colorful melon to this salad, toss in 1 cup cubed cantaloupe or seedless watermelon.

PINEAPPLE-CHIPOTLE
ICE POPS

SERVES 6 • GLUTEN FREE • VEGETARIAN • NO COOK

1 pound frozen unsweetened pineapple chunks, thawed

3 tablespoons agave nectar

1 tablespoon lime juice

½ teaspoon minced canned chipotles en adobo

1 Put pineapple (and any juice), agave nectar, and lime juice in blender or food processor; puree, stopping to scrape down sides at least once. Add chipotles and pulse again to combine.

2 Divide mixture among 6 (⅓-cup) ice pop molds. Cover molds with tops and insert wooden craft sticks. Freeze until completely frozen, 8 hours or up to 1 week.

2 SmartPoints value

Per serving (1 ice pop): 68 Cal, 0 g Total Fat, 0 g Sat Fat, 5 mg Sod, 18 g Total Carb, 15 g Sugar, 1 g Fib, 0 g Prot.

COOK'S TIP

Chipotle and smoky adobo chile peppers make a wonderfully sweet and savory combination in these refreshing ice pops.

*Dreamy Raspberry
Ice Pops and
Pineapple-Chipotle
Ice Pops (see recipe
on page 219)*

DREAMY RASPBERRY
ICE POPS

SERVES 6 • GLUTEN FREE • VEGETARIAN • NO COOK

1½ cups fresh or frozen raspberries

1 (6-ounce) container raspberry fat-free yogurt

½ cup water

¼ cup honey

1½ teaspoons lemon juice

2 teaspoons raspberry liqueur (optional)

1 Combine all ingredients in blender or food processor and puree. Push puree through strainer; discard seeds.

2 Divide mixture among 6 (⅓-cup) ice pop molds. Cover molds with tops and insert wooden craft sticks. Freeze until completely frozen, 6 hours or up to 1 week.

4 SmartPoints value

Per serving (1 ice pop): 89 Cal, 0 g Total Fat, 0 g Sat Fat, 18 mg Sod, 21 g Total Carb, 19 g Sugar, 2 g Fib, 2 g Prot.

COOK'S TIP

If you don't have ice pop molds, make these in paper cups: Spoon the mixture into 3-ounce paper cups and cover each with foil. Make a small slit in the foil and insert a wooden craft stick. Freeze as directed. Remove the foil and tear away the paper cups to serve.

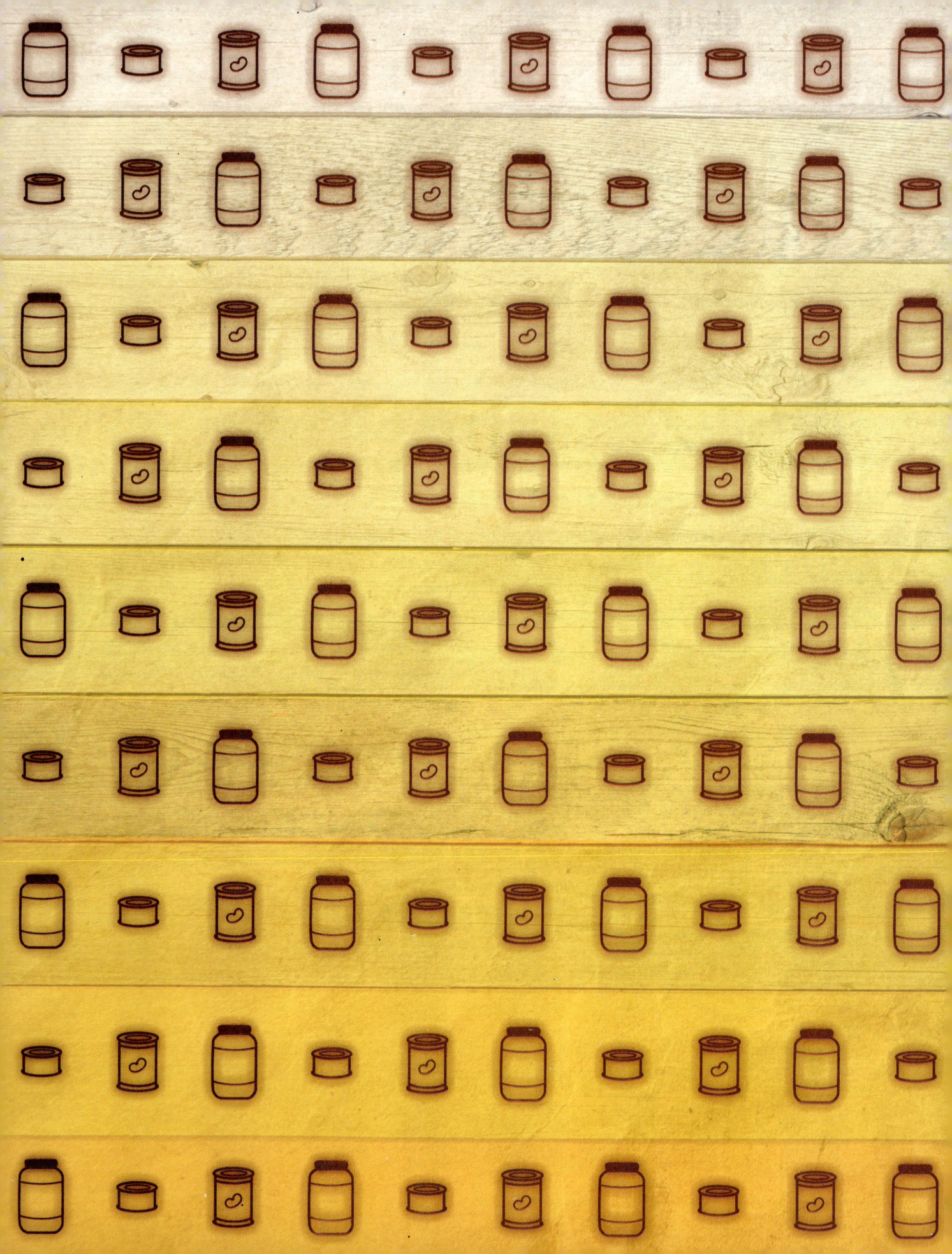

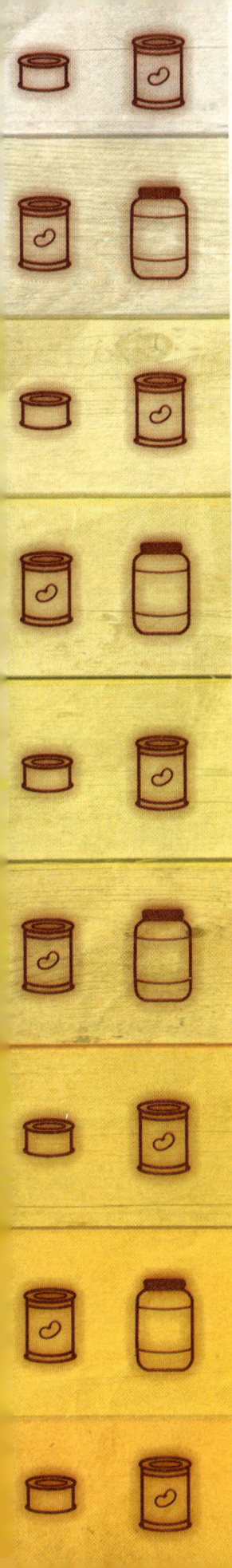

QUICK MEALS WITH FRIDGE & PANTRY STAPLES

BAKED CHICKEN BURRITOS

SERVES 4

1 teaspoon canola oil

1 green bell pepper, chopped

1 zucchini, chopped

8 ounces roasted skinless boneless chicken breast, diced

½ cup frozen corn kernels, thawed or fresh

½ small onion, minced

¼ cup plain fat-free yogurt

¼ teaspoon ground cumin

¼ teaspoon chili powder

¼ teaspoon salt

4 burrito-size fat-free whole wheat tortillas

1 cup fat-free salsa

1 Preheat oven to 350°F. Spray 9 x 13-inch baking pan with nonstick spray.

2 Heat oil over medium heat in medium nonstick skillet. Add bell pepper and zucchini and cook, stirring, until softened, 3–4 minutes. Transfer to large bowl and stir in chicken, corn, onion, yogurt, cumin, chili powder, and salt.

3 Place one-fourth of chicken mixture in center of each tortilla. Fold in sides of tortillas and then roll closed from bottom. Place burritos, seam side down, in baking pan; cover with salsa. Bake until burritos begin to brown and filling warms through, 15–20 minutes.

6 SmartPoints value

Per serving (1 burrito): 264 Cal, 3 g Total Fat, 1 g Sat Fat, 928 mg Sod, 36 g Total Carb, 8 g Sugar, 7 g Fib, 21 g Prot.

UP THE PROTEIN

*Add beans or cheese to these burritos if you like:
A ¼ cup of rinsed and drained canned red beans or
⅓ cup shredded fat-free Cheddar rolled into each burrito
will increase the per-serving SmartPoints value by 1.*

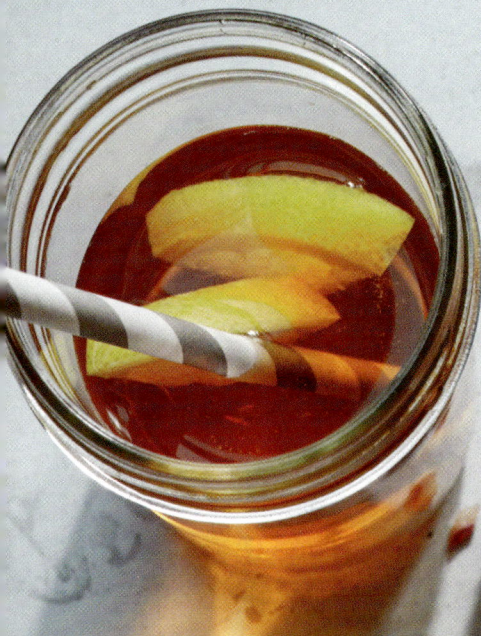

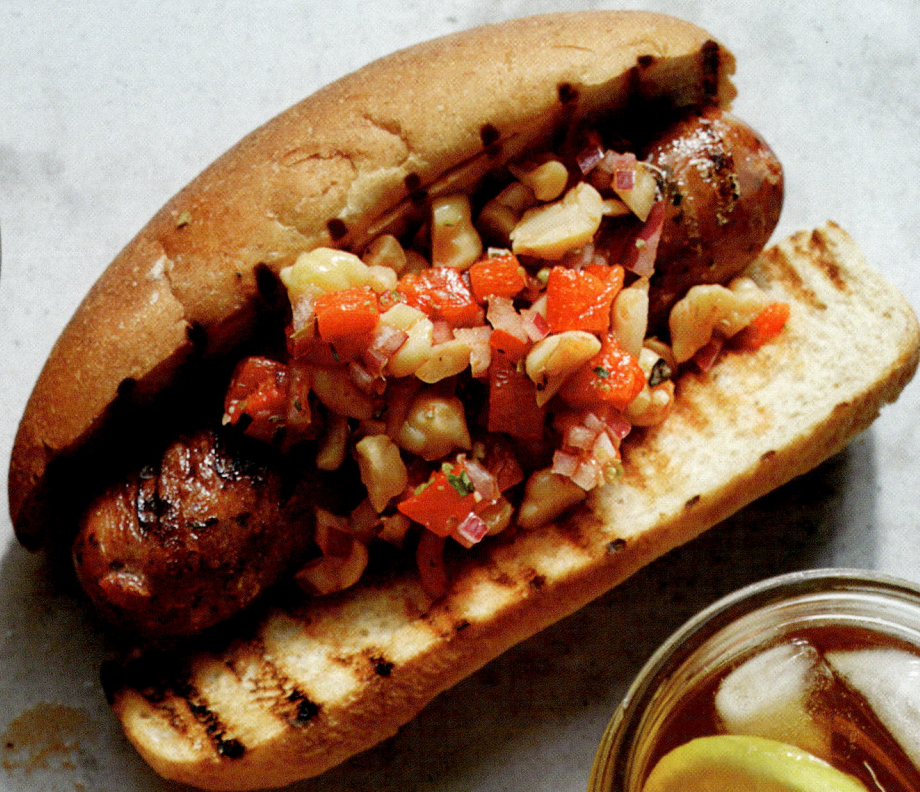

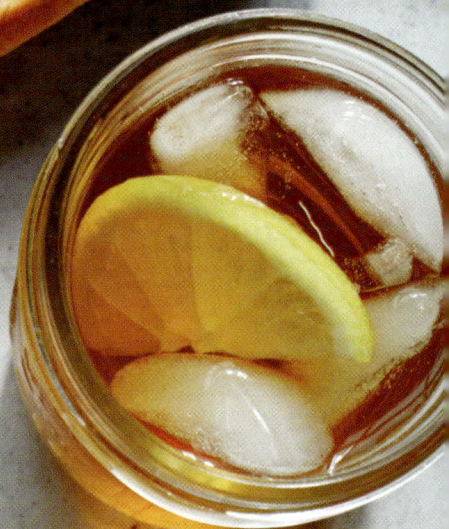

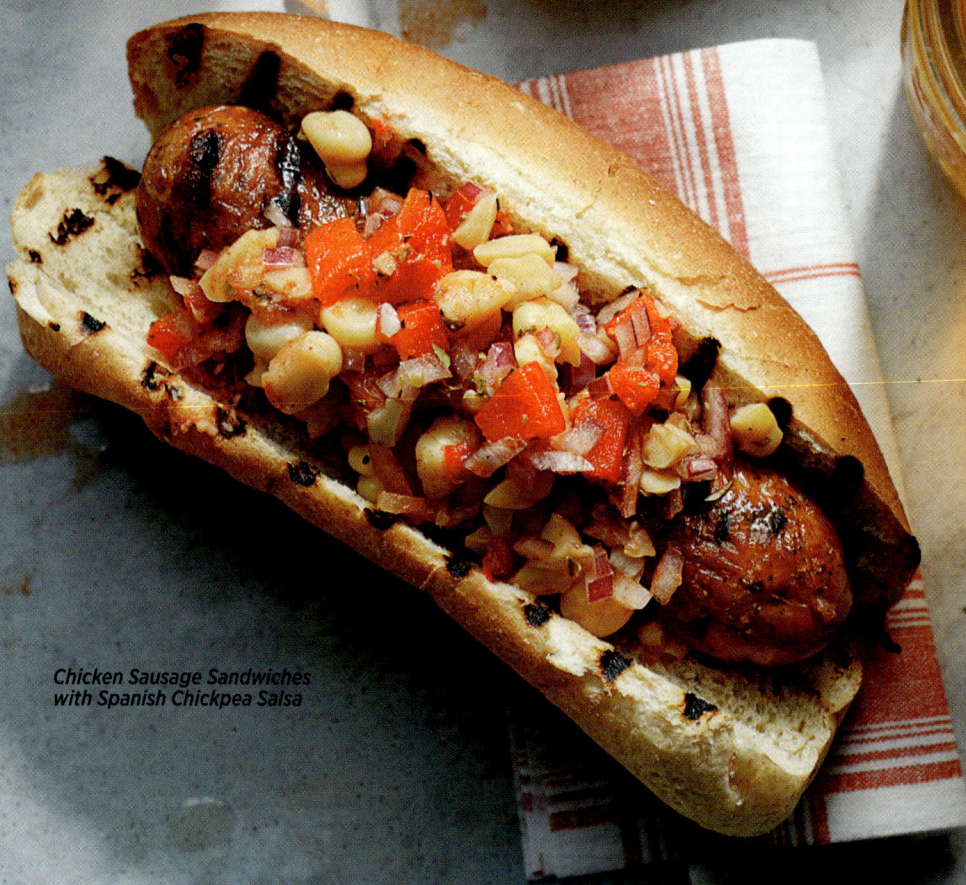

Chicken Sausage Sandwiches with Spanish Chickpea Salsa

CHICKEN SAUSAGE SANDWICHES WITH SPANISH CHICKPEA SALSA

SERVES 4 • UNDER 20 MINUTES

⅓ cup canned pimientos, drained and chopped

⅓ cup canned chickpeas, rinsed and drained

1 tablespoon finely chopped red onion

2 teaspoons sherry vinegar

½ teaspoon smoked paprika

½ teaspoon dried oregano

4 (3-ounce) cooked spicy chicken chorizo or other spicy chicken sausages

4 reduced-calorie whole wheat hot dog buns

1 Combine pimentos, chickpeas, onion, vinegar, paprika, and oregano in small bowl; mash with fork until chickpeas are slightly broken up. Set aside.

2 Place ridged grill pan over medium-high heat. Grill sausages, turning as needed, until grill marks appear and sausages are heated through, about 5 minutes. Grill buns until lightly toasted, about 1 minute.

3 Place sausages in buns; top each with about 2½ tablespoons chickpea salsa.

6 SmartPoints value

Per serving (1 sausage sandwich): 221 Cal, 7 g Total Fat, 2 g Sat Fat, 791 mg Sod, 23 g Total Carb, 4 g Sugar, 5 g Fib, 18 g Prot.

UP THE PROTEIN

Pimentos, sherry vinegar, and smoked paprika give this salsa a wonderful Spanish flavor. If you like, top each sandwich with 2 tablespoons shredded Manchego cheese for an additional 2 SmartPoints per serving.

CUBAN CHICKEN AND PINEAPPLE SALAD

SERVES 4 • GLUTEN FREE • UNDER 20 MINUTES • NO COOK

¼ cup lime juice

1 tablespoon olive oil

½ teaspoon ground cumin

½ teaspoon salt, or to taste

¾ pound cooked skinless boneless chicken breast, cut into chunks

1¼ cups fresh pineapple chunks

1 cup matchstick-cut jicama

⅓ cup coarsely chopped fresh cilantro

¼ cup very thinly sliced red bell pepper

2 scallions, thinly sliced

Stir lime juice, oil, cumin, and salt together in large bowl until blended. Add chicken, pineapple, jicama, cilantro, bell pepper, and scallions and toss to coat.

3 SmartPoints value

Per serving (about 1¼ cups): 218 Cal, 7 g Total Fat, 1 g Sat Fat, 359 mg Sod, 12 g Total Carb, 7 g Sugar, 3 g Fib, 27 g Prot.

UP THE PROTEIN

Add 1 cup black beans to the salad for an additional 1 SmartPoints per serving.

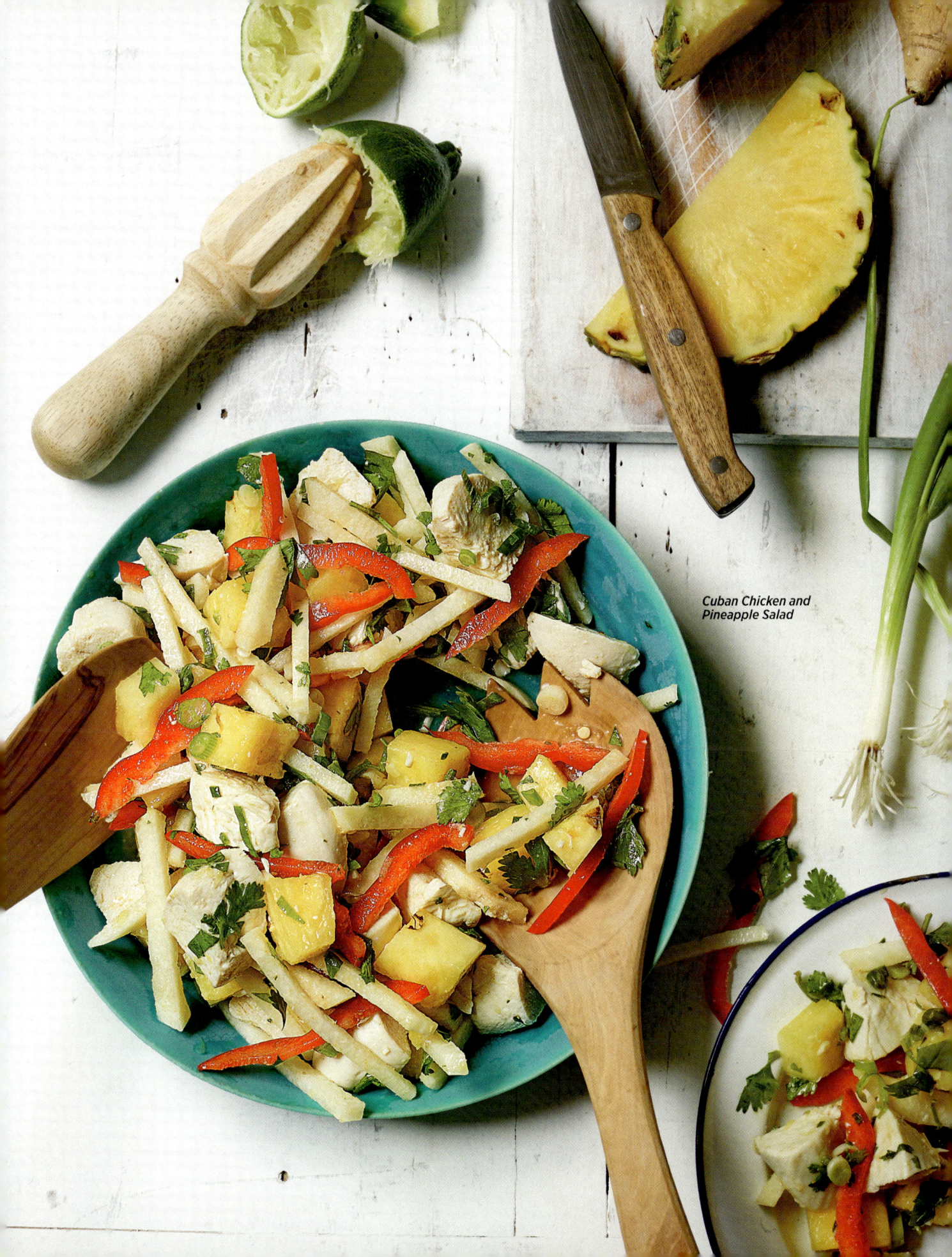

Cuban Chicken and Pineapple Salad

TURKEY-APPLE SALAD WITH RASPBERRY VINAIGRETTE

SERVES 4 • GLUTEN FREE • UNDER 20 MINUTES • NO COOK

2 cups cooked skinless turkey breast, sliced, shredded, or chopped

2 celery stalks, chopped

1 apple, cored and diced

½ cup golden seedless raisins, chopped

1½ tablespoons raspberry vinegar or apple cider vinegar

2 teaspoons olive oil

½ teaspoon ground coriander

¼ teaspoon salt

¼ teaspoon black pepper

4 cups very thinly sliced romaine lettuce

Combine turkey, celery, apple, and raisins in large bowl and toss. Whisk vinegar, oil, coriander, salt, and pepper together in small bowl. Add dressing to turkey mixture; toss to combine. Arrange lettuce on 4 plates and top with turkey salad.

5 SmartPoints value

Per serving (1¼ cups turkey salad and 1 cup lettuce): 194 Cal, 4 g Total Fat, 1 g Sat Fat, 224 mg Sod, 23 g Total Carb, 16 g Sugar, 3 g Fib, 19 g Prot.

UP THE PROTEIN

For a heartier salad, add a large grated carrot and some chopped hard-cooked egg. One large hard-cooked egg per serving will increase the SmartPoints value by 2.

SMOKED TURKEY AND SCALLION QUESADILLAS

SERVES 4 • UNDER 20 MINUTES

8 small (6-inch) whole wheat tortillas

¾ pound sliced deli smoked turkey breast

3 scallions, thinly sliced

1 cup shredded reduced-fat pepper Jack cheese

¾ cup fat-free salsa

1 Lay 4 tortillas on work surface and top evenly with turkey, scallions, and pepper Jack. Top with remaining tortillas.

2 Spray large cast-iron skillet with nonstick spray and set over medium heat. Place one quesadilla in skillet and cook until lightly browned, 2–3 minutes. Spray with nonstick spray and turn over with spatula. Cook until cheese melts, about 2 minutes longer. Transfer to plate and keep warm. Repeat with remaining quesadillas. Cut each quesadilla into 4 wedges and serve with salsa.

7 SmartPoints value

Per serving (1 quesadilla and 3 tablespoons salsa): 266 Cal, 8 g Total Fat, 5 g Sat Fat, 977 mg Sod, 27 g Total Carb, 3 g Sugar, 3 g Fib, 26 g Prot.

COOK'S TIP

Love guacamole? Top each quesadilla with 2 tablespoons store-bought guac for an additional 2 SmartPoints per serving.

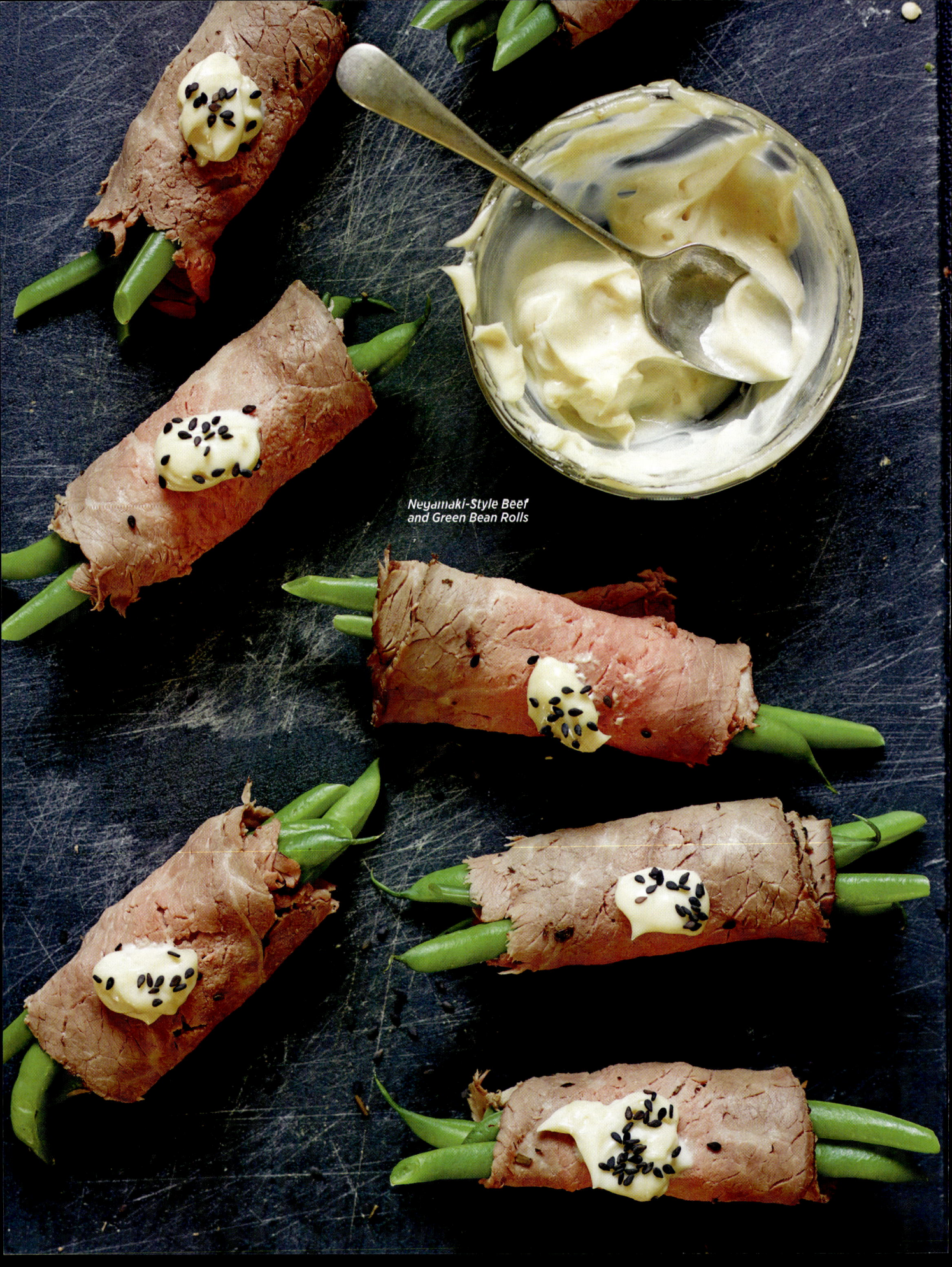

Negamaki-Style Beef and Green Bean Rolls

NEGAMAKI-STYLE BEEF AND GREEN BEAN ROLLS

SERVES 4 • GLUTEN FREE • UNDER 20 MINUTES

48 green beans (10 ounces), trimmed

¼ teaspoon salt

3 tablespoons reduced-fat mayonnaise

¾ teaspoon wasabi paste

Pinch black pepper

12 slices (¾ pound) lean sirloin roast beef, trimmed

½ teaspoon black sesame seeds

1 Bring large saucepan of salted water to boil. Add green beans and cook until bright green and crisp-tender, about 5 minutes. Drain in colander under cold running water until cooled. Pat dry and sprinkle with ⅛ teaspoon salt.

2 Meanwhile, combine mayonnaise, wasabi paste, remaining ⅛ teaspoon salt, and pepper in small bowl; set aside.

3 Fold tops and bottoms of each slice of beef toward center, making even-length strips, each about 2½ inches wide. Place 4 green beans on one end of each strip and roll beef around beans. Divide rolls among 4 plates, sprinkle with sesame seeds, and top with dollop of wasabi sauce.

3 SmartPoints value

Per serving (3 rolls and 1½ teaspoons wasabi sauce): 172 Cal, 7 g Total Fat, 2 g Sat Fat, 288 mg Sod, 6 g Total Carb, 3 g Sugar, 2 g Fib, 21 g Prot.

COOK'S TIP

For a perfect warm weather entrée, serve these savory rolls with chilled soba noodles (a ½-cup serving cooked soba has a SmartPoints value of 1). Sprinkle the noodles with a little soy sauce and top with grated carrot if you wish.

OPEN-FACE ROAST BEEF SANDWICHES WITH HORSERADISH

SERVES 4 ● UNDER 20 MINUTES ● NO COOK

2 tablespoons prepared horseradish, drained

2 tablespoons light sour cream

4 slices pumpernickel bread

4 (1-ounce) slices lean sirloin roast beef, trimmed

1 Kirby cucumber, thinly sliced

12 small sprigs mâche or watercress

Black pepper to taste

Stir horseradish and sour cream together in small bowl. Spread evenly over one side of each bread slice. Top each with 1 slice beef, folding the beef as necessary to fit on the bread. Top evenly with cucumber slices and mâche. Sprinkle each sandwich generously with pepper.

4 SmartPoints value

Per serving (1 open-face sandwich): 150 Cal, 4 g Total Fat, 1 g Sat Fat, 248 mg Sod, 17 g Total Carb, 1 g Sugar, 3 g Fib, 12 g Prot.

UP THE PROTEIN

If you like, add an extra slice of roast beef to each sandwich and increase the per-serving SmartPoints value by 1.

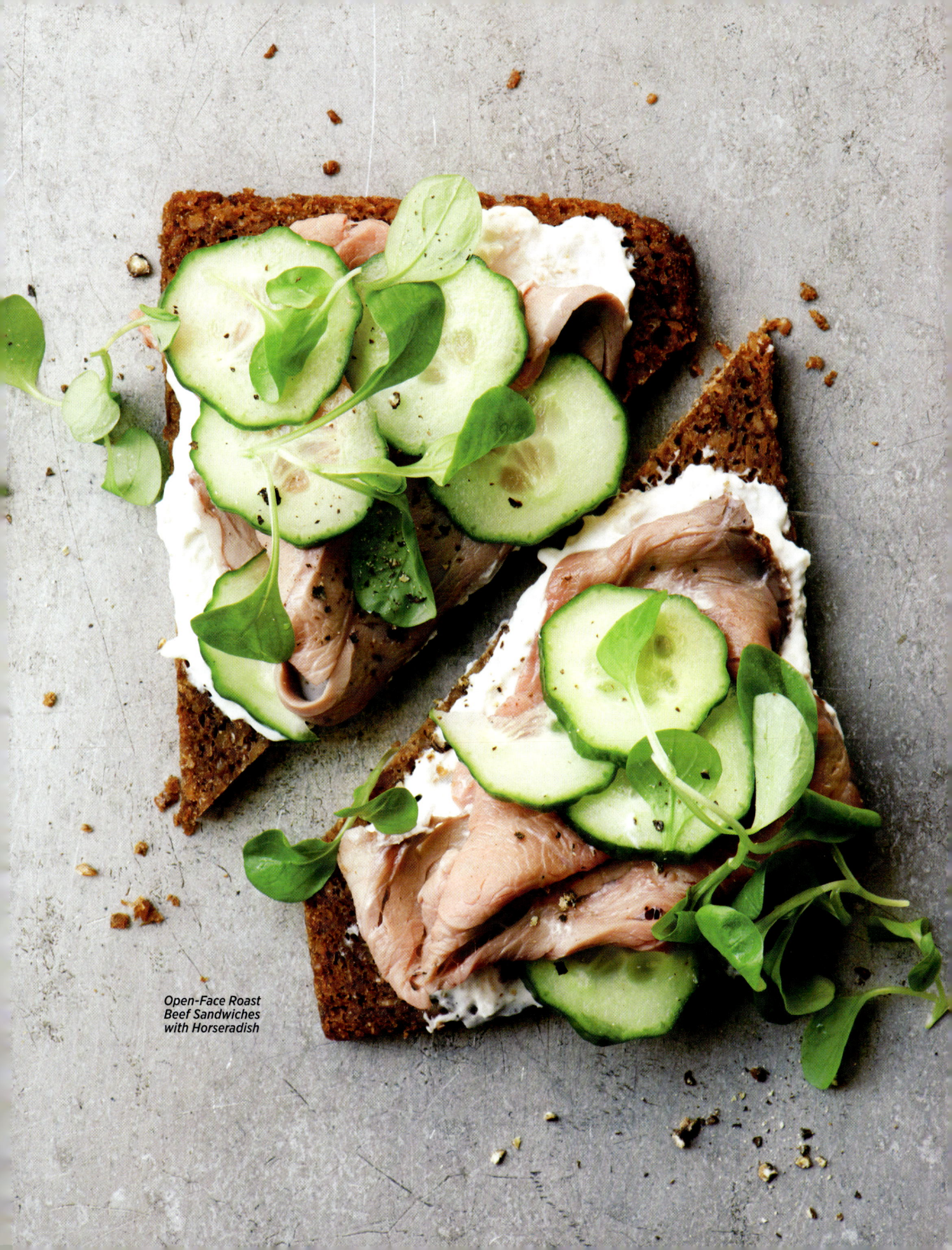

Open-Face Roast
Beef Sandwiches
with Horseradish

LEAN HAM SANDWICHES WITH EDAMAME SPREAD

SERVES 4

3 cups water

4 ounces shelled frozen edamame

⅛ teaspoon salt, or to taste

⅛ teaspoon black pepper

1 tablespoon lemon juice

1 tablespoon reduced-fat whipped cream cheese

½ teaspoon wasabi paste (optional)

8 slices light multigrain bread

8 ounces thinly sliced lean reduced-sodium ham

1 Bring water to boil in medium saucepan; cook edamame until tender, about 5 minutes. Drain, reserving ½ cup cooking water.

2 Combine edamame, salt, pepper, lemon juice, cream cheese, and wasabi paste (if using) in food processor; pulse until smooth, pausing occasionally to scrape down sides of bowl and adding 1–2 tablespoons reserved cooking water each time to achieve spreadable consistency. Spoon edamame spread into container, cover, and cool in refrigerator.

3 When edamame spread is cool, spread about 1 tablespoon on each slice of bread. Top half of bread slices with ham, dividing evenly. Cover with remaining bread slices.

6 SmartPoints value

Per serving (1 sandwich): 225 Cal, 6 g Total Fat, 1 g Sat Fat, 1,000 mg Sod, 22 g Total Carb, 1 g Sugar, 5 g Fib, 19 g Prot.

COOK'S TIP

Got leftover edamame after making this recipe? Try adding them to soups and salads; ½ cup of cooked shelled edamame has a SmartPoints value of 3.

SALMON MELTS WITH GARLIC-HERB CHEESE

SERVES 4 • UNDER 20 MINUTES

1 (14¾-ounce) can wild salmon, drained

2 tablespoons reduced-fat mayonnaise

1½ tablespoons capers, drained

1 tablespoon chopped fresh chives

1 teaspoon grated lemon zest

4 teaspoons lemon juice

2 light multigrain English muffins, split and toasted

¼ cup light garlic-and-herb cheese dip

1 cup pea shoots or micro greens

1 Preheat broiler. Line broiler pan or small baking sheet with foil.

2 Place salmon in medium bowl. Flake with fork and pick out and discard any large pieces of bone or skin. Add mayonnaise, capers, chives, lemon zest, and lemon juice and toss lightly with fork to mix. Spoon salmon mixture onto muffin halves. Top each with 1 tablespoon cheese dip.

3 Place muffins on prepared pan. Broil 5 inches from heat until cheese browns lightly, about 2 minutes. Top each evenly with pea shoots.

6 SmartPoints value

Per serving (1 sandwich): 239 Cal, 9 g Total Fat, 2 g Sat Fat, 726 mg Sod, 13 g Total Carb, 1 g Sugar, 3 g Fib, 25 g Prot.

UP THE PROTEIN

Double the amount of cheese dip you use for an additional 1 SmartPoints value per serving.

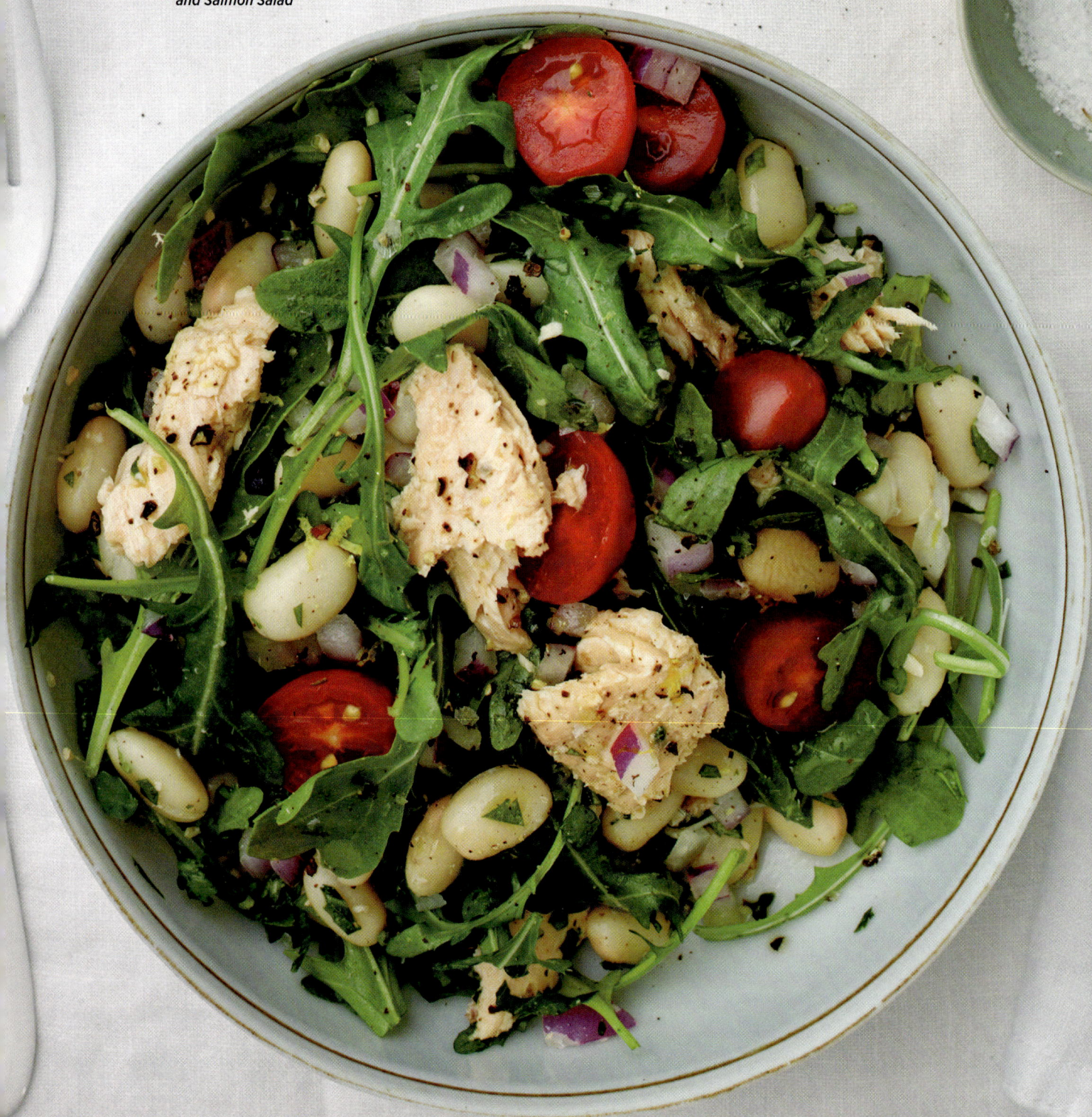

White Bean, Citrus, and Salmon Salad

WHITE BEAN, CITRUS, AND SALMON SALAD

SERVES 4 • GLUTEN FREE • UNDER 20 MINUTES • NO COOK

1 (16-ounce) can wild salmon, drained

1 (15-ounce) can white beans, drained and rinsed

1 small red onion, diced

6 cups baby arugula

¼ cup chopped fresh parsley

1 teaspoon finely grated lemon zest

1 teaspoon chopped fresh thyme

3 tablespoons lemon juice

1 tablespoon olive oil

½ teaspoon salt

½ teaspoon black pepper

1 Place salmon in large bowl. Flake with fork and pick out and discard any large pieces of bone or skin.

2 Add remaining ingredients and toss gently to combine.

7
SmartPoints value

Per serving (about 1½ cups): 309 Cal, 9 g Total Fat, 1 g Sat Fat, 753 mg Sod, 26 g Total Carb, 2 g Sugar, 6 g Fib, 30 g Prot.

COOK'S TIP

Salmon and beans pair wonderfully with citrus in this no-cook meal. If you like, add halved grape or cherry tomatoes for more color.

QUICK PROVENCAL SEAFOOD STEW

SERVES 4 ● UNDER 20 MINUTES

1 (15-ounce) can chicken broth

1 large onion, chopped

1 (15-ounce) can cannellini beans (white kidney), rinsed and drained

1 (14-ounce) can diced tomatoes with juice

1 (5½-ounce) can water-packed tuna, drained and flaked with fork

1 (6½-ounce) canned chopped clams, drained

¼ teaspoon dried oregano

¾ teaspoon salt

¼ teaspoon black pepper

¼ cup chopped fresh basil

Lemon wedges for serving

1 Heat ¼ cup broth in medium saucepan over medium-high heat; add onion and cook, stirring, until tender, about 5 minutes.

2 Add beans, tomatoes, tuna, clams, and oregano; stir in remaining broth and simmer 5 minutes. Stir in salt, pepper, and basil. Serve with lemon wedges.

5 SmartPoints value

Per serving (about 1½ cups): 250 Cal, 2 g Total Fat, 0 g Sat Fat, 911 mg Sod, 29 g Total Carb, 2 g Sugar, 6 g Fib, 29 g Prot.

COOK'S TIP

Using canned staples helps this stew come together in minutes, but if you'd like to add some fresh veggies, you should! Include diced carrots and diced zucchini with the onion, or try a finely diced 8-ounce potato for an additional 1 SmartPoints value per serving.

TUNA AND NEW POTATO SALAD WITH BASIL DRESSING

SERVES 4 ● UNDER 20 MINUTES

¾ **pound small red potatoes**

¼ **cup chopped fresh basil**

2 **tablespoons red-wine vinegar**

1 **tablespoon lemon juice**

2½ **teaspoons olive oil**

4 **teaspoons Dijon mustard**

½ **teaspoon salt**

¼ **teaspoon black pepper**

4 **small tomatoes, cut into wedges**

½ **cup roasted red peppers (water-packed), cut into chunks**

1 **(12-ounce) can water-packed solid white tuna, drained and broken into chunks**

4 **cups sliced romaine lettuce leaves**

1 Prick potatoes with tip of paring knife. Place in microwavable bowl; cover bowl with plastic and vent one corner. Microwave on High until potatoes are tender, about 5 minutes. Set aside to cool slightly, then cut into 1-inch cubes.

2 Whisk basil, vinegar, lemon juice, oil, mustard, salt, and pepper together in large bowl. Add potatoes, tomatoes, and roasted pepper to bowl with dressing; toss to coat. Gently stir in tuna. Spoon tuna mixture over lettuce and serve.

4 SmartPoints value

Per serving (1¼ cups tuna mixture and 1 cup lettuce): 205 Cal, 4 g Total Fat, 1 g Sat Fat, 725 mg Sod, 24 g Total Carb, 6 g Sugar, 4 g Fib, 20 g Prot.

UP THE PROTEIN

For a Niçoise-style salad, add some cooked, chopped green beans and some sliced egg to the salad. Half a peeled hard-cooked egg per serving will increase the SmartPoints value by 1.

CHILI DOGS WITH CHEDDAR CHEESE

SERVES 4 • UNDER 20 MINUTES

4 fat-free beef-and-pork hot dogs

4 reduced-calorie hot dog buns

1 (15-ounce) can low-fat chili

¼ cup finely chopped red onion

½ cup shredded low-fat Cheddar

1 Preheat oven to 350°F.

2 Place hot dogs in buns; top each with about ¼ cup chili, 1 tablespoon onion, and 2 tablespoons Cheddar cheese. Lightly spray cheese with nonstick spray.

3 Wrap hot dogs in foil; place on baking sheet and bake until warmed through and cheese is melted, about 15 minutes. Serve hot.

7 SmartPoints value

Per serving (1 chili dog): 256 Cal, 4 g Total Fat, 1 g Sat Fat, 1,156 mg Sod, 35 g Total Carb, 7 g Sugar, 8 g Fib, 20 g Prot.

COOK'S TIP

Want a vegetarian version of this recipe? Use meatless fat-free hot dogs, usually called veggie dogs, and the per-serving SmartPoints value will drop to 6.

SUPER-EASY SLOW-COOKER THREE BEAN CHILI

SERVES 10 • VEGETARIAN

1 large onion, finely chopped

1 garlic clove, finely chopped

2 (15-ounce) cans reduced-sodium black beans, rinsed and drained

2 (15-ounce) cans reduced-sodium kidney beans, rinsed and drained

2 (15-ounce) cans reduced-sodium pinto beans, rinsed and drained

2 (15-ounce) cans diced tomatoes with chiles

1 (15-ounce) can tomato sauce

1 (1¼-ounce) package chili spice seasoning mix

1 (14-ounce) package frozen corn kernels, thawed

1 tablespoon lime juice, or to taste

½ cup fresh cilantro leaves, chopped

1 Combine onion, garlic, black beans, kidney beans, pinto beans, tomatoes, tomato sauce and chili spice seasoning mix in slow cooker. Cover and cook on Low 4–6 hours or High 2–3 hours.

2 Add corn and cook 1 hour longer. Stir in lime juice and cilantro just before serving.

7 SmartPoints value

Per serving (1⅓ cups): 280 Cal, 2 g Total Fat, 0 g Sat Fat, 1,256 mg Sod, 55 g Total Carb, 8 g Sugar, 16 g Fib, 16 g Prot.

COOK'S TIP

This vegetarian chili is a cinch to prepare thanks to supermarket staples. Leftovers make excellent burrito or taco fillings.

BAHN MI-STYLE VEGGIE BURGERS

SERVES 4 • VEGETARIAN • UNDER 20 MINUTES

¾ **cup shredded carrot**

4 radishes, thinly sliced

¼ **cup rice vinegar**

4 frozen soy-protein veggie burgers (2 grams or less fat per burger)

¼ **cup fat-free mayonnaise**

1 teaspoon grated lime zest

½ **teaspoon Sriracha, or to taste**

4 light sandwich thins, toasted if desired

4 small Boston lettuce leaves

1 Kirby cucumber, thinly sliced

½ **cup lightly packed fresh cilantro leaves**

1 Combine carrot, radishes, and vinegar in small bowl; marinate for 15 minutes. Drain well.

2 Meanwhile, cook burgers according to package directions. Mix mayonnaise, lime zest, and Sriracha in small bowl. Spread mayonnaise mixture on cut sides of sandwich thins. Top bottoms of thins with lettuce leaves, cucumbers slices, burgers, carrot mixture, and cilantro. Cover with sandwich tops.

6 SmartPoints value

Per serving (1 burger): 252 Cal, 6 g Total Fat, 1 g Sat Fat, 755 mg Sod, 37 g Total Carb, 6 g Sugar, 10 g Fib, 16 g Prot.

UP THE PROTEIN

Add a sliced hard-cooked egg to each sandwich for an additional 2 SmartPoints per serving.

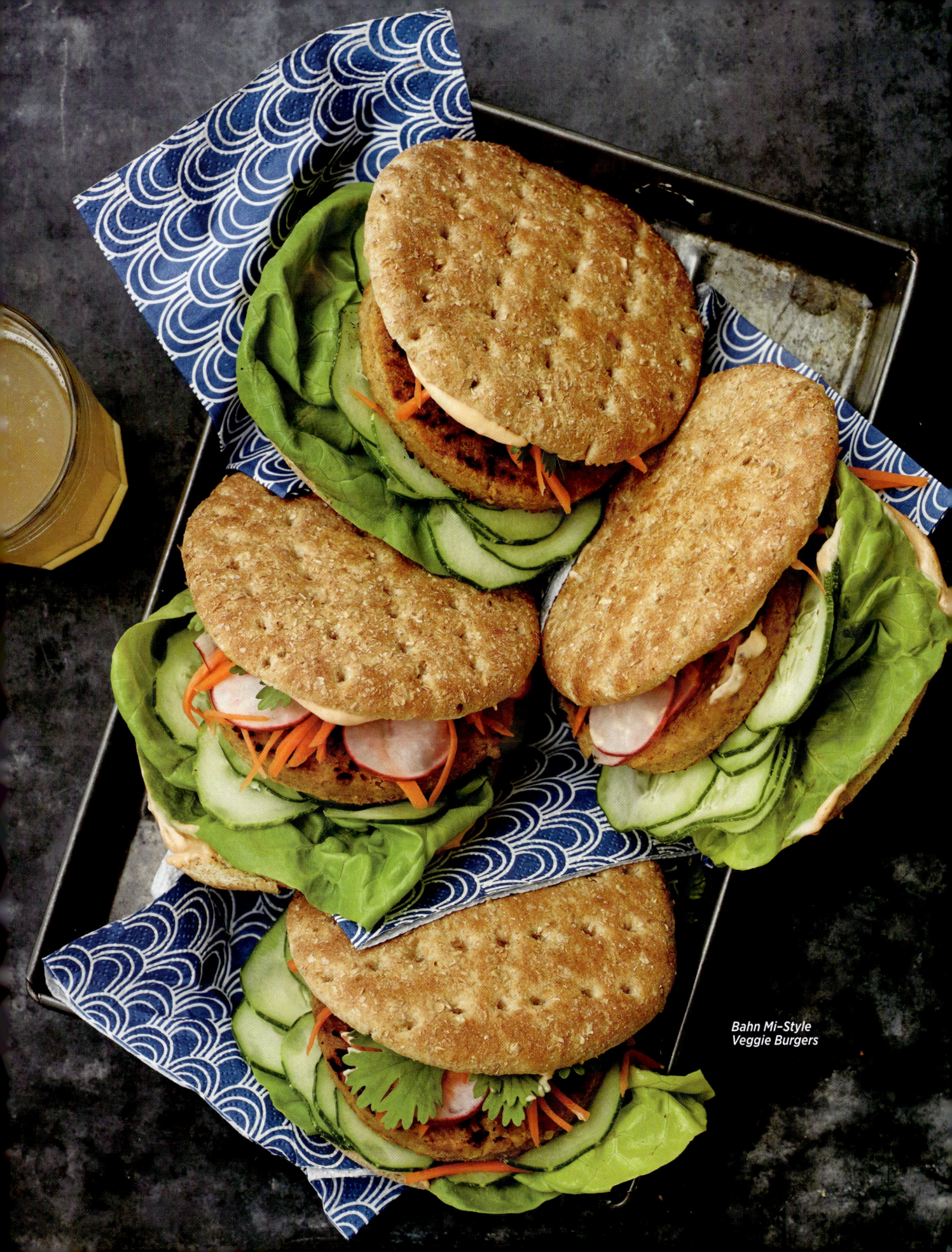

Bahn Mi-Style Veggie Burgers

Kale Caesar Salad with Grilled Shrimp, page 154

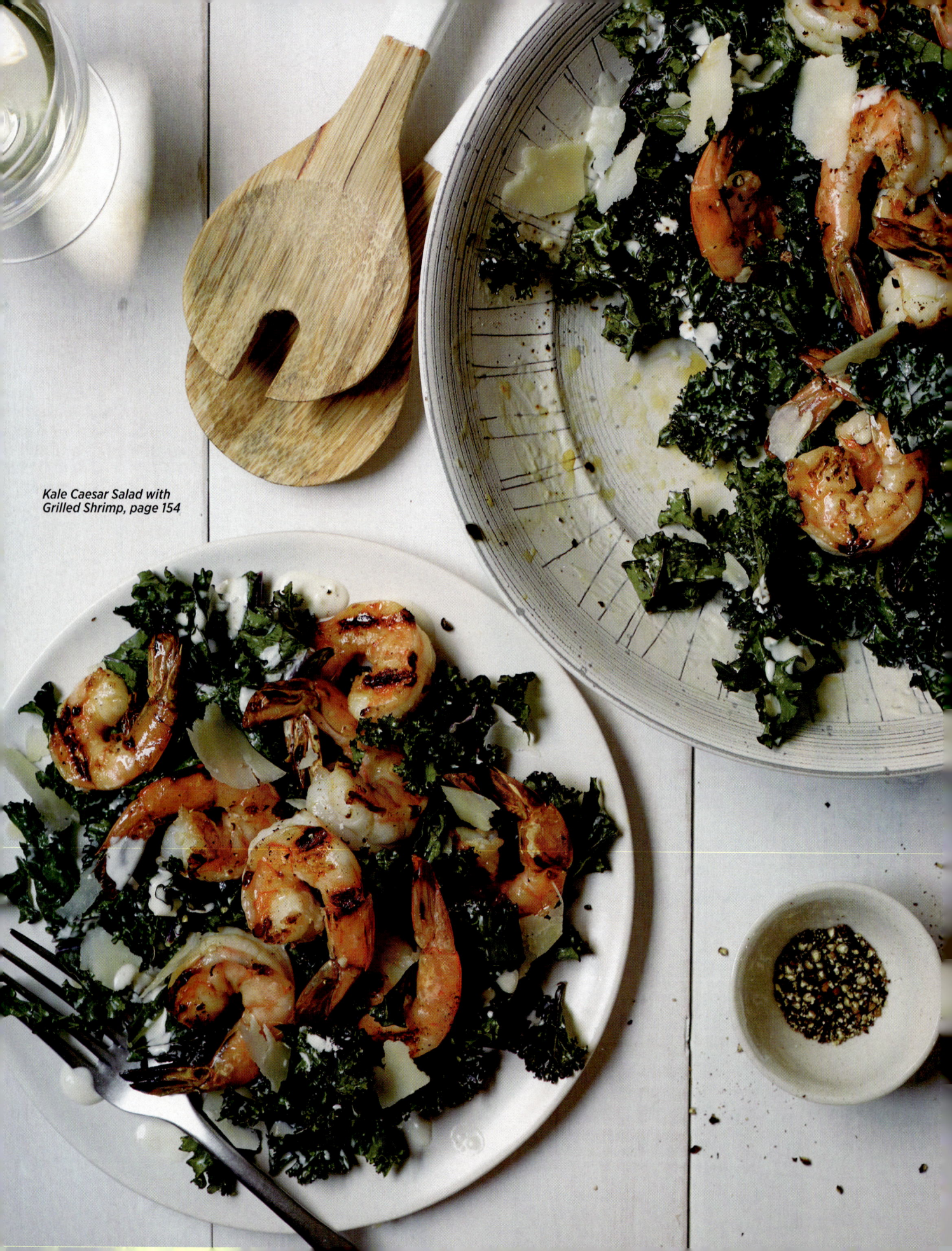

RECIPES BY SMARTPOINTS VALUE

1 SMARTPOINTS

Blueberry-Cheesecake Yogurt Bark, 214
Broiled Pineapple with Candied Ginger
    Yogurt Cream, 212
Maple-Pecan Grilled Bananas, 211
Tropical Cheesecake Tarts, 204

2 SMARTPOINTS

Baked Pears with Chocolate and Raspberry Sauce, 209
Brilliant Fruit Salad with Lemon-Vanilla Syrup, 217
Chili-Crusted Grilled Sea Scallops with Zucchini, 158
Figs Stuffed with Honey and Goat Cheese, 215
Pineapple-Chipotle Ice Pops, 219
Steamed Sole and Broccoli with Black Bean Sauce, 140
Tuna with Fennel, Oranges, and Mint, 133

3 SMARTPOINTS

Barbecue Pork with Fresh Kimchi, 112
Bell Peppers with Chickpea Mash, Eggs, and Harissa, 182
Broccolini and Goat Cheese Frittata, 10
Cajun Shrimp Sauté, 162
Cantonese-Style Whole Branzino, 136
Cuban Chicken and Pineapple Salad, 228
Cuban-Style Braised Fish, 146
Curried Lentils with Butternut, Kale, and Coconut, 190
Garlic-Seared Shrimp with Smoked Paprika, 153
Grilled Mahimahi with Lemon-Herb Aïoli, 142
Homemade Turkey Sausage with Scrambled Egg Whites, 4
Lemon-Sage Roast Turkey Breast, 66
Maple-Lemon Fruit Parfaits with Yogurt, 29
Mojo-Grilled Scallops and Shrimp, 157
Fresh Manhattan Clam Chowder, 163
Mozzarella, Basil, and Roasted Pepper Omelette, 13
Negamaki-Style Beef and Green Bean Rolls, 233
Pear Crisp with Star Anise, 205
Roasted Pork Tenderloin, 110
Shakshouka (Tomato-and-Egg Stew), 8
Spaghetti Squash Bolognese with Mushrooms, 106
Summer Fruits with Limoncello, 218
Tandoori Chicken with Cucumber-Scallion Raita, 62
Turkey with Apples, Fennel, and Barley, 68
Vegetable-Stuffed Sole with Dill Butter, 139

4 SMARTPOINTS

Apricot-Cherry Clafouti, 199
Bacon-and-Swiss Quiche, 27
Brown Rice California Rolls, 159
Chicken Breast Sauté Puttanesca Style, 39
Chicken Tikka Masala, 48
Chicken-and-Spinach Phyllo Pie, 60
Classic Pan-Fried Flounder, 141
Dreamy Raspberry Ice Pops, 221
Fresh Strawberry Crêpes, 210
Greek Frittata with Feta and Dill, 11
Greek Portobello-Chickpea Burgers, 186
Grilled Chicken with Minty Melon-Feta Salad, 43
Haddock and Potato Stew with Saffron, 148
Italian Beef and Lentil Slow-Cooker Stew, 99
Italian Wedding Soup with Turkey Meatballs, 74
Kung Pao Shrimp, 151
Mexican-Spiced Shredded Chicken with Hominy, 53
Mini Shepherd's Pies, 100
Open-Face Roast Beef Sandwiches with
    Horseradish, 234
Peruvian Chicken with Avocado and Red Onion
    Salad, 40
Sesame Chicken and Broccoli Stir-Fry, 44
Sirloin Spoon Roast with Gravy and
    Thyme Potatoes, 84
Slow-Cooker Lamb Stew with Leeks and
    Carrots, 123
Slow-Roasted Pork in Mole Sauce, 111
Strawberry Napoleon, 206
Tangy Spinach Florentine Soup with Chicken, 56
Tempeh and Snow Peas in Orange Sauce, 180
Thai Tuna Burgers, 134
Tomatoes Stuffed with Tabbouleh Egg Salad, 30
Tuna and New Potato Salad with Basil Dressing, 241
Turkey-Stuffed Cabbage Leaves, 70

5 SMARTPOINTS

Angel Food Cake with Peach-Bourbon
    Sauce, 200
Breakfast Veggie Casseroles, 14
Creamy Fruit-Topped Waffles, 21
Easy Chicken Tortilla Soup, 57
Easy Oven-Barbecued Brisket, 87

RECIPES THAT WORK WITH THE SIMPLY FILLING TECHNIQUE

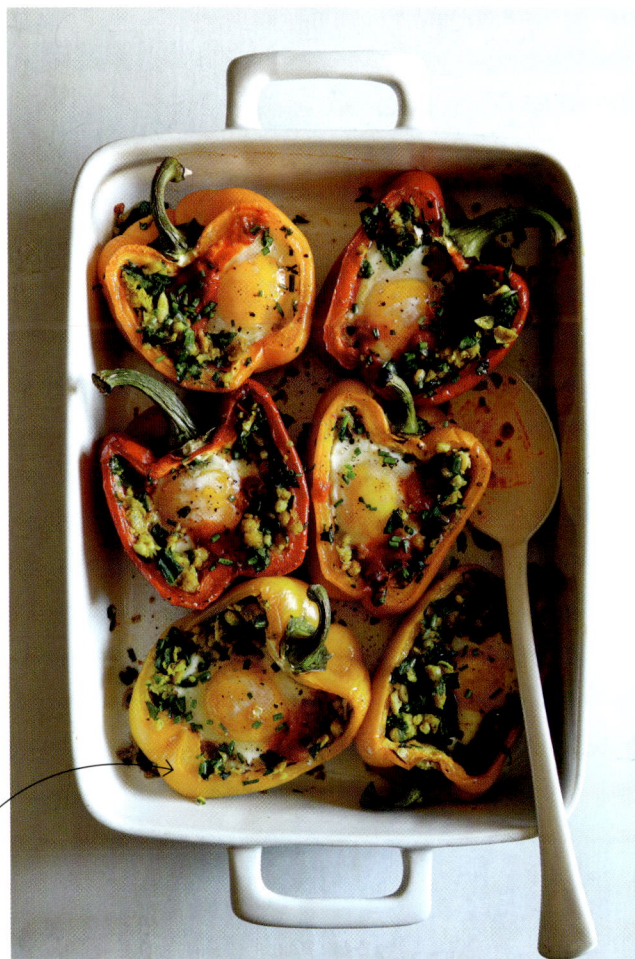

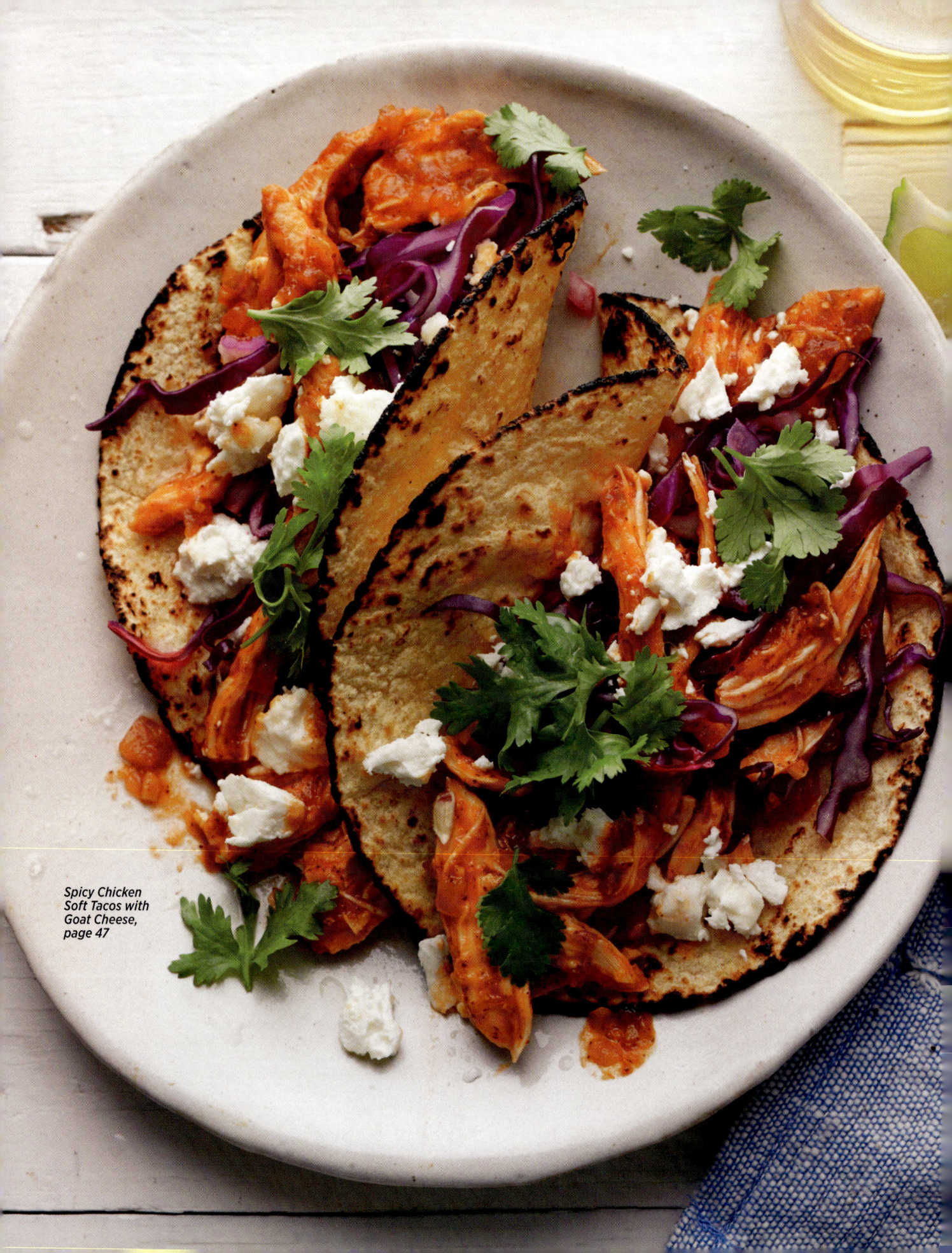

*Spicy Chicken
Soft Tacos with
Goat Cheese,
page 47*

BOOK INDEX

MEASUREMENT EQUIVALENTS

If you are converting the recipes in this book to metric measurements,
use the following chart as a guide.

TEASPOONS	TABLESPOONS	CUPS	FLUID OUNCES
3 teaspoons	1 tablespoon		½ fluid ounce
6 teaspoons	2 tablespoons	⅛ cup	1 fluid ounce
8 teaspoons	2 tablespoons plus 2 teaspoons	⅙ cup	
12 teaspoons	4 tablespoons	¼ cup	2 fluid ounces
15 teaspoons	5 tablespoons	⅓ cup minus 1 teaspoon	
16 teaspoons	5 tablespoons plus 1 teaspoon	⅓ cup	
18 teaspoons	6 tablespoons	¼ cup plus 2 tablespoons	3 fluid ounces
24 teaspoons	8 tablespoons	½ cup	4 fluid ounces
30 teaspoons	10 tablespoons	½ cup plus 2 tablespoons	5 fluid ounces
32 teaspoons	10 tablespoons plus 2 teaspoons	⅔ cup	
36 teaspoons	12 tablespoons	¾ cup	6 fluid ounces
42 teaspoons	14 tablespoons	1 cup minus 2 tablespoons	7 fluid ounces
45 teaspoons	15 tablespoons	1 cup minus 1 tablespoon	
48 teaspoons	16 tablespoons	1 cup	8 fluid ounces

VOLUME	
¼ teaspoon	1 milliliter
½ teaspoon	2 milliliters
1 teaspoon	5 milliliters
1 tablespoon	15 milliliters
2 tablespoons	30 milliliters
3 tablespoons	45 milliliters
¼ cup	60 milliliters
⅓ cup	80 milliliters
½ cup	120 milliliters
⅔ cup	160 milliliters
¾ cup	175 milliliters
1 cup	240 milliliters
1 quart	950 milliliters

LENGTH	
1 inch	25 millimeters
1 inch	2.5 centimeters

OVEN TEMPERATURE			
250°F	120°C	400°F	200°C
275°F	140°C	425°F	220°C
300°F	150°C	450°F	230°C
325°F	160°C	475°F	250°C
350°F	180°C	500°F	260°C
375°F	190°C	525°F	270°C

WEIGHT	
1 ounce	30 grams
¼ pound	120 grams
½ pound	240 grams
¾ pound	340 grams
1 pound	480 grams

NOTE: Measurement of less than ⅛ teaspoon is considered a dash or a pinch. Metric measurements are approximate.